Understanding

Human Behavior

A Guide for Health Care Providers

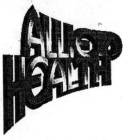

Understanding

Human Behavior

A Guide for Health Care Providers

Sixth Edition

Mary Elizabeth Milliken, B.S.N., M.S., Ed.D.

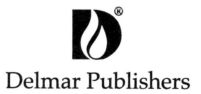

Delmar Publishers

an International Thomson Publishing company I(T)P®

Albany • Bonn • Boston • Cincinnati • Detroit • London • Madrid
Melbourne • Mexico City • New York • Pacific Grove • Paris • San Francisco
Singapore • Tokyo • Toronto • Washington

NOTICE TO THE READER

Cover Design: Juanita Brown

Delmar Staff
Publisher: Susan Simpfenderfer
Acquisition Editor: Marlene Pratt
Developmental Editor: Jill Rembetski
Editorial Assistant: Sarah Holle

COPYRIGHT © 1998
By Delmar Publishers
and International Thomson Publishing Company

The ITP logo is a trademark under license.

Printed in the United States of America

For more information, contact:

Delmar Publishers
3 Columbia Circle, Box 15015
Albany, New York 12212-5015

International Thomson Publishing Europe
Berkshire House
168-173 High Holborn
London, WC1V 7AA
England

Thomas Nelson Australia
102 Dodds Street
South Melbourne, 3205
Victoria, Australia

Nelson Canada
1120 Birchmount Road
Scarborough, Ontario
Canada, M1K 5G4

International Thomson Editores
Campos Eliseos 385, Piso 7
Col Polanco
11560 Mexico D F Mexico

International Thomson Publishing GmbH
Konigswinterer Strasse 418
53227 Bonn
Germany

International Thomson Publishing Asia
221 Henderson Road
#05-10 Henderson Building
Singapore 0315

International Thomson Publishing—Japan
Hirakawacho Kyowa Building, 3F
2-2-1 Hirakawacho
Chiyoda-ku, Tokyo 102
Japan

1 2 3 4 5 6 7 8 9 10 XXX 03 02 01 00 99 98 97

Library of Congress Cataloging-in-Publication Data

Milliken, Mary Elizabeth.
    Understanding human behavior : a guide for health care providers /
Mary Elizabeth Milliken. — 6th ed.
        p.   cm.
    Includes bibliographical references and index.
    ISBN 0-8273-8221-9
    1. Allied health personnel and patient.   2. Allied health
personnel—Psychology.   I. Title.
    [DNLM: 1. Professional-Patient Relations.   2. Allied Health
Personnel.   3. Behavior.   W 21.5 M654u 1998]
R727.3.M55 1998
610.69' 53—dc21
DNLM/DLC
for Library of Congress   97-13707
                                                                                    CIP

Contents

Preface

INTRODUCTION

Understanding Human Behavior: A Guide for Health Care Providers was written to assist students in health occupations education programs to learn basic principles of human behavior. These principles will give them a basis for increased self-understanding and improved interpersonal relationships. With technological advances in diagnostic and therapeutic procedures, it is easy for a health care provider to focus on procedures and routines. Patients, however, want personalized care that conveys respect for the patient as a person.

Patients' expectations are more likely to be met when each health care provider strives for effective interaction with each patient. By consciously attending to each interaction with patients, the health care provider will experience greater job satisfaction.

ORGANIZATION

This textbook is organized to proceed from relatively simple information to more complex concepts, from the known to the unknown, and from self to others in a variety of interpersonal situations. For that reason, Units 1 through 22 are designed for *sequential study*. Each section builds on the previous section; within each section, each unit builds on the preceding unit. Units 23 through 26 are *not* sequential. In fact, Unit 25 may be assigned early in the course of study to help students learn ways of managing the stress that inevitably accompanies the role of student and introduction to the clinical setting.

Section I provides an orientation to the role of health care provider, the importance of accepting each patient as a worthwhile human being, the challenge of striving for self-understanding, and guidelines for personal and professional growth. Section II presents information about various influences on human behavior: basic physical and psychological needs, developmental factors and role of the social environment, emotions and their power to influence behavior, and adjustment as a composite of all these factors. Section III presents more complex concepts, with emphasis on applications to self and to one's life situation: threats to adjustment, developmental tasks of various life stages that challenge adjustment, common defense mechanisms and their purposes, inner conflict, and the challenge of dealing with frustration. Section IV emphasizes the application of these learnings to interactions with others, especially patients. Section V provides opportunities for practicing effective communication, both nonverbal and verbal. Through follow-up discussions, each student will identify changes needed to eliminate ineffective or negative communication habits and set goals for improving communication skills. Section VI provides an introduction to death education through the discussion of loss as a part of living, the importance of the grief process to emotional/mental health, and the dying process as an opportunity for growth. Section VII is designed to provide an informational foundation for evaluating various approaches to health care, including holistic health care and selected nonmedical therapies.

Throughout Section VII the terms "orthodox medicine," "conventional medicine," and "allopathic medicine" are used interchangeably to refer to current medical practice in the United States. The terms "alternative therapy," "complementary therapy," and "nonmedical therapy" refer to therapeutic approaches that are not currently included in orthodox medical care. Some of these therapies are, however, included in practices of physicians who embrace a holistic approach to health care.

Section VII consists of four units. Unit 23 provides a historical overview of health care practices in order to show that many nonmedical therapies, as well as current orthodox practices, have historical roots. Unit 24 examines the concept of healing, particularly the mind/body connection and the influence of beliefs, will to live, and intention on the course of illness. Unit 25 introduces specific techniques for management of stress, emphasizing the value of stress management in both therapy and health maintenance. Unit 26 provides guidelines for evaluating alternative therapies, an informational overview of several alternative therapies, and sources of information for those who wish to learn more about specific therapeutic methods.

Although Unit 25 may be assigned early in the Health Occupations curriculum to help students learn stress management techniques, Section VII as a whole is best used as an advanced area of study for those who are concluding the health occupations program of study and are about to assume the role of health care provider. It is hoped that the study of Section VII will facilitate the transition from student to practitioner and prepare the new graduate to deal with future dynamics of the health care system.

FEATURES OF THE SIXTH EDITION

The sixth edition of *Understanding Human Behavior* is characterized by the following changes:

- **New content** in relevant units: empowerment; sleep as an essential physical need, the sleep cycle, REM sleep; influences on one's sense of self; differences in the emotional needs of men and women; the health effects of negative emotions; guilt; types of love, importance of learning to love; variations in expression of emotions, mood swings; role of emotions in adjustment; threats to adjustment; ToughLove; organizational structure, horizontal and vertical communication; issues related to death, euthanasia, suicide, assisted suicide, rights of patients and families, involvement of the courts in medical decisions, DNR orders, advance medical directives and liability; Healing Touch, Homeopathy.

- **Extended discussion** of social and cultural issues that are threats to adjustment and to physical/mental health: domestic violence, child abuse, spousal abuse, discrimination and harassment, violence and accidents, victims and survivors.

- **New topics** related to the blurring distinction between physical and mental/emotional disorders, between "eccentric" behavior and undiagnosed disorders.

- **Communication as a thread** that runs through several units, from introduction of basic principles of communication through specific techniques, culminating in practice sessions.

- **Expanded or updated content** on heredity; nutrition, especially in prenatal development; emotions; substance abuse and codependency; losses in specific life periods, advance medical directives; the holistic perspective on health care.

- **Suggested Readings** for every unit; provision of Internet sources of information for selected topics. Replacement of previous "Suggested Readings" with more recent publications; retention of some older references because they are "classics" (introduced new concepts or techniques and still present a specific point of view better than subsequent publications).

- **Revision** of selected drawings and illustrations.

- **Key words** appear as boldface when explained or defined.

USING THE TEXT

Learning objectives for each unit should be used by the student to gain a sense of direction—what is to be achieved through study of the unit. The review questions should be used as a self-check to determine which objectives have been achieved and which topics should be reviewed to enhance achievement.

Assignments at the end of each unit are designed to assist students to achieve the unit objectives. Some assignments require application of information from the unit to the solving of a relatively simple problem. Others present complex situations that require study, then selection of one or more principles of human behavior. A number of assignments require observation of people in various settings to identify examples of specific types of behavior. Thus, beginning practice in observing and interpreting behavior and implementing appropriate responses as a means of improving human relations is provided through the assignments.

The instructor will schedule activities in class to (1) clarify the meaning of concepts presented in the text, (2) share examples of observed behavior patterns, (3) analyze patient/health care provider situations, and (4) practice applying principles of human behavior to real and hypothetical situations. Some of these activities will be led by the teacher; some will provide an opportunity for members of the class to lead a discussion or problem-solving session. The value of the course will depend upon (1) the extent to which the student uses assignments to prepare for class activities, (2) involvement of the student in class activities, and (3) continuous striving for improved human relations skills.

No one every fully masters human relations skills. Those who sincerely want to relate effectively to others must become lifelong students of human behavior. They must consciously practice human relations skills in order to improve their sensitivity to the possible meaning of observed behavior and select appropriate responses. The immediate challenge is to gain as much as possible from this course, as a foundation for the lifelong challenge of developing a high level of skill in human relations.

ABOUT THE AUTHOR

Mary Elizabeth Milliken, B.S.N, M.S., Ed.D., is a graduate of Duke University School of Nursing. Her graduate study at North Carolina State University at Raleigh concentrated on both education and psychology. She has practiced nursing in a variety of settings, served as instructor, then coordinator of a practical nursing education program, was curriculum specialist for health occupations in the North Carolina Department of Community Colleges, and has been a consultant on curriculum and effective teaching. From 1971 to 1987 she served as Coordinator of Health Occupations Teacher Education at The University of Georgia in Athens.

ACKNOWLEDGMENTS

Many health occupations instructors have contributed to the improvement of *Understanding Human Behavior,* either through written critique or personal contact with the author. Students in a variety of health occupations programs have shared their views with the author. Throughout the history of *Understanding Human Behavior,* students and instructors of health occupations educational programs have suggested topics and provided situations that could be used to illustrate various concepts related to human behavior. My children contributed examples as they struggled with adolescence, peer/parental/teacher relationships, and the challenges of assuming adult responsibilities. The contributions of Scott to the sixth edition have been extensive: retrieving files each time the old computer "lost" them, updating computer components to accommodate the demands of *Understanding Human Behavior,* coaching the author through the frustrations of giving up the familiarity of *MS DOS Word* and learning to use the innumerable icons and buttons and menus of *Word for Windows,* and sharing his Internet expertise to enable the author to locate up-to-date information and determine the availability of needed references in near-by libraries.

The illustrations have evolved with expanding text content. The original illustrator was Bill Pugh of the N.C. Department of Community Colleges, who provided the drawings for Units 1–16 (the first edition). For the fourth edition, Bill Staton prepared original artwork and modified several of the original drawings. Subsequent revisions included photographs taken at St. Mary's Hospital in Athens, GA, Athens Regional Medical Center, Newton County Hospital in Covington, and Georgia Regional Hospital-Atlanta. Health professionals enrolled in an educational media class assisted with photographs for the fourth edition; Shirley J. Harrell Harris was especially helpful in that endeavor. New illustrations for the fifth edition were provided by Elmer Moreira, Robert King of The Chicago School of Massage Therapy, Cathy Young of the American Holistic Nurses' Association, Dwight C. Byers of Ingham Publishing, Inc., Michael Reed Gach of the Acupressure Institute, Dr. C. Norman Shealy, Dr. Herbert Benson, Bantam Doubleday Dell Publishing Group, Inc., and Delmar staff. Illustrations for the sixth edition include contributions from Project Safe in Athens, GA, Dr. Larry Hudson, the Menninger Clinic, Minnesota Domestic Abuse Intervention Project, Worley-Shoemaker Artist Management (Dr. Lerner's photograph), and Mary Neville (Dr. Myss' assistant). Certain illustrations borrowed from other Delmar publications contribute interest and clarity to numerous topics; the contribution of these authors to the sixth edition is appreciated.

All of these contributions, as well as the never-failing support and helpfulness of editors in the Allied Health Team of Delmar Publishers are gratefully acknowledged.

REVIEWERS

Joan Claire Chabriel
Former Coordinator
Nursing Assisting Program
Blake Business School
New York, NY

Bonnie Lou Deister, M.S., B.S.N., R.N., C.M.A-C
Chairperson
Medical Assisting and Paramedics Departments
Broome Community College
Binghamton, NY

Rebecca S. Livigni, R.N.
Medical Assisting
Akron Medical & Dental Institute
Cuyahoga, OH

Carol Nelson, R.N., M.S.N.
Practical Nursing Program
Spokane Community College
Spokane, WA

Bonnie J. Perrin, C.M.A.
Baldwin Park Adult School
Baldwin Park, CA

Mary Trumble
Practical Nursing Program
Ridgewater College,
Hutchinson Campus
Hutchinson, MN

Section I

On Becoming a Health Care Provider

In this section, some of the challenges, responsibilities, problems, and satisfactions of being a health care provider are introduced. People from all walks of life have health problems. You, as a health care provider, will be challenged to learn how to serve each person effectively, within the role for which your course is preparing you. Section I is designed to help you become aware of the realities of a health career and also help you learn ways to succeed, both as a student and as a health care provider.

Challenges and Responsibilities of Health Care Providers

OBJECTIVES

Upon completion of this unit, you should be able to:

- Compare the satisfaction gained from the approval of others with that of knowing you have performed well.
- List three challenges for health care providers.
- Explain the value of high standards for a health care provider.
- List two responsibilities of a student.
- Explain your responsibilities as a health care provider.
- Explain the relationship between your achievement standards as a student and your future performance standards as a health care provider.
- Use effective study habits to improve learning.
- Set personal standards for achievement as a student and for performance as a health care provider.
- Explain the meaning of empowerment.

KEY TERMS

Accomplishment	Satisfaction	Challenge
Empowerment	Standards	Mediocre
Excellence	Self-confidence	Self-reliant

So you have decided to become a health care provider. Congratulations! Your decision will place you within a large group of people who are providing very important services to others. You will acquire new knowledge and develop new skills as you proceed through your educational program. Much satisfaction can be yours, both through your educational achievements and through your career as a health care provider. You will be able to take your place in the community as one who is making a significant contribution to society. You will be respected by your friends, especially those who do not have the benefit of your education and those who are not prepared, as you will be, to fulfill important responsibilities.

A career in the health field differs in many ways from careers in other fields. There are many satisfactions to be experienced. There are many challenges to be met. There are heavy responsibilities to be fulfilled. The purpose of this unit is to help you be aware of these satisfactions, challenges and responsibilities as they relate to you as a student and as a future health care provider.

SATISFACTIONS

Approval Versus Inner Satisfaction

We all admire and envy those who can do something extremely well; each of us would like to be the kind of person who is admired by others. We get a lift from expressions of approval, yet this good feeling is only temporary. The athlete may enjoy hearing the cheers of the crowd when performing well, but the deepest satisfaction comes from the performance itself, from knowing that you performed with great skill. True **satisfaction** is an inner feeling of pride in doing something well, regardless of whether or not the performance is applauded by others.

As a health care provider, you will find your greatest satisfaction in trying to give each patient appropriate care. By striving to meet each patient's needs to the best of your ability, you will complete the day with an inner feeling of pride. The opposite approach—to view your work as a series of assigned procedures to be completed so that you can get off work or go on break—results in finishing the day by saying "Whew, I'm glad that's over!" Stop now and give a moment's thought to a very important question: How will you approach your work? As a **challenge** that may provide much satisfaction and a sense of accomplishment? Or, as work you have to do to get a paycheck?

Setting Goals for Inner Satisfaction

Skillful performance can provide **self-confidence** and a deep sense of satisfaction that is not dependent on praise from others. Continuous striving to improve one's performance, to do each task well, and to do better today than yesterday is the means of achieving a high level of skill. Even though we would all like to be admired for our performance, many of us settle for mediocrity because it requires less effort to "just get by" than to do well. You have probably heard the saying, "If a job is worth doing at all, it is worth doing well." The time required to do a task sloppily is usually about the same as the time required to do it well, although doing the task correctly may require a little

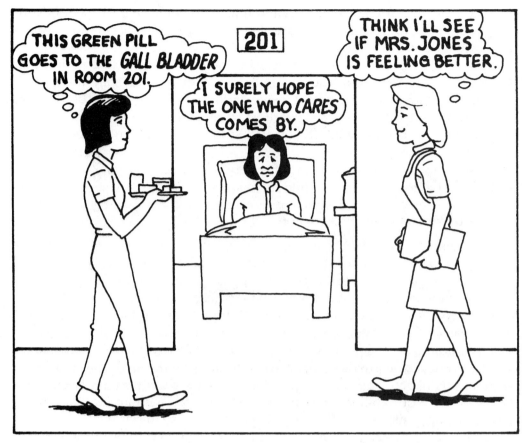

Think of each patient as a person, rather than a diagnosis.

more effort. **Excellence** lies in that little bit of extra effort. *In the health field, that little bit of extra effort may make the difference between safe and unsafe practice.*

Will the habits you form as a student carry over into your performance as a health care provider? You may be sure that they will! So, now is the time to set **standards** of excellence for yourself and begin to establish the habits that will lead to skillful performance, self-confidence, and pride in your work.

THE CHALLENGE

Setting Standards of Performance

Only you can set the standards that will guide your performance over the coming years. Many times there will be the opportunity to take a shortcut. Sometimes a piece of equipment will be contaminated; obtaining sterile materials to complete the procedure will require extra effort and time. You are the only one who will know whether or not sterile technique was violated and the contaminated equipment was used—unless, of course, the patient develops a serious infection as a result of your poor technique. Your standards of performance serve as your conscience and determine whether or not you experience the inner satisfaction that comes from knowing the job was well done.

Habits formed as a student will affect performance throughout your career. When making that little bit of extra effort to "do it right" has become a habit, doing it correctly no longer seems an effort; it becomes an essential part of your performance. Thus, excellence as a health care provider will depend upon setting high standards of performance for yourself and establishing the habit of making that extra bit of effort while still a student. Then, when someone takes a shortcut or settles for a mediocre performance, you can take pride in thinking, "I wouldn't do it that way, even though it does save a few steps."

Excellence and Patient Safety

In the health field, all care providers should strive for excellence. Why? Because anything less than excellence can endanger the patient. The nurse should give the correct medicine to each patient 100% of the time. The medical assistant should use faultless technique in 100% of the situations that require asepsis. The laboratory assistant should report test results correctly 100% of the time. The dental assistant should sterilize instruments correctly 100% of the time. The ambulance attendant should move the accident victim correctly 100% of the time. *Performance that is less than 100% correct can have disastrous effects for the patient.* Should the patient benefit from health care or be the victim of it?

Meeting Patient Needs

As a health care provider, you will find many fascinating challenges. Your work will be with human beings, and each one is different as a person and as a patient. *The greatest challenge in the health field is to provide for each patient the health care that promotes the patient's well-being.* This requires concern about the patient as a person, rather than as someone for whom a specified procedure must be carried out as part of the physician's therapeutic plan.

Attending to each patient as a person is not only a challenge, it is also a responsibility—one that provides enrichment and opportunities to grow as a person and as a health care provider.

RESPONSIBILITIES

As a Student

You are presently involved in activities designed to prepare you to function as a health care provider in some specific role. At the moment, your primary concern

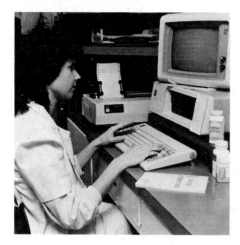

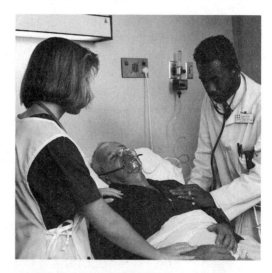

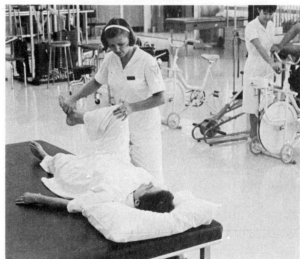

High performance standards
ensure patient safety and
effective care.

is with performance as a student; remind yourself frequently that your performance as a student *will* affect your performance as a health care provider.

Your first responsibility as a student, then, is to take full advantage of every opportunity to learn. Try to see the purpose in each assignment. When you become aware of the purpose of an assignment, you will look at it as an *opportunity to learn*, rather than as a chore to complete.

Your second responsibility is to decide what standards will guide your performance. This is related to the previous discussion about excellence, but now

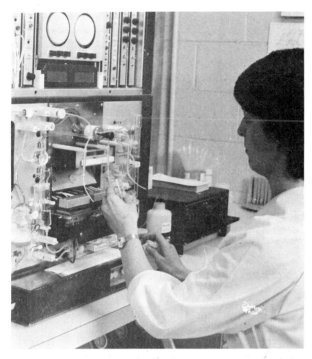

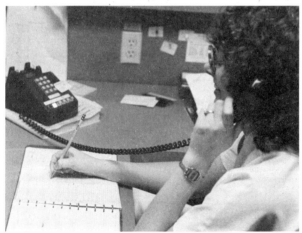

High performance standards
ensure patient safety and
effective care. (Continued)

you should think about standards in relation to your performance as a student. Your school has set a certain grade as passing; let us say 70 is passing in your program. Suppose, through habit, you say to yourself, "I'll study this material until I know it well enough to make 75." In many courses of study, a grade of 75 is acceptable; in such courses, a deficiency in the student's knowledge of subject matter is not likely to cause harm to someone else.

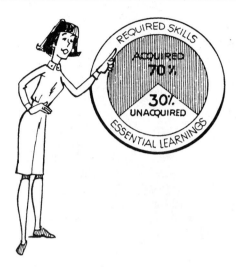

Is "just passing" good enough for students in a health care preparatory program?

As a Health Care Provider

In a health occupations course, the implications of "just passing" are more serious. Any gaps in knowledge and performance skills can affect every patient served. Will your future services to patients be of "just passing" quality? Or do you wish to give the best service you are capable of giving? If your educational program is preparing you to provide health services, can you be content to learn only 70% of what your teachers expect you to learn? Can you be content to develop your skills just enough to get a passing grade in a laboratory course? Can you automatically change your standards and established habits after graduation?

Achievement as Progress

If you set high standards for achievement now, then these high standards will carry over into performance as a health care provider. In setting standards for achievement, plan to *do your best*, rather than trying to be the best student in the class.

How can you do your best? Not by wasteful study procedures, such as putting in many hours of study when you are too tired to benefit or taking pages and pages of notes that mean nothing to you after they "get cold." Instead, work out a study routine and establish the habits that work best for you. This may take some experimenting, but you can establish a routine that enables you to learn with a minimum of time and effort. In order to get started, consider the following guidelines:

- Let your family and friends know that you have set aside a certain time of day as your study period. Do not allow them to violate your schedule by interrupting you. Phone calls can be returned when you have finished studying. Most family problems can wait until you are through studying. This is *your* time; do not let it become someone else's time.

- At the beginning of each study period, write out a list of specific things you need to complete; then, rank the items in order of importance. Complete the #1 (most important) task first, then move on to #2. If one of the tasks is something you dislike but must get done, let it be #1 so that you get it out of the way. Most of us tend to put off unpleasant tasks as long as possible; sometimes we never quite get around to them! "I didn't have time to do that" often means "I didn't want to do that, so I kept putting it off."

- If your list of study assignments is too long to complete today, set up tomorrow's list; then put the items on that list out of your mind until tomorrow. Give your full attention to today's list.

- Use the objectives stated by your instructor and in the textbook as guides to what you are expected to learn. Refer to the objectives of this text; note what you will *be able to do* after you have finished this chapter. How many of those objectives could you demonstrate at this time? You are able to demonstrate the first six if you acquired the important ideas from the preceding paragraphs. The paragraphs to follow deal with objectives seven and eight.

If you cannot demonstrate the first six objectives, give your attention to the following guidelines, so that you will learn to gain more from your reading. Then review this chapter until you have achieved each of the objectives.

- Form the habit of testing yourself to decide whether or not you have achieved an objective. First, write out the ideas involved. For example, test your achievement of the objective, "Explain your responsibilities as a health care provider" by writing out, in your own words, a description of these responsibilities. Then check your description against the textbook. Add to or correct what you have written. With practice you will be able to test yourself by running the information through your mind rather than writing it out. Finally, use the Review and Self-Check at the end of each unit as a final check on whether or not you have learned the main ideas of the unit. By following these steps as you study each unit, you will soon develop study skills that increase learning and decrease the amount of study time required.

- When reading the text, look up from the printed page at intervals and mentally run through the main ideas of the paragraphs you have just read. Note paragraph headings, as these help to set your mind for what you are about to read. Also, refer at intervals to the objectives so you can be alert for information that is related to specific objectives. Remember, the objectives can help you separate important ideas from those that are less important.

- When you have a lengthy assignment, pace yourself. Set a realistic goal for the first hour's effort; then spend an intensive 60 minutes completing that part of the assignment. Next, take about 15 minutes for a change of activity. By alternating study periods with physical activity, the effectiveness of each study period can be increased. In other words, an hour of study followed by 15 minutes of walking in the fresh air, followed by another 45 minutes of studying will be more productive for most people than a solid two hours of "plugging away" at the books.

- At intervals during your study period, take four very long, slow breaths; hold each for a count of 4 before exhaling. Then do several stretching exercises and two or three head rolls. You should return to your studying refreshed and with a clear mind.

- When you are studying material that includes totally new information, try to relate it to something you have already learned or to some past experience (e.g., Uncle Joe's broken leg that gave him such a bad time was a comminuted fracture of the tibia).

- Your nervous system can only handle a certain amount of new information at one time. This is a physiological limitation we all have. If we learn to work *with* it instead of against it, we can accomplish more. When you begin to feel overwhelmed with new material, review about five to seven main ideas and think of ways to use the information. Then, do something else for a while to give your mind time to process the new information. After a lapse of time (maybe an hour, maybe a day or two), review those same ideas and try to think of new examples and other applications. By then the ideas will be very familiar—you will be comfortable with them—and you will be ready to study additional new information.

- If you tend to be "uptight" much of the time, learn a relaxation routine or meditation procedure (see Unit 25). By taking about twenty minutes a day to relax completely, you can avoid a buildup of tension that may interfere with your performance—and with your health if the tension persists over a period of time.

- As you acquire information or develop the performance skill described in a learning objective, consciously congratulate yourself. Recognize that you have reached a stepping-stone to becoming a health care provider. Enjoy a sense of achievement.

- Measure your achievement in terms of progress toward your goal of becoming a qualified practitioner in the health field. Take pride in each forward step. Avoid thinking of achievement as a "good grade." Avoid comparing your progress with the progress of others in your class. You are competing with the *you* of yesterday, not with your classmates. Where are you now as compared to last month? Last year? How much have you achieved since you entered this health care program?

- Take pride in your achievements, but also be honest with yourself about areas in which you need to improve. By investing additional effort in your areas of weakness, you can convert those, too, into achievements.

Attitudes and Interest

The foregoing suggestions will help you form favorable attitudes toward your studies. Your attitudes influence the interest you have in your assignments and in various learning experiences. Your interest affects your achievement; that is, you learn more easily and perform better when you are interested in what you are doing. This is reflected in a familiar saying, "The difference between a dull job and an interesting job is the person doing it."

There will be times of discouragement during your course of study. There will also be times when you experience the satisfaction that comes from doing well. You will have a sense of **accomplishment** as you draw on your knowledge to solve problems and use your skills to provide patient care that reflects the highest standards.

Empowerment

Every adult should control most aspects of his/her life. During adolescence, learning to make decisions (i.e., take control) is an important developmental task; if this is not learned, the individual enters adulthood poorly equipped to cope with life problems. Adolescent girls are more likely than boys to fail in completing this task. Parents, teachers, boyfriends and others often make decisions for young girls and expect girls to accept these decisions without question. Boys, on the other hand, are more likely to be encouraged to make decisions, because "taking charge" is a major aspect of the macho image. If you entered adulthood with a tendency to let your parents, spouse, friends, or anyone else make decisions for you, it is time to recognize what is happening: you are giving away your power—the power to be a **self-reliant,** responsible adult.

When you are planning to eat out with a friend, who decides which restaurant? Do you usually say, "Oh, I don't care. You choose." Does your spouse or boyfriend give you a choice? If you are not involved in small decisions that affect you, how can you expect others to include you in big decisions? For example:

> *Kate is a dental hygienist whose earnings are about equal to her husband's. Each payday, she gives her check to her husband because "he handles our finances." They have only one car, so Kate usually waits as much as an hour for her husband to pick her up. She insists on keeping the car this week so she can do some errands after work. Yesterday her husband waited 45 minutes for her to pick him up. Today, he announces proudly, "Well, I bought you your own car." He has purchased a compact car with 125,000 miles on it. Kate has a strong dislike for compact cars, believing that a midsize car is safer. Buying a car is a major decision, yet Kate's husband did not see any need to involve her in that decision. Kate has given away her power; it will take much effort to renegotiate this relationship so that she is empowered to participate in decision-making.*

How does **empowerment** affect you? Suppose you have informed the family that your study hour will begin at 9 o'clock each evening. During the second day of this plan, your teen-ager calls you to the phone at 9:15; the caller is your sister-in-law who talks about her problems for a full half-hour. Two days later, your ten-year-old opens the door at 9:30 and says, "I need a note for my teacher about the field-trip next Monday." Each time you permit these violations of your study hour, you are giving away your power. You gave your two children the power to interrupt your study hour. You gave your sister-in-law the power to use up thirty minutes of your study time for her own purposes. You probably responded to these requests because you are accustomed to meeting the needs of others, even if doing so interferes with your own needs.

Suppose you have completed eight months of your one-year program when your spouse complains that you are "spending too much time at that school." The complaints also include such things as not having home-made cakes any more and "you don't watch TV with me like you used to." Your spouse says you should quit the program and go back to your part-time job at the fast-food restaurant. You really hated that job! How will you handle this situation? If you quit the program, you *give your spouse the power* to control your occupational choice. *Your own empowerment* requires that *you* make the decision, based on what *you really want*. If you insist on completing the program, it may be necessary to negotiate a compromise. This might require you to find more time to be with the family, and family members to give you more help with homemaking tasks. If you leave the program in order to please your family, you are letting others control your life.

If you allow others to make decisions for you because you just do not like to make decisions, then you are *avoiding the adult task of taking responsibility for your life.* If you allow others to make decisions that affect your life in order to avoid arguments, then you are "de-selfing," which Dr. Harriett Lerner describes as betraying oneself or sacrificing one's own wishes in order to preserve harmony (Lerner, 1985). The apparent harmony of such a relationship exacts a high price in terms of resentment, feelings of being trapped, powerlessness and hopelessness.

If this pattern applies to your life situation, you can start reclaiming your power by requiring others to respect your needs. For example, after informing all members of your family that a certain time period is your study time, do not permit any violations to occur. Remind those who interrupt you that you are not available during study hour. If you are consistent, the interruptions will eventually stop. Then you can use the same approach to another of your needs. You may choose to make the next decision about where to eat or which movie to see, instead of allowing someone else to make that decision. You may wish to inform your spouse or a friend that you are to be involved in any decisions that affect you. This type of change will not occur rapidly; be content with small changes initially. But by persisting, you will eventually gain more control over your life.

Empowerment may or may not be a problem in your own life. As a health care provider, however, you will need to be aware of the importance of empowerment to self-esteem and a sense of well-being. Patients who are dependent on others for their personal needs may feel much anger about their helplessness. Many patients need help in regaining some control over their life situations. By respecting their wishes and involving patients in decisions, *when appropriate,* you contribute to feelings of empowerment.

MAKING A DECISION

Standards of performance are personal. Teachers can say that a certain grade is necessary, but it is your decision about the desired level of achievement that influences your performance. Even more important, the standards that guide your performance as a student will carry over into your performance as a health care provider.

Choosing to enter this educational program for the health field was an important decision in your life. Now, it is time to make another decision— what kind of health care provider will you be? Excellent? **Mediocre?** Or "just passing"? Remember, the standards of performance that will characterize you as a health care provider will be influenced by the standards you set for yourself now.

References and Suggested Readings

Lerner, Harriet G. *The Dance of Anger.* New York, NY: Harper & Row Publishers, 1985. Chapter 1, "The Challenge of Anger," pp. 1–16.

REVIEW AND SELF-CHECK

Complete the following statements, using information from Unit 1.

1. True satisfaction comes from _____ .

2. Three challenges for a health care provider are _____ ,
   _____ , and _____ .

3. High standards are important for a health care provider because _____
   _____ .

4. Your responsibilities as a student include _____
   and _____ .

5. Four habits that will help you study effectively are
   _____

   _____

   _____

   _____

ASSIGNMENT

1. Use Worksheet A at the end of this unit to develop a tentative study plan.
   Try this plan for two weeks. If it seems to be effective, continue to use it.
   If it is not effective:
   a. List problems that interfered with the effectiveness of the plan.
   b. Modify the plan by changing the schedule, the place where you study,
      or any other details involved in "the problems." Try the modified
      plan for one week. If you continue to have problems, repeat steps a
      and b until you have a workable study plan.

If other people are part of the problem, try to involve them in developing the "improved plan" to increase the probability of getting their cooperation. For example, a six-year-old may find numerous reasons for needing his mother's attention as soon as she disappears into her room for the study hour. By discussing mother's need to study so that she can become a health care provider, the six-year-old may begin to accept some responsibility for "helping" mother become a health care provider. The mother should negotiate so that "everybody is a winner."

For example, she could agree to read to the six-year-old for thirty minutes in exchange for an hour of uninterrupted study. The child gets the mother's attention, and mother gets to study. Needless to say, both parties must fulfill their parts of the agreement.

2. Complete each of the following using Worksheet B at the end of this unit.
    a. List the things you *have to do* each day.
    b. List the things you *have to do* each week, but not every day.
    c. List the things you *have to do* occasionally.
    d. Beside each item in a, b, and c write the name of someone who could do that task for you, at least some of the time.
    e. Beside any items that have no names, write out the possible result of that task not getting done at all. (Be honest with yourself. What will *really* happen if the car doesn't get washed *today?*)

3. Revise the lists in Assignment 2 to include only those tasks that you, and you alone, must perform. Consider whether or not some of the daily tasks could be done on alternate days or perhaps weekly. Consider whether or not some of the weekly tasks could be done alternate weeks or once a month.

4. Use Worksheet C at the end of this unit to plan your daily schedule for one week. Give your student role a high priority in this schedule, instead of letting it play "second fiddle" to all the responsibilities you fulfilled before becoming a student.

5. Try your schedule for one week, then:
    a. List the "time-wasters" you experienced during the week.
    b. List the "energy wasters" you experienced during the past week. Beside each, write out a justification; if you cannot justify the energy spent, resolve to eliminate that activity from your life.

c. List three times you allowed someone else to control your time. (For example, a neighbor insisted that you go shopping with her. When you indicated that you needed to study, she responded, "You never spend time with me anymore." So, feeling guilty, you spent an entire afternoon doing what she wanted to do and came home too exhausted to study.) Consider how you could have controlled the situation.

NOTE: Your instructor may schedule a group discussion to help members of the class share ideas on how to maintain control of your time without alienating your family and friends.

d. Recheck your weekly schedule. Be sure you have given a reasonable balance of time to your various roles: as a member of the family, a student in a health occupations program, and an individual who requires activity, sleep, rest, recreation, and has various other needs to be met. Resolve to (1) give attention to each of these important aspects of your life, (2) hold to a minimum any time and energy wasters that interfere with your performance.

Stick to your plan. You are now taking control of your life. And, becoming a *self-reliant person* is a major step toward becoming a *reliable health care provider!*

6. During the next week, pay attention to the times you have an opportunity to make a decision but delegate the decision-making power to someone else. Develop a list of the types of situations where you give away your power.

7. Review the list you developed in #6. Consider ways you could regain your own empowerment in each situation. How many of these situations are merely a matter of your being more assertive? How many of these situations will require negotiating a different relationship with someone (spouse, significant other, parent)?

8. Develop your own Empowerment Plan.
    a. List the types of situations in which you will insist on being involved in decisions.
    b. Select one type of situation for practicing decision-making (experiencing empowerment).
    c. Number the items on the list according to priority. The simpler situations (e.g., where to eat, which television show to watch) should have high priorities. When you have gained confidence (are feeling

somewhat empowered), then you are ready to attempt the more difficult situations that involve your relationship with someone who is accustomed to making decisions for you.

9. Refer to "Key Terms" at the beginning of this unit. Write out the meaning of each in your own words; consult the glossary or a dictionary for any words you cannot define.

WORKSHEET A

Study Plan

Time	Monday	Tuesday	Wednesday	Thursday	Friday	Saturday	Sunday
6 A.M.							
7							
8							
9							
10							
11							
12 Noon							
1 P.M.							
2							
3							
4							
5							
6							
7							
8							
9							
10							
11							
12 Mn							

WORKSHEET B

Tasks I Have to Do

Every day:

Once a week:

Occasionally:

WORKSHEET C

Daily Schedule for Week of _____

Time	Monday	Tuesday	Wednesday	Thursday	Friday	Saturday	Sunday
12:00 Mn							
1:00 A.M.							
2:00							
3:00							
4:00							
5:00							
6:00							
7:00							
7:30							
8:00							
8:30							
9:00							
9:30							
10:00							
10:30							
11:00							
11:30							
12:00 Noon							

Daily Schedule (Cont'd)

Time	Monday	Tuesday	Wednesday	Thursday	Friday	Saturday	Sunday
12:30 P.M.							
1:00							
1:30							
2:00							
2:30							
3:00							
3:30							
4:00							
4:30							
5:00							
5:30							
6:00							
6:30							
7:00							
8:00							
9:00							
10:00							
11:00							

Unit 2

The Philosophy of Individual Worth

OBJECTIVES

Upon completion of this unit, you should be able to:

- Explain the philosophy of individual worth.
- Explain why cultural bias can affect the quality of patient care.
- List five examples of cultural differences that could contribute to misunderstandings between a patient and a health care provider.
- Apply the philosophy of individual worth to relationships with patients and their families.

KEY TERMS

Affluent	Values	Individual worth
Culture	Customs	Socioeconomic
Philosophy	Prejudice	Unique
Superstitions	Cultural bias	

A health care provider comes in contact with people from many different backgrounds. Some patients have never known anything but poverty. Some have come from other countries or from homes in which the **customs** of other nationalities are followed. Some have been reared in a religious faith with beliefs very different from those of you and your friends.

If you have had little contact with people from other **cultures** or from other **socioeconomic** levels of society, your first reaction may be to view these people not only as "different" but also as less acceptable than people who are like you and your friends. However, it is not a health care provider's right to judge people or to vary the quality of services because the patient is "different."

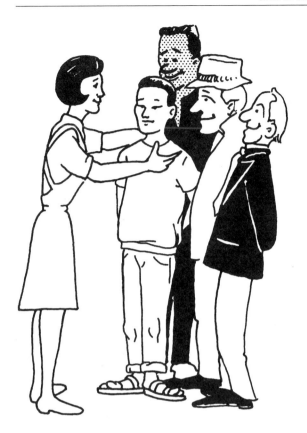

Everyone has worth and is entitled to respect as a human being.

MEANING OF INDIVIDUAL WORTH

The philosophy of **individual worth** is the belief that *everyone, regardless of personal circumstances or personal qualities, has worth and is entitled to respect as a human being.* For health care providers this means that the quality of service does not vary because of the patient's race, nationality, religion, sex, age, economic level, occupation, education, diagnosis, or any other characteristic.

Each patient is an individual. Each should receive health care that takes into consideration both the person's individuality and the specific health problem. The **philosophy** of individual worth has many implications for patient care. A health care provider who does not accept the philosophy of individual worth may interact differently with patients from another culture than with patients from his/her own culture. Yet the health care provider would probably be unaware of any differences in care he/she is giving that patient.

THE HEALTH CARE PROVIDER AND SOCIOECONOMIC CLASS

Cultural Bias

Each socioeconomic class within a society has its own customs, standards of living, **values,** interests, and other characteristics that distinguish it from other socioeconomic classes. Members of one class generally do not understand the differences between their own class and other classes. The health care provider's expectations regarding patient behavior may be unrealistic for patients from a different cultural background or socioeconomic level. The tendency to make negative judgments about a person because of the culture or class from which that person comes is called **cultural bias.**

Most health care providers are members of the middle class. They did not grow up as a member of an extremely wealthy family, nor did they live in poverty. Although there is great diversity within the middle class, members also have much in common. And one thing most of them have in common is a lack of understanding about poverty and about **affluence.** But the health care provider encounters patients from all socioeconomic groups. It is especially important that health care providers not allow their middle class beliefs and value systems to influence the care they give patients from other socioeconomic levels and other cultures.

The Patient from the Poverty Class

People who have never lived in poverty find it difficult to understand those whose lives center around survival. People who live in poverty have a daily routine that is quite different from the daily activities of middle-class people. They may lack running water in the home; to some, the modern toilet may seem strange and frightening. Badly decayed teeth may mean poor diet, lack of knowledge about oral hygiene, and perhaps ignorance of such things as toothbrushes and fluoride toothpastes. Deodorants are a luxury for those who do not know today where tomorrow's dinner will come from. The language of the poverty group may include words you regard as "bad," yet these words may be the patient's only means for expressing personal needs.

Information about the human body, health practices, and modern methods of diagnosis and treatment are unknown to many people, in spite of widespread health education programs in the schools, on television and radio, and in the newspapers. People who do not have factual information are likely to believe the **superstitions** of their culture just as firmly as you believe the information in a textbook. In fact, their beliefs may be closely tied in with love and respect for their parents, since such beliefs are passed down from one generation to the next. The teachings of your parents are important to you; and so it

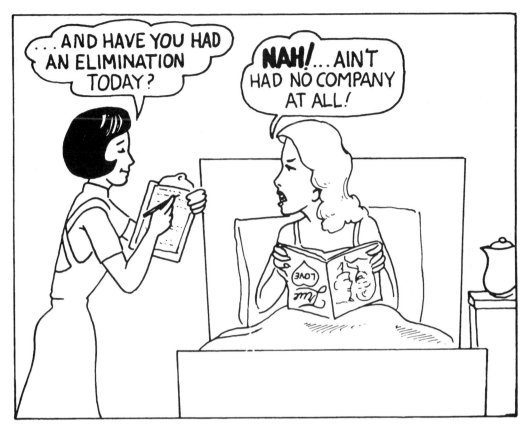

The vocabulary of health care providers may be foreign to some patients.

is with others, even though those teachings may be different from what you think is "right." If you do not respect beliefs of persons from a culture different from yours, you are showing cultural bias.

The Patient from the Affluent Class

Consider a patient who is from the upper socioeconomic level. This patient does not have financial problems. The material necessities of life are assured. Perhaps this person is accustomed to the best of service and, through habit, expects to receive good service. Perhaps this person's wealth represents much hard work and successful competition in the business world. Perhaps it is inherited wealth, and this person has known a life of ease without having to struggle for material comforts.

Good health, freedom from pain, and escape from disabling accidents cannot be assured by wealth. Does a wealthy patient seem unwilling to put up with an inconvenient illness? Is impatience exhibited when there is a delay in receiving an expected service? Is there evidence of rebellion against being a patient? Illness interrupts and alters patterns of living and does not respect the important matters that may await one's attention.

Even the wealthy have problems. Though different from those of the poverty group, their life problems may be very demanding. Therefore, the health care provider should not conclude that the wealthy patient should lie back and be a "good patient" because he/she does not have to worry about how to pay the medical bills.

Expectations of Health Care Providers

Each patient, regardless of socioeconomic status, age, race, religion, or national origin, is entitled to the best care you can give. Each is a human being with feelings, hopes, problems, habits, and needs. All of these factors contribute to the uniqueness of each personality.

Can you as a health care provider expect people from other economic levels of society to have the same beliefs, attitudes, hygienic habits, health practices, and understandings that you have? Are they either less worthy or more worthy as human beings because their lifestyles are different from yours?

IMPLICATIONS FOR HEALTH CARE PROVIDERS

Feelings About Patients

The degree to which you accept the philosophy of individual worth will influence your practice as a health care provider. You may need to overcome **prejudice** in order to apply this philosophy to your daily work. You may even have difficulty in understanding some patients, especially those whose cultural background is different from yours. Your responsibility as a health care provider is to know your role and, within that role, to serve each patient effectively. Avoid making value judgments about a patient or allowing your feelings to interfere with the quality of care you provide that person.

The Challenge

One of the greatest challenges in a health career is to provide health services to those who are from a different culture or economic level. Try to understand these patients in terms of their background; try to see situations as they see them. You can fulfill your role as a health care provider and at the same time adapt to the special needs of each patient. The example you set is important in teaching health habits. Your choice of words is important in helping the patient

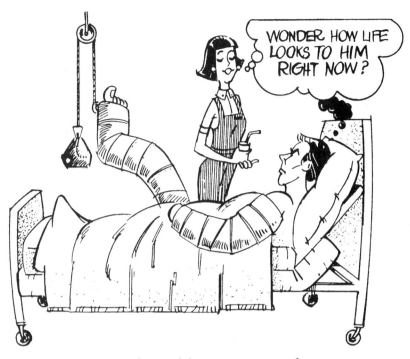

Try to understand the patient's point of view.

understand your meaning. Your sincerity and interest can influence a patient's attitude toward the entire health care system.

Studying a Situation

It is not easy to serve all patients equally well. Sometimes there is a strong desire to escape—to carry out an assigned task and leave the patient as quickly as possible. If you find yourself trying to avoid a patient or to leave the room quickly, that situation needs thoughtful study. Why do you find this patient difficult to serve? Does this patient remind you of someone you dislike? Have you tried to understand this patient's personal and health needs? Have you tried to see the situation as the patient sees it? If you make a habit of studying such situations, applying knowledge about some of the many influences on human behavior, you will grow in your ability to form effective relationships with your patients.

APPLYING A PHILOSOPHY OF INDIVIDUAL WORTH

It is easy to give lip service to the philosophy of individual worth. It is quite difficult to practice it day after day when there is a busy schedule and a wide variety of patients to take care of, unless you form certain ways of thinking about your patients. The following suggestions provide a starting point for developing and applying a philosophy of individual worth to your relationships with patients:

- Accept each patient as he or she is—an individual with a ***unique*** *personality.*

- Recognize that each person tries to meet his or her needs with patterns of behavior that have developed over a lifetime; these patterns cannot be changed readily.

- Make a conscious effort to understand each patient's behavior.

- Expect that many of your patients will not behave as you want them to behave.

- Do not expect a sick person to adapt to you. As a health care provider and as a well person, you should adapt to the patient.

- Consider each patient with a cultural background different from yours as an opportunity for you to learn about the influence of customs, beliefs, values, religious practices, and socioeconomic level on human behavior.

References and Suggested Readings

Backer, Barbara A., Hannon, Natalie R., and Gregg, Joan Young. *To Listen, To Comfort, To Care.* Albany, NY: Delmar Publishers Inc., 1994. "Role Expectations," pp. 53–57.

Tamparo, Carol D. & Lindh, Wilburta Q. *Therapeutic Communications for Allied Health Professions.* Albany, NY: Delmar Publishers Inc., 1992. "The Therapeutic Process," pp. 10–13.

REVIEW AND SELF-CHECK

Complete the following statements, using information from Unit 2.

1. The philosophy of "individual worth" is the belief that _____

   _____

   _____.

2. The following are examples of cultural differences that could contribute to a misunderstanding between a health care provider and a patient:

    a. _____

    b. _____

    c. _____

    d. _____

    e. _____

Circle the letter of the phrase that correctly completes the statements below.

1. A health care provider who accepts the philosophy of individual worth
    a. is not prejudiced.
    b. provides safe patient care.
    c. is likely to interact differently with patients from various cultures.
    d. is likely to interact the same with patients from various cultures.

2. The term "cultural bias" means
    a. that people are prejudiced.
    b. that people tend to make negative judgments about persons from another culture.
    c. that people from different cultures have different health practices.
    d. that people from different cultures have difficulty understanding each other.

ASSIGNMENT

1. Think about someone you know whose background is different from your own; list five ways in which this person's lifestyle is different from yours.

2. Think about each of the following situations; then write a possible explanation for each patient's behavior.
    a. Mrs. M. has a private room. Her gowns appear very expensive and there are luxury cosmetics on her dresser. She is hospitalized for diagnostic studies. After the second day, she appears to lack interest in grooming; her hair is uncombed and she has not applied any makeup.

b. Mrs. J. is a ward patient. She shows no interest in the food on her tray, has a messy unit, and shows no interest in other patients in the ward. The doctor carefully explained the plan for Mrs. J.'s care, but she fails to follow the doctor's instructions.

c. Johnny has been admitted through the clinic for a tonsillectomy. When the laboratory technician tries to draw a blood sample, Johnny kicks and screams. When he is being prepared for the operating room, a string with a small bag attached is found around his neck. He tries to prevent this from being removed, saying he will die if it is taken off.

3. Look up each of the following key terms in the glossary or a dictionary. Then write the meaning in your own words.

affluent	customs	socioeconomic
belief	philosophy	superstitions
cultural bias	prejudice	values

4. Participate in a class discussion about examples of cultural practices related to:
   - Beliefs
   - Eating habits and/or food selection
   - Hygienic practices
   - Attitudes about sickness
   - Attitudes toward health care
   - Expectations of health care providers
   - Beliefs about death

5. In your own words, explain the meaning of "individual worth."

6. Write a brief description of a situation involving you and someone from a different culture. Was there any evidence of misunderstanding or distrust? If so, try to identify one or more cultural differences that may have contributed to the misunderstanding or distrust.

Unit 3

Striving for Self-Understanding

OBJECTIVES

Upon completion of this unit, you should be able to:

- List three responsibilities of the learner.
- Explain why learning is defined as "a change in behavior."
- List five essentials for developing one's potential.
- Identify one's life role and appropriate behaviors for each role.
- Explain why role confusion is dangerous for a health care provider.
- List five guidelines for personal growth.

KEY TERMS

Continuous	Ethics	Habits
Learning	Potential	Procrastinate
Recurrence	Repertoire	Role
Self-understanding	Similarities	Traits

Today you are enrolled in a course of study that will lead to your becoming a health care provider. In the near future you will graduate and assume a position in an agency that provides health services to the community. What changes are needed before you, the student of today, can become you, the health care provider of tomorrow?

YOU, THE STUDENT

Obviously, you must acquire knowledge, learn to apply it appropriately to a wide variety of situations, and develop skill in performing certain procedures. Your teachers have organized for you a meaningful sequence of learning experiences. They will guide your step-by-step progress toward a future **role** in the field. Your teachers, however, cannot do the whole job. The desire to learn, willingness to make the necessary effort, and determination to gain as much as possible from each learning experience must come from you.

Learning Versus Memorizing

Learning has been defined as a *change in behavior.* If you can answer the questions on a test, but do not apply that information in appropriate clinical situations, have you *really* learned? Do you approach assignments as though you are a tape recorder, storing information that can be played back on demand? Such an approach to study is not true learning.

Developing Mental Skills

Do you constantly ask yourself how a new idea can be used? Does new information guide you in selecting appropriate behavior for situations where that information is relevant? If you can answer "Yes" to these questions, then you are truly learning. You are using mental processes such as thinking, reasoning, selecting, decision-making, and evaluating for conscious control of your behavior.

Developing Your Potential

Think of yourself for a moment as a person who loves music, but does not have a musical instrument or teacher. Suddenly, your family obtains a piano, and a gifted piano teacher moves next door. After an appropriate period of study under the guidance of your teacher, you become an excellent pianist. Thus, through a combination of the right circumstances and effort, your **potential** for becoming a pianist has been fulfilled and you *are* a pianist.

This period as a student is your opportunity to develop your potential as a health care provider. The circumstances for learning are being provided in the form of many learning experiences, each designed to help you acquire new knowledge and develop skills. The effort necessary to develop your potential can only come from you.

Let us now explore some of the ways you can strive to develop your potential for learning. These same approaches, applied to your future career, will help you develop your potential for becoming a health care provider.

TAKING A NEW LOOK AT YOURSELF

The immediate task is to undertake a study of yourself. "But," you say, "I already know myself." Do you really? If you do, you are a rare person indeed. True **self-understanding** is difficult to achieve. Even a beginning effort—just taking an honest look at yourself—may make you decide on some changes. The ability to be honest with yourself is absolutely necessary for achieving self-understanding.

Willingness to Change

The first question to ask yourself is, "Am I willing to make changes in myself?" When someone criticizes you, do you nurse your hurt feelings or express anger toward your critic? Do you reject the criticism? Or, do you see criticism as a possible indication that you need to change some aspect of your behavior? Willingness to change is necessary so that you can learn and grow as a person. Remember, learning was defined earlier as a change in behavior.

Strengths and Weaknesses

Your next question might be, "What are my strengths and my weaknesses?" To develop your potential, you must know your weak points, for these will need your attention and greatest effort. For example, do you have a habit of putting off a task until the last minute? This habit can lead to many undesirable results: being late to class, not being prepared for a test, not practicing a skill until you have achieved a high level of proficiency. By correcting a tendency to **procrastinate,** you can spare yourself the emotional strain of doing things at the last minute. You may even escape the irritation others express when your last-minute efforts inconvenience them.

An honest appraisal of your personal **traits,** including your work **habits,** is the key to planning ways of developing your potential. If you eliminate those behaviors that interfere with good performance, you will improve your ability to perform well in a variety of situations.

Adapting to New Conditions

A third question to ask yourself is, "How well do I adapt to change?" Are you still clinging to habits formed early in your school years? If so, these habits are probably not working very well in your present educational program. No longer can you depend on the teacher. No longer can you expect the teacher to go over the same material until you have passively absorbed it. Time is short, and there is much to be learned before you qualify as a health care provider. *You* must assume primary responsibility for learning.

Perhaps you once worked in the hospital as an aide. Now you are preparing for a different role. Will the habits you formed as an aide be acceptable in your new role? You will need to develop new habits appropriate to your new role and, possibly, to higher standards of performance.

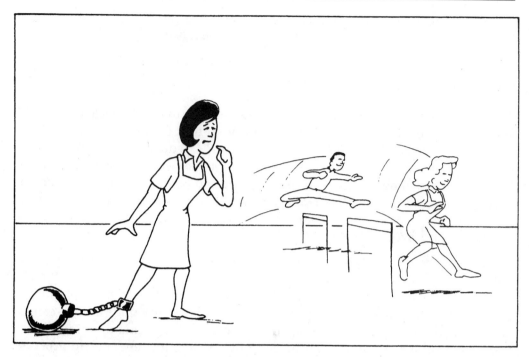

Old habits can hold you back.

Using Experience to Learn

A fourth question is, "Do I learn from my experiences?" Let us take a look at how two people reacted to an embarrassing experience. When Mary and Sue gave oral reports, they both showed signs of nervousness and performed poorly. For each of them, this was a very embarrassing experience.

Mary reviewed the situation, admitted to herself that she had put little effort into this assignment, and made plans to be well-prepared for the next oral report. She decided to have her information better organized, to study the material until she understood it, to prepare good notes, and to rehearse her presentation until she could present the report with minimal use of notes.

Sue, on the other hand, used the same approach to prepare her next oral report, which proved to be another poor performance. She was no better prepared for the second report than she was for the first. In addition, she was developing a fear of oral reports that would have a negative effect on her future efforts to speak in front of others.

Mary used her experience constructively, making careful plans to prevent a **recurrence** of this particular embarrassment. With additional practice, Mary will give oral reports with confidence. Sue, on the other hand, allowed the experience to create self-doubt and fear of oral reports. Do you think she will develop either skill or confidence? Which of these students will grow as a person? Are you a Mary or a Sue, in relation to learning from experience?

Role Perception

A fifth question to ask yourself is, "What is my role?" The present program of study will help you understand your future role as a health care provider. For every role there are appropriate and inappropriate ways of behaving. Whether a particular manner of behavior is appropriate depends not only on the specific *type* of health care provider you are preparing to become, but also on the *level* of that role in relation to other health team members.

Certain behaviors that are appropriate for personnel in a nursing service may not be appropriate for personnel in a different service. Also, there are differences in nursing service roles based on level. Nursing assistants, licensed practical nurses, registered nurses, head nurses, and supervisors all have specific roles within nursing. There are numerous roles within the hospital laboratory: pathologist, medical technologist, clinical laboratory assistant, laboratory aide, and others. These roles of laboratory personnel are distinct from those of nursing service personnel. The same is true of other hospital departments: physical therapy, radiology, food service, and others. In the dental field, dentists, dental hygienists, dental assistants, and dental laboratory technologists are all concerned with oral health. Their roles have **similarities,** but vary according to the specific functions and educational preparation of each.

Knowing one's role is essential to effective functioning; it is also essential to self-understanding. Most roles within the health field require accepting instructions from someone at the next higher level. If you do not like "taking orders," then you may not be happy as a health care provider. If you feel anger or distrust toward persons in authority, you are likely to resent the **ethics** of the health field, the policies of your health agency, and relationships with those on the health team who have responsibility for giving instructions, making assignments, and evaluating performance. On the other hand, if you can accept a defined role, function within that role to the fullest extent of your educational preparation, and accept the limitations of the role without feeling "put down," then you are likely to find much satisfaction as a health care provider.

YOU, A PERSON WITH SEVERAL LIFE ROLES

How many roles do you play? Probably several. You are a student now and hope to have a role as a health care provider in the future. You may be a husband, father, wife, mother; or you may be living in your parents' home, still in a dependent role. Even if you are living on your own, you still have the role of child to your parents, if they are living, in addition to the other roles in your life.

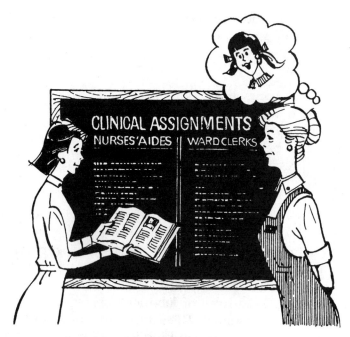

Each life role requires certain behaviors.

Role and Relationship With Others

There are similarities in the child-parent relationship and the teacher-student relationship during the school years. In a health occupations education program, the teacher-student relationship is between two adults, even though one adult is a student. What difficulties in role perception might occur if the student is a mature, fifty-year-old person, and the teacher is a twenty-five-year-old health professional?

Making a Distinction Between Roles

The roles you play at home, in your church activities, as a health occupations student, and as a neighbor are all different. To some extent, each role requires different behavior patterns. Do not confuse the health care provider role with other roles in your personal life. Some friends may try to get "free medical advice"; but the role of friend and the role of health care provider are different. Medical practice acts, which are state laws, make it illegal for nonphysicians to diagnose and prescribe. Therefore, this type of role confusion is dangerous.

GUIDES FOR GROWTH

Becoming an effective health care provider is a process that extends over a period of time. It requires **continuous** effort throughout one's career.

Value of Self-Study

In undertaking a self-study, you will be making an investment in your own future. Hopefully, this study will start you on a lifetime process of striving for personal growth. You should continuously evaluate your habits and modify those that do not get the desired response from others. There will always be some people with whom you do not "hit it off," but you can learn to relate to most people in ways that promote understanding and minimize unfavorable feelings. As you become skillful in using a large **repertoire** of human relations skills, you will grow in self-understanding, in tolerance, and in your ability to accept others as they are.

Value of Studying Human Behavior

Note that the sequence of growth is from understanding self to understanding others. Therefore, *the ability to understand others is limited until you have begun to understand yourself.*

Human behavior is very complex. In any situation, the behavior of a person is influenced by many different factors. The remainder of this course will introduce some of these influences. Striving to understand oneself and others must be based on knowledge about human behavior in general.

Striving for Personal Growth

Now let us summarize some ways you can try to understand yourself and set goals for personal growth and achievement as a student and health care provider.

- Recognize that learning occurs only if you make the effort to learn, if you are willing to change, and if you recognize opportunities for learning.

- Study yourself in relation to specific traits, such as willingness to change, ability to be honest with yourself, and readiness to correct weaknesses and change habits.

- Identify your strengths and make full use of them to achieve your goals.

- Identify your weaknesses—the traits or habits you need to change in order to be more effective in your roles.

- Study your various roles in terms of desirable behavior. Identify differences, such as habits used at home that are not appropriate at school: interpersonal relations between a parent and child that are not appropriate between the health care provider and a pediatric patient; relations between friends that are not appropriate between a hospital employee and a patient.

- Study your ability to make distinctions between different life roles and change behaviors accordingly.

- Study your tendency to use old habits in new situations. Do you allow habits to determine your behavior in any situation? Do you need to improve in adapting your behavior to each situation?

- Mentally review past experiences to understand how your own behavior contributed to the outcome. Consider the important question, "Would the outcome of that experience be improved if I had behaved differently?" This practice can serve as a "rehearsal" for future similar experiences.

References and Suggested Readings

Anderson, Carolyn. *Patient Teaching & Communication in an Information Age.* Albany, NY: Delmar Publishers Inc., 1990. "Self-Knowledge," pp. 29–33.
Tamparo, Carol D. & Lindh, Wilburta Q. *Therapeutic Communications for Allied Health Professions.* Albany, NY: Delmar Publishers Inc., 1992. "What Is Your Style?," pp. 16–17; "Professional Application," pp. 17–18.

REVIEW AND SELF-CHECK

Complete the following statements, using information from Unit 3.

1. In order to acquire the knowledge and skills needed as a health care provider, the health occupations student must _____ , _____ , and _____ .

2. Learning is defined as "a change in behavior" because _____ _____ .

3. In order to develop one's potential, it is necessary to:

   a. _____

   b. _____

   c. _____

   d. _____

   e. _____

4. The health care provider role and the role of friend/neighbor require different behaviors because _____ .

5. List five guidelines to follow as you undertake a program for developing your potential.

   a. _____

   b. _____

   c. _____

   d. _____

   e. _____

6. Compare the meanings of "habits" and "traits." _____

   _____

   _____

   _____

ASSIGNMENT

1. List some changes you have made in daily habits since you entered this health occupations program. Think of one additional change that may improve one of your life roles. Write out a description of the change and the steps necessary for making it part of your habitual behavior.

2. List the roles you play in addition to being a student.

3. Identify one habitual behavior in each of your roles that is not a desirable (or effective) behavior for your student role.

4. Identify one habitual behavior in your personal life that is not an acceptable behavior with patients or coworkers.

5. List five actions or behaviors that are appropriate in a friend/friend relationship, but are not appropriate in a health care provider/patient relationship.

6. Recall some unpleasant memory: an embarrassing experience, a failure, a situation in which a misunderstanding occurred, or one in which you behaved in a manner that you now recognize as inappropriate. Mentally review the situation and proceed with the following steps.
   a. Picture yourself in the actual setting.
   b. Who was there?
   c. What did other people say or do?
   d. What did you say or do?
   e. What happened after your behavior (whatever you said or did)?
   f. Was the consequence of your behavior a result of what you said or did? (Careful! Be honest with yourself in answering this question. Don't refuse to acknowledge that you brought about the consequences by inappropriate behavior. On the other hand, don't blame yourself for consequences over which you had no control.)
   g. How did you feel about the undesirable consequences at the time? (Again, be completely honest with yourself.)
   h. How do you now feel when you think about this experience?
   i. Now, reconsider the situation to learn from it. What behavior on your part might have brought about a more desirable consequence? Is the experience something that might occur again in the future? What will you say (or do) if a similar situation occurs in the future?

NOTE: We cannot change the past. So, it is pointless to continue feeling angry, embarrassed, or guilty about something that cannot be changed. If you are "haunted" by past experiences that arouse negative feelings, you should talk with a professional counselor to learn how to resolve these feelings; otherwise, they can interfere with your present and future adjustment.

The purpose of this exercise has been to help you learn from a past experience. Everyone has unpleasant memories that recur at times, arousing the same negative feelings that were experienced at the time. When reflecting upon that experience, you can eliminate to a large extent (and perhaps completely) the emotional response associated with the memory of that situation. Trying to extract a lesson from the experience may prepare you to deal effectively with some future situation. The advantages of using the above exercise are twofold: (1) elimination of a recurring, unpleasant memory and (2) preparation, through mental rehearsal, for a future similar experience.

Striving to Understand Human Behavior

Health care providers deal with people whose lives have been complicated by illness. The reactions people exhibit toward illness and hospitalization must be understood and accepted by health care providers as behavioral responses to a stressful situation.

The interpersonal skills of health care providers are important to the patient. The health care provider who can build rapport with patients increases confidence in the health team, promotes faith in the treatment plan, and is more likely to gain the patient's full cooperation in tests necessary for diagnosis. If a health care provider is unable to develop rapport, then the opposite may occur. The patient may have negative feelings toward members of the health team, may distrust them, and may not comply with the health care plan. The skillful health care provider can recognize behavior indicative of negative feelings and attitudes and make an effort to correct them. Section II explains some of the many factors that are basic influences on human behavior.

Unit 4

Influences on Behavior

OBJECTIVES

Upon completion of this unit, you should be able to:

- List five ways people are alike.
- Define heredity, chromosome, and gene.
- Define dominant, recessive, and sex-linked traits.
- List five possibilities that determine whether or not a particular trait will be inherited.
- Name four dimensions of the developmental process.
- Name two types of environment that influence a child's development.
- Name three important influences on development during childhood.
- Name three early childhood learnings that influence behavior in adult life.
- List four ways that one's interests influence behavior.
- Name the primary influence of one's value system on behavior.
- Define "standards of behavior."
- Compare responsibility for behavior during childhood and the adult period of life.
- Define "rapport."

KEY TERMS

Addiction	Embryo	Congenital
Chromosomes	Genes	DNA
Ethnic	Genotype	Genetics
Hereditary	Phenotype	Rapport
Prenatal	Standards of behavior	Teratogens
Value systems	Nurturing	

Human behavior is extremely complex. No one can hope to understand behavior completely, but it is helpful to know about some of the many factors that influence behavior.

HOW PEOPLE ARE ALIKE

All of us are alike in many ways. We have certain basic physical needs; we also have certain basic psychological needs. We have interests and value systems. We each have a unique hereditary endowment. We have all developed in a definite sequence that is characteristic of the human species. Behavior is influenced by factors that all people have in common and also by individual differences.

HOW PEOPLE ARE DIFFERENT

Each person forms certain behavior patterns for trying to meet basic physical and psychological needs. Each person develops their own certain interests. Each of us has a value system that influences our life choices. In striving to understand behavior, then, it is necessary to be aware of ways people are alike, ways people are different, and factors that influence the learning of behavior patterns. Three major forces interact to create a specific individual: heredity, the developmental process, and the environment.

HEREDITY

Each person is a unique individual. At the time of conception, **hereditary** traits are inherited from the mother and father to form a unique combination of traits. Since thousands of traits are involved, the possible combinations are limitless. That is why we say that no two people have exactly the same heredity, except in the case of identical twins. You are undoubtedly learning about heredity in other courses. Therefore, our concern here is to emphasize that *each person, from the time of conception, is endowed with a one-and-only combination of traits that will affect that individual throughout life.*

The Physiology of Heredity

At the time of conception, 46 **chromosomes** are organized into 23 matched pairs (23 from each parent). There are two sex-linked chromosomes: X for females and Y for males. The combination of chromosomes from the two parents provides the individual's **genotype,** a unique set of inherited traits. The **phenotype** is the result of all genes that, in combination, provide traits that determine the individual's physical appearance.

Genes are locations, more than a thousand on each chromosome. The total number of genes has been estimated at 50,000 (Burke, 1992). Each gene is composed of molecules of a protein called deoxyribonucleic (de-oxy-ribo-nu-cle-ic) acid **(DNA).** DNA is made up of four basic molecules, and each gene is made up of strings of these molecules arranged in a particular sequence. The molecules may be thought of as letters and their arrangement as words made up of those letters. The "words" are actually larger protein molecules, and each has a specific function—control of a specific cellular activity. The discovery of DNA and subsequent discovery of molecular sequences on strands of DNA were exciting scientific breakthroughs. This led to rapid development of human **genetics** as a scientific field of inquiry and the discovery of much new information on heredity.

The Genetic Basis for Individuality

A particular characteristic of an individual may be due to:

- One specific gene,
- The sequential arrangement of molecules on each gene,
- A particular pair of genes,
- A group of genes interacting with each other, or
- The influence of environmental factors on a gene or genes.

Some traits are expressed, meaning that the individual will definitely manifest that trait. Other traits are unexpressed but predispose that individual to manifest the trait under certain conditions. For example, a person may have the gene for a specific hereditary disease but will develop the disease only if the life situation includes certain conditions. A person who has the gene for a disease but does not develop symptoms is a carrier; that gene can be passed on to the children, who may manifest the disease.

Like chromosomes, genes are paired so that a given trait is determined by the contribution of either or both parents. A dominant trait will be expressed, even if inherited from only one parent; a recessive trait will manifest only if matched with a recessive gene from each parent. Some traits are sex-linked, meaning they are inherited through the X chromosome of the mother or are linked to the Y chromosome of the father. For example, red/green color blindness is expressed only in males but is inherited from the mother because the gene for color-blindness is carried on the mother's X chromosome.

Implications for Health Care

Genetics, the study of heredity, has expanded rapidly and is making significant contributions to medicine. Research to locate the genetic basis of diseases is ongoing, with new findings announced at increasingly frequent intervals.

A genetic disorder is one that results from an individual's genetic make-up. It may be apparent at birth, may appear as a developmental disorder, or may appear later in life as a disease or health problem. A single-gene disorder is due to the absence or alteration of one gene specific to that trait. Tests are available for many single-gene disorders, such as cystic fibrosis, hemophilia, and red/green color blindness.

A multifactorial disorder is one involving variations in several genes. Obviously, identifying several defective genes is more complex than identifying a single gene. There are also chromosomal disorders; for example, persons with Down Syndrome have three, rather than two, copies of chromosome 21. Chromosomal disorders affect about seven out of every thousand live births and are responsible for about fifty percent of spontaneous abortions during the first trimester (MS Encarta, 1993–1995).

Gene therapy is emerging as a specialty in medicine; therapy consists of modifying a defective gene in order to treat or prevent a specific disease. Genetic testing is already in use to identify certain single-gene disorders, confirm a diagnosis, identify carriers, and identify persons who are at risk for developing a disease, although currently free of symptoms.

From the moment of conception, then, an individual has a unique combination of **hereditary** traits, a blueprint that will guide growth, development, and numerous processes throughout that individual's life. Some genes are so specific that their traits cannot be modified by environmental influences or therapy. Other genes require pairing (one from each parent) in order for a trait or disorder to develop. Some genes are sex-linked—specific to the X or Y chromosome. Some genes provide a trait that will manifest only if environmental conditions foster its development.

Genetic Testing

Genetic testing is expensive. It also involves certain risks that should be made known to anyone who is considering genetic testing. Insurance companies and employers (or potential employers) can demand the results of genetic testing. There are examples of people who were denied insurance or lost their jobs when genetic tests indicated the presence of a gene for some specific disease (e.g., breast cancer, Huntington's Disease). Whereas a negative test can relieve one's anxieties, a positive test has profound psychological effects on the individual and his/her loved ones.

If your parent died at age forty-nine of Huntington's Disease, you may or may not develop this incurable disease. Genetic testing could remove this terrible cloud over your life if you do not have the specific gene. On the other hand, if you do have the gene, you will be faced with the certainty of developing the disease, probably during your forties. Would you choose to live with uncertainty? Or would you want to know, even if a positive test might cost you your job, insurance coverage, and relationships with those who cannot face the prospect of caring for you through a long illness. A positive approach to knowing that you have the gene would be to acknowledge your own mortality, accept that you will not have a long life, use your remaining years of health to live life to the fullest, and make end-of-life decisions while you are still in good physical and mental health.

Heredity establishes the basic physical/mental/emotional make-up and all the personality traits of each individual. But many other influences determine how these ingredients will be molded as the individual grows and develops from a helpless baby into an adult. One important difference is the built-in developmental rate, a **hereditary** factor. Thus, physical development proceeds at one rate for Johnny and at another rate for his brother Joe. The study of a child must always consider the apparent rate of development.

THE DEVELOPMENTAL PROCESS

Prenatal Influences

The developmental process is subject to tremendous environmental influence, even during the **prenatal** period. Ideally, the mother's body provides the **embryo** with a physical environment that is favorable to healthful development. This prenatal environment is affected by the mother's general health, her nutritional status, pathogenic organisms such as those causing syphilis or measles, and the presence in her blood of any substance that is toxic to the embryo.

The results of recent research indicate that the mother's daily habits have tremendous influence on the embryo. Even moderate use of tobacco, alcohol, and coffee can cause birth defects. Certain drugs, called **teratogens,** are known to cause **congenital** defects. Addictive substances used by a pregnant woman pass through the placenta to the baby. During the 1980s, cocaine **addiction** among women gave rise to a new type of patient—the "crack baby," a newborn baby addicted to cocaine. With increasing evidence that the pregnant woman's lifestyle has profound effects on the fetus, it is now clear that every expectant mother must avoid numerous substances if she is to have a healthy baby.

The role of nutrition during the prenatal period is currently acknowledged as critical to healthy prenatal development. For example, a serious congenital

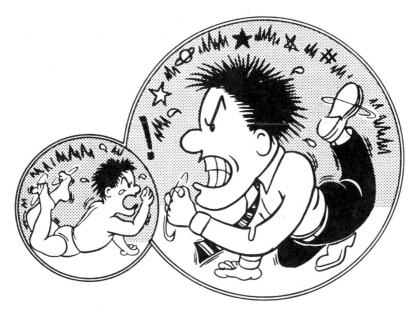

Physically a man—emotionally a little boy.

anomaly, spina bifida, is now known to be caused by a deficiency of folic acid. This developmental failure in the embryo occurs very early, so if a woman supplements her diet with folic acid *after* learning that she is pregnant, it is already too late to prevent this neural tube defect. The importance of folic acid is indicated by the new government requirement that it be added to certain commercial foods.

Every woman who may become pregnant should be concerned about nutrition, especially adequate intake of vitamins and minerals. With increasing evidence that the expectant mother's nutrition and use of certain substances has profound effects on the developing embryo/fetus, it is apparent that expectant mothers should maintain a healthful lifestyle and abstain from the use of substances that can harm the fetus.

Aspects of Development

The developmental process involves physical, emotional, intellectual, and spiritual dimensions. There is an interrelationship among these various dimensions, but the development of one can proceed faster than another. The conditions of an individual's life may promote maximum physical development, yet fail to promote emotional or intellectual growth. The conditions that affect each aspect of development are different. An ideal environment promotes optimal physical, emotional, intellectual and spiritual development. Most of us, however, have

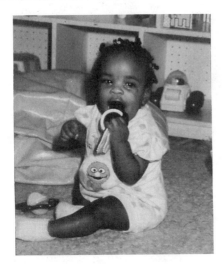 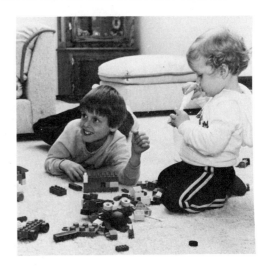

Attitudes, beliefs, and expectations learned as an infant and toddler influence behavior throughout life.

not been privileged to grow and develop in an ideal environment. The effects of environmental influences on the developmental process are discussed later in this unit in relation to specific periods of the life span.

ENVIRONMENT

The environment is another major influence on development and the expression of certain hereditary potentials. Much has been written about the relative importance of heredity and environment. With increasing knowledge about heredity and with growing awareness of the power of the physical and social environment to affect the developmental process, the debate becomes rather pointless. It is now apparent that the interaction of many forces determines the traits of an individual. Heredity provides the basic ingredients and the blueprint, but environmental factors and events that affect the developmental process determine what aspects of the blueprint will be expressed as traits. The result—a unique person who reflects both how people are alike and how people are different.

Physical Environment

Environment in its broadest sense means many things. The physical environment includes home conditions, climate, community conditions, means for meeting physical needs, and resources for developing one's potential. The boy who lives in a large city has a physical environment greatly different from the boy who lives on a farm. The air he breathes is polluted rather than fresh; the vegetables obtained from the store are not as fresh as those picked directly from the farm. Generally, the city boy has more technological resources available for developing certain talents. On the other hand, he may not have an opportunity to learn to ride a horse. All aspects of the physical environment affect personality. Some personality traits tend to develop in one kind of environment, whereas a different environment fosters the development of other traits.

Social Environment

The social environment involves people. A baby's experiences provide important first learnings about the world and people. The baby may learn that the world is a friendly place—that one can depend on others to correct such discomforts as hunger, cold, and a wet diaper. Or, the baby may learn the world is a hostile place—that one cannot rely on others to relieve hunger and cold. These infant experiences lay the foundation for future relations with other people: distrust or trust, expectations of comfort and **nurturing** from others, or resignation to discomfort without help from others.

INFLUENCES ON DEVELOPMENT DURING CHILDHOOD

The basic heredity of a child, plus environmental influences, exert a powerful influence on development.

The Preschool Years

Throughout the early years, a child continues to learn about people and the world. If these learnings are favorable, the child develops a sense of security and finds the world a place for exploring and satisfying curiosity. There are happy experiences and unhappy ones, but comfort is available when unhappy experiences occur. If the learnings of early childhood are unfavorable, the child learns to distrust other people and tends to fear new experiences or strange places. These early life experiences establish attitudes, beliefs, and expectations that may continue to influence behavior throughout life.

The School Years

When the child enters school, the physical and social environments are greatly extended. If development has proceeded according to schedule, the child is ready for this expansion of experience. If the physical or social environment of early life inhibited some aspect of development, then the child may not be ready to benefit fully from school. Early school experiences may be so unsatisfying that they inhibit development of one or more dimensions.

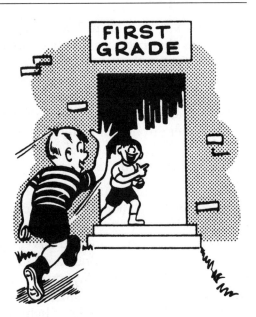

Early learnings influence readiness for new experiences.

First-graders show marked differences in development and in behavior patterns. These differences reflect both hereditary and environmental influences. Some children readily adapt to being with a group of their own age; others hang back, afraid to join the group. Some see the teacher as absolute authority, to be obeyed without question; others show rebellion toward authority. Still others voice their opinions freely and may even expect to have a choice of whether or not to follow the teacher's instructions. Some first-graders are quite self-reliant; others depend on the teacher for assistance with every task. Some are bubbling with ideas and participate fully in every activity; others sit quietly and participate only when urged. These differences are not accidental. They are the result of early influences on patterns of behavior.

Social Influences on Development

The home environment is of great importance in the young child's development. How well does the family provide for the child's physical needs? What health practices are followed? Is the home atmosphere democratic or authoritarian? Do the parents "wait on" the child, or do they allow the child to develop self-reliance gradually? Is there an anxious parent who repeatedly warns the child about getting hurt?

The child's home may include an abusive parent. Child abuse is widespread; many abusive parents were themselves abused as children. The abuse may be physical, mental or emotional. Mental and emotional abuse may be inflicted verbally (for example, with put-downs or guilt-arousing statements) or by specific actions (isolation, darkness). Physical abuse may be in the form of beatings or sexual activities. When a child is abused sexually, the abuser is most often a relative or family friend, someone the child trusts (or fears). All too often the abuser makes the child feel responsible for what happened; or the abuser convinces the child that the two of them have a secret that must not be shared with anyone. The abuser may even threaten to harm the child if this "secret" is revealed to anyone. The abused child has a heavy burden. In addition to physical trauma, the child has to deal with fear, anger, and guilt. And unless they get help, abused children may grow up to become abusive parents. This reflects the lifelong influence of adults on a child's future.

The child may belong to a minority group. Or, be labeled "different" as a result of being the only individual of a particular culture in the peer group. If so, does the family maintain the lifestyle of the **ethnic** culture? How much rejection has the child experienced? Is the child's religion different from that of most classmates? What misunderstandings might this create?

What is the neighborhood environment? Is it safe or full of hazards for children? Are there opportunities for a wide variety of experiences? Are there relatives and neighbors who care about the child, or is the social climate of the neighborhood hostile? Are the parents from another country? If so, do they require the child to behave in ways appropriate for that country, but inappropriate in the present community?

Role models are powerful influences on children. Every adult in a child's world has the potential to serve as a role model, whether they be within the home (immediate or extended family), the neighborhood, the church, or at school. Role models influence children in many ways—value system, parenting style, career choice. The role model's influence may be positive or negative. It may last a lifetime or it may be temporary. A child may have only one role model or may adopt different role models at various life stages. An adult may even be unaware that he/she is serving as a role model for a specific child.

CHANGING INFLUENCES DURING LIFE

Early learnings continue to influence behavior throughout life, often without the individual's awareness. On the other hand, one can learn to recognize certain early influences on behavior and, where desirable, modify the behavior patterns that have resulted. *Whereas a child is the helpless victim of developmental influences, an adult can become self-directing.* The adult can recognize an undesirable behavior pattern and choose to change it. An adult can seek to understand the basis for a particular behavior and, with such understanding, resist or eliminate that early influence. An adult can leave an unhealthy situation and seek a more favorable environment. These options are not available to a child, who is trapped in a specific living situation. It is now acknowledged that many runaway children are trying to escape abusive home situations.

Modifying Early Learnings

Prejudice is one example of early learning that can influence a person's behavior throughout life unless the individual chooses to examine behavior patterns and their apparent origins. Prejudice is usually learned early in life from those people around us. In its most common form, prejudice consists of negative feelings toward people from a different race or subculture. If parents and their friends speak in unkind terms about members of another race, the child is influenced to develop negative feelings also. The child may exhibit hostility or disrespect toward members of another race. As adults, however, we do not have to cling to such early learnings. We can re-examine our attitudes in light of new knowledge and personal experience. Often, we find that our prejudice does not hold up against rational examination. As adults, we can modify early learnings and take control of our own behavior, attitudes, and beliefs.

An example of unexamined prejudice is the behavior of people who belong to one of the "hate groups." The leaders of such groups depend on "us versus them" thinking to arouse strong feelings and mobilize people to behave as the leaders wish them to behave. Televised reports of demonstrations show people who are controlled by their emotions, rather than by clear thinking. And those emotions probably have their roots in early learnings that have not been re-examined during adulthood. People who blindly accept the hate policies of a group, or even of a government, are allowing others to do their thinking, determine their beliefs, and control their behavior. Throughout adult life, one should continuously evaluate and modify beliefs and **value systems.**

Interests

Interests also influence behavior. They determine where we direct our attention. They even enter into the decisions we make, the activities we pursue, the occupations we choose, and the types of recreation we select for our leisure time. People who have many interests are well prepared for forming effective relationships with a variety of people. Those who have only their work and hours of television-watching do not have much to offer others in the way of interesting companionship. Developing a variety of interests, is one way to become a more interesting person, find greater satisfaction in living, and form satisfying relationships.

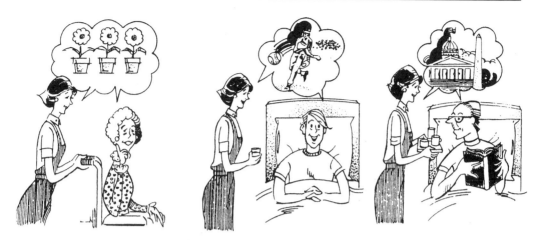

Having a variety of interests helps in forming effective relations with different people.

Value Systems

A value system is the degree of importance we attach (largely unconsciously) to various beliefs, ideas, or material things. Each person's value system has a strong influence on behavior. Each of us has a value system, even though we may not be conscious of it. Did you give up going to a movie in order to do an assignment for today? Then you placed a higher value on some aspect of being a student—responsibility, achievement, or perhaps duty—than you did on recreation, at least as far as this one sample of your behavior is concerned. Did you return the extra dime you received as change at the grocery store? Then you placed a higher value on honesty than on "getting the best of the other fellow." Did you cheat on that last test in order to improve your grade? Then you placed a higher value on a grade than on honesty or true learning.

The value system includes many things: character traits such as honesty and truthfulness, personal achievement, the symbols of achievement, love and friendship, material possessions, religion, recreation, work, and family living. Each person's value system begins to form early in life, influenced by the rewards or punishments that followed specific types of behavior. Throughout life, the value system exerts a powerful influence on behavior, particularly when there is a choice to be made. Your enrollment in this educational program indicates that you value education enough to attend classes and do your assignments. If one of the young women in the class has a boyfriend urging her to quit school and marry him, she will be influenced not only by the feeling she has for him but also by the place education occupies in her value system. Does the value she places on her education outweigh the value she places on immediate marriage?

Standards of Behavior

Standards of behavior consist of our own personal rules and regulations, our own "dos" and "don'ts," that are part of our self-concept. There is a close relationship between one's value system and one's standards of behavior. They are both learned early in life and continually modified according to life experiences.

Standards of behavior should never be modified impulsively, especially if it involves lowering one's standards. Teenagers are often subjected to pressure from their friends to abandon home teachings and adopt the groups' code of behavior. This can be a difficult decision for a young person, since peer acceptance is very important during adolescence. Sometimes, as an adult who is dealing with a difficult decision, one needs to examine *consciously* the standards of behavior, values, and beliefs that usually control one's behavior. Identification of these influences may facilitate making a decision. Or, becoming clear about these influences may result in modifying a certain value or belief and the specific behavior that it supports.

There is a difference between current standards and those of the previous generation. Standards of behavior, therefore, are a frequent source of misunderstanding between parents and adolescents. There are also wide differences in standards of behavior from one subculture to another. Standards of behavior, including sexual behavior, vary between socioeconomic levels. Middle-class families tend to have the most rigid codes of behavior. Yet even within a particular socioeconomic level, there are wide variations from one family to another.

ASSUMING RESPONSIBILITY FOR BEHAVIOR

You should now be aware that human personality is the result of many ingredients. It is continuously molded by the environment and by life experiences. It is always subject to further change as a result of future life situations.

As children, our early learnings were determined by circumstances beyond our control. As adults, we have a choice. We can continue to live without consciously directing our lives, or we can take control. We can foster certain aspects of our personalities and play down other aspects. We can learn to make sound decisions. We can learn to recognize ineffective behaviors that may prevent us from reaching our goals. Thus, we can become relatively self-directing instead of living by patterns of thought and behavior established during childhood. Even more important, as adults we can think through various issues, decide what our values are, set our own standards of behavior, and accept or reject the values and standards proposed to us by others.

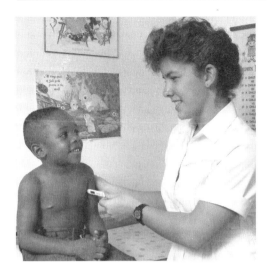
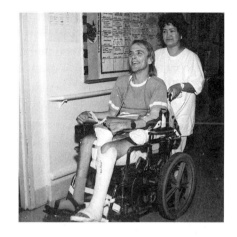
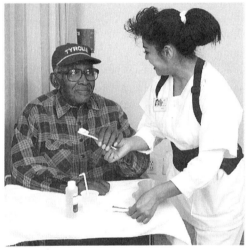
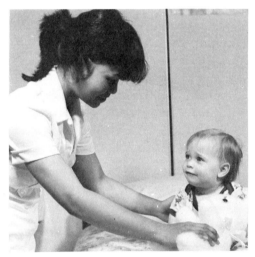

Accept each patient in accordance with his or her stage of development.

THE HEALTH CARE PROVIDER AND THE PATIENT

As a health care provider, you will find great satisfaction in your work if you make a conscious and continuous effort to study behavior—your own and that of other people.

You will be meeting people from many different backgrounds. With some, it will be easy to establish a pleasant relationship, one in which the patient believes that *you understand* and that *you are sincerely concerned.* Such a relationship is called **rapport.**

There will be some patients with whom you find it difficult to communicate. Perhaps the patient's behavior arouses unfavorable feelings in you. Perhaps you just do not find the patient "interesting" as a person. Such a patient is likely to perceive you as "indifferent" or "cold." As long as this climate exists between you and the patient, rapport will not be established. It is easy to project blame or label the patient "difficult." The patient's behavior, however, may be a reaction to your unconscious rejection of the patient.

Any patient who has been labeled "difficult" needs special attention from the health team. The behaviors that cause the patient to be labeled "difficult" may actually be signs that the patient's needs are not being met. But, on the other hand, the pleasant, agreeable patient may be covering up true feelings and may have just as much need for understanding and concern. In other words, as a health care provider, you will need to apply interpersonal skills to *establish rapport with each patient* as an individual. Some patients will be more of a challenge than others, but all need your understanding and sincere interest if you are to make a positive contribution to their health care.

References and Suggested Readings

Burke, Shirley R. *Human Anatomy and Physiology in Health and Disease.* Albany, NY: Delmar Publishers Inc., 1992. "Genetics," pp. 428–431.

Fong, Elizabeth, Scott, Ann Senisi, Ferris, Elvira, and Skelley, Ester G. *Body Structures & Functions;* Eighth Edition. Albany, NY: Delmar Publishers Inc., 1993. "Genetics" and "Types of Mutations," p. 306; "Lethal Genes," pp. 306–307; "Human Genetic Disorders," pp. 307–310.

Kalman, Natalie & Waughfield, Claire G. *Mental Health Concepts;* Third Edition. Albany, NY: Delmar Publishers Inc., 1993. Chapter 3, "Understanding Self and Others," pp. 36–63.

MicroSoft Corporation. *Microsoft® Encarta® 96 Encyclopedia.* © Funk Wagnalls Corp., 1993–1995.

Ornstein, Robert. *The Roots of the Self: Unraveling the Mystery of Who We Are.* New York, NY: HarperCollins Publishers, 1993. Chapter 1, "Introduction: The Puzzle of Individuality," pp. 1–12; Chapter 2, "From the Cell to the Self," pp. 25–32.

Source of Additional Information

National Cancer Institute: 1–800–422–6237. Free booklet "Understanding Gene Testing."

REVIEW AND SELF-CHECK

Complete the following statements, using information from Unit 4.

1. List five ways that people are alike.

    a. _____

    b. _____

    c. _____

    d. _____

    e. _____

2. Define the following words and phrases in your own words, using infor-
    mation in Unit 4.

Heredity	DNA	Recessive trait
Chromosome	Dominant trait	Sex-linked trait
Gene		

3. List five possibilities (pertaining to genes) that determine whether or not
    a particular trait will be inherited.

4. The two major influences on a person's development are _____

    _____ and _____.

5. Four dimensions of the developmental process are _____ ,

    _____ , _____ and _____ .

6. Two components of environment that influence development are the

    _____ environment and the _____ environment.

7. List three learnings of the early childhood period that influence behavior
    throughout life.

    a. _____

    b. _____

    c. _____

8. Three important influences on a child's early development are:

   a. _____

   b. _____

   c. _____

9. The influence of interests on behavior includes:

   a. _____

   b. _____

   c. _____

   d. _____

10. The term "standards of behavior" refers to _____

    _____ .

11. Choices available to an adult but not available to a child include:

    a. _____

    b. _____

    c. _____

    d. _____

12. Rapport exists between a caregiver and patient when _____

    _____ .

ASSIGNMENT

The following exercises are designed to give you an opportunity to apply some of the ideas discussed in Unit 4.

1. Using the following format, develop your family genetic chart as a guide to the possible contributions of heredity to your present and future health. Add additional lines as needed to list all members of your

RELATION	CURRENT AGE OR AGE AT DEATH	CAUSE OF DEATH	HEALTH PROBLEMS
Father			
Grandfather			
Grandmother			
Uncles			
Aunts			
Mother			
Grandfather			
Grandmother			
Uncles			
Aunts			
Sisters			
Brothers			

extended family. Add any cousins who have significant health problems, birthmarks, or congenital conditions.

2. Mary grew up in a home where standards of behavior were quite rigid. Her requests for permission to do something were often met with the question, "What would people think?" As an adult, Mary often feels anxiety about the opinions of others.

   You, too, are affected in many ways by early learnings. List five learnings from your own childhood that still influence your behavior.

3. Refer to the list you made in Assignment 1. Which of these early learnings are no longer appropriate guides to your behavior? State why they are no longer appropriate.

4. List ten things that are important to you. Number them from 1 to 10 in order of importance—*1* most important and *10* least important. Describe a decision that may be influenced by this order of values.

5. Don is an only child. He has finished school and started his first job. He has been dating Cindy for two years and wants to get married. His parents want him to wait until he is older and has accumulated some money. How will Don's value system influence his decision?

6. Joan is hopeful that she will be admitted to a dental assistant educational program next month. Joan's mother wants her to take a secretarial course. How can Joan consciously use her interests and value system to make a wise choice?

7. List five of your interests. State how each interest will be helpful to you as a health care provider.

8. Mrs. J. is filling out an application form for a nursing education program. She lists reading as a hobby. When discussing the application with Mrs. J., the director of the program asks what books she has read recently. Mrs. J. is unable to name the last book she read. In fact, she has not read a book for several years.

    Mrs. J. is not realistic about herself. She sees herself as a person who reads books as a hobby, yet she does not take the time to read a book. Her idealized self is a person who reads books; her true self is a person who does not read books. Consider your idealized self as an obstacle to understanding your true self, and also as a goal toward which the true self can strive. If you are not in the habit of seeing yourself as you are, there may be wide differences in the values, interests, and standards of behavior of your idealized self as opposed to your true self. Consider this possibility, as you study yourself in relation to interests, in the following exercise.

    a. Review the list of interests you made for Assignment 6. Estimate the amount of time you have spent on each interest during the past seven days.

    b. Place a star by those interests to which you have devoted as much as five hours. (Reading assignments for your health occupations course do not count as evidence of reading as one of your interests!)

    c. Place an "X" by those interests about which you are sufficiently informed to carry on a conversation with someone who is knowledgeable on that subject.

    d. Evaluate your interests in terms of variety, keeping in mind that it is not really one of your interests *unless you devote time to it and are informed about it.*

    e. Select one activity for increasing the breadth of your interests. Plan how you will learn about this activity and develop the skills of that activity during the next six months.

9. Prepare a written plan for improving your ability to establish rapport with patients. The instructor will tell you how this plan is to be evaluated.

Unit 5

Physical Needs

OBJECTIVES

Upon completion of this unit, you should be able to:

* List the five levels of human needs as proposed by Maslow.
* Explain why Maslow stated these needs as a hierarchy.
* List and explain four influences on the formation of behavior patterns.
* List five physical needs that are essential to survival.
* Accept the behavior of others as the result of past experiences and/or striving for need-satisfaction.

KEY TERMS

Biorhythms	Substitution	Variability
Circadian rhythms	Consequence	Dependency
Compensation	Necrosis	REM sleep
Hierarchy		

All of us have certain basic needs. In having such needs and inner forces that drive us to satisfy these needs, we are all alike. In the ways we attempt to satisfy these needs, we are all different. We are also different in the goals we set. What satisfies one person does not satisfy another. The tremendous **variability** in human behavior patterns makes the study of human behavior a continuing challenge.

A number of psychologists and sociologists engaged in the study of human behavior have described these needs in various ways. The most useful approach for our purpose is the model provided by a psychologist. Professor Abraham Maslow. This model is known as Maslow's Hierarchy of Needs. The term hierarchy means arranged in a specific order or rank.

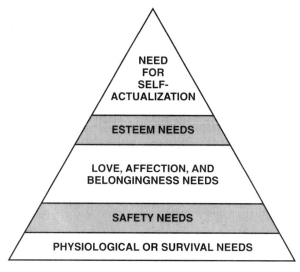

Maslow's hierarchy of needs

MASLOW'S HIERARCHY OF NEEDS

In Maslow's hierarchy, human needs for survival are primary; the need for safety is secondary. Following in sequence are needs related to love and belonging, the need for esteem and the need for self-actualization. These five levels of human needs are shown in hierarchical arrangement in the above diagram.

According to Dr. Maslow, each level of need must be satisfied before an individual is ready to strive for satisfaction of the next higher level of need. The highest level refers to full development of one's human potential. The remainder of Section II will focus on needs relevant to the first four levels. Unit 5 is devoted to the physical needs, which are related to levels 1 and 2.

ESSENTIAL PHYSICAL NEEDS

Meaning

Some physical needs are essential to life; others contribute to comfort and satisfaction. The physical needs that are essential to life are oxygen, water, food, protection, and sleep. These needs are not only essential to the life of the total organism, but also to the survival of individual cells. For example, a body part that does not receive a continuous supply of oxygen and nourishment will die. If this body part is a vital organ, then the individual will also die. If, however, the body part is a finger, the affected finger can be surgically removed and the individual will survive, minus the finger. Death of tissues in a limited area is called **necrosis.** It is usually due to lack of an adequate blood supply that deprives the cells of oxygen and nourishment. As you work in the health field, you may see patients with necrosis of some body part or area.

Deprivation

Death due to suffocation, drowning, starvation, or dehydration occurs when the body is deprived of oxygen, food, or water. Frostbite and injuries (from accidents, ferocious animals, or a human attacker) illustrate the importance of protection.

Lack of oxygen can be fatal in a matter of minutes. Lack of water first leads to an imbalance in body chemistry. If the lack of water continues, severe dehydration develops, vital functions cease, and death occurs.

Lack of food can be tolerated for longer periods of time because the body can store digested nutrients in certain body tissues. Prolonged lack of nourishment leads to utilization of these stored materials, with consequent shrinking or wasting of body tissues. If lack of nourishment continues until the body reserve is exhausted, then death from starvation occurs.

The time element does not apply to protection in the same sense that it applies to lack of oxygen, food, and water. The importance of protection is related to the presence of potential harm as well as the ability of the individual to avoid it.

Sleep is essential to life and health, but people are more inclined to deprive themselves of sleep than of water, food, and air. The body's demand for sleep can be resisted, or even ignored, more easily than hunger, thirst, and the need for oxygen. Yet ignoring one's need for sleep is a form of body abuse, and the price can be high. For this reason, health care providers need to be informed about the sleep mechanism and its relationship to health.

THE SLEEP CYCLE

Numerous body functions involve specific rhythms or cycles, known collectively as **biorhythms.** The frequency of these rhythms ranges from fractions of a second to months or years; **circadian rhythms** are based on the 24-hour period that makes up one day. The need for sleep is regulated by the brain's circadian pacemaker, influenced by the earth's electromagnetic fields.

Sleep consists of two phases that alternate throughout the sleep period: **REM (rapid eye movement) sleep** and non-REM sleep. The latter phase is a period when most body processes slow down, the muscles are relaxed, and the eyes are relatively still. This phase includes four stages of progressively deeper sleep. Following a complete cycle of the four stages, the REM phase begins. In this phase, there is an increase in mental activity, dreaming occurs concurrently with bursts of rapid eye movement, breathing is irregular, and pulse and blood pressure rise and fall. In normal young adults, the first non-REM phase lasts about 90 minutes and is followed by about 15 minutes of REM sleep. The frequency and duration of REM sleep periods increase during the final hours of sleep, especially between the sixth and eighth hours.

The dreaming that occurs during REM sleep is thought to be a major factor in stress management. The entire sleep period is a time when the brain cleanses itself of the day's accumulated sensory input and prepares for the next day's mental activity; it is also the time when the brain replenishes its stock of neurotransmitters. Although people vary in the amount of sleep they need to awaken rested and refreshed, less than eight hours of sleep deprives the body of some periods of REM sleep. Research conducted in sleep laboratories has revealed that deprivation of REM sleep has the same effects as sleep deprivation.

The effects of sleep deprivation emphasize the essential aspect of sleep and rest. After the loss of one night of sleep, a person has poor concentration and coordination; usually irritability is increased. Anyone who is deprived of sleep for several days will experience hallucinations and exhibit psychotic behavior.

Sleep deprivation is an increasing problem in American society. The temptations of late night television programming and the lure (some say "addiction") of the Internet are causing large numbers of people to get as little as two or three hours of sleep per night. Eventually, continued sleep deprivation will exact a price.

Some health care providers work a double shift; those who regularly work the night shift may experience twenty-four to thirty hour periods without sleep before or after their days off. These people should make a special effort to ensure adequate sleep and rest, for both personal health and protection of patients from errors due to lack of sleep and fatigue.

Satisfaction of Physical Needs

The physical needs have an important characteristic that sets them apart from psychological needs—*they can be satisfied in only one way.* An abundant supply of oxygen cannot make up for a lack of food. Abundant food stored within body tissues cannot provide survival for the worker who has just been buried in a cave-in and has no supply of oxygen. The need for sleep can be satisfied only by sleeping; though eating may enable one to delay going to sleep, food cannot satisfy the body's need for sleep. *Each essential physical need can be met only by a specific substance or condition.* Neither **substitution** nor **compensation** is possible. This will become more meaningful as we explore comfort needs in the next section and the social and emotional needs of people in the following topics.

COMFORT AND SAFETY NEEDS

There are also physical needs that are highly desirable but not essential to life. These needs are related to comfort and a sense of well-being. Labor-saving devices, soundly built homes, running water, comfortable clothing, and automatic heat seem like essential needs to those who are accustomed to them. Though some of these comforts are not essential for survival, they do meet safety needs and contribute to health and well-being.

PHYSICAL NEEDS AND BEHAVIOR

Results of Behavior

Each person has specific ways for trying to meet needs. The baby cries when hungry but is dependent on others to provide nourishment. Throughout childhood each of us learned which behaviors were successful or unsuccessful in meeting our needs within the home and in the subculture. The child tends to repeat any behavior that results in satisfaction of a need and to abandon behaviors that do not get results. Behavior patterns are established on the basis of **consequences**—what happens following a specific behavior.

Cultural Influences

A city person purchases food at the grocery store, but is dependent upon a complex system of marketing and distribution to keep a supply available. A rural person may purchase only staples and depend on a garden and perhaps livestock from a nearby farm to provide most of the family's food. A rural family living at a subsistence level may depend upon hunting or fishing for food. A family living in poverty in a large city may depend upon the welfare department for food. The pattern of striving that is learned from childhood on is influenced by the customs and practices of the family, neighborhood and community. The pattern of striving is also influenced by individual factors, such as the desire to obtain the comforts of life and the value placed on conforming to group standards.

Self-Reliance Versus Dependency

Some people are largely self-reliant in obtaining food, clothing and shelter. Some people depend on others to provide their basic needs. Dependency may involve so much of the person's life that any change is extremely upsetting. The farm wife whose husband is hospitalized with a serious illness may seem to you to be unnecessarily upset. Actually she is realizing that unless her husband recovers in time to plant or harvest the crops, their family will be without income for a year. Patient and family reactions to illness are closely tied to the role of each member and their life situation.

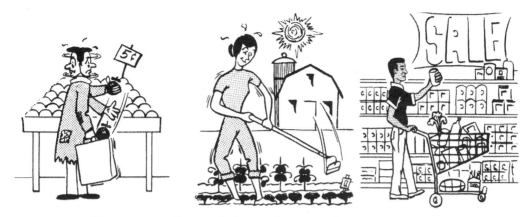

Our life situation influences behavioral patterns for meeting basic needs.

UNDERSTANDING BEHAVIOR IN TERMS OF PHYSICAL NEEDS

There are certain physical needs that people must meet in order to survive. There are other needs that make people more comfortable, enable them to live with less struggle, or free them from routine tasks so they may do other things that are more satisfying. In having these needs, people are alike. In the specific ways they strive to meet these needs, people are different. But each person strives in ways that have been learned by imitating members of one's subculture and from personal experiences. Each person tends to repeat the behavior that has been successful in satisfying a particular need. This repetition becomes established as a behavior pattern.

Most people meet their needs in ways acceptable within the laws, customs, and religious beliefs of their group. Some people choose or are forced by circumstances to violate the laws or customs of the group in order to satisfy their needs. These people too may be striving in their own way—the only way they know. Here too, the health care provider's philosophy of individual worth can be applied to understanding, rather than judging, a patient.

References and Suggested Readings

Hauri, Peter, Ph.D. & Linde, Shirley, Ph.D. *No More Sleepless Nights.* New York, NY: John Wiley & Sons Inc., 1990.

Kalman, Natalie & Waughfield, Claire G. *Mental Health Concepts;* Third Edition. Albany, NY: Delmar Publishers Inc., 1993. "Hierarchy of Needs," pp. 66–67.

Meredith, Dennis. "How to get your ZZZZZzzzz: Sleep therapy." *Duke Magazine,* March–April, 1996, pp. 2–5.

Tamparo, Carol D. & Lindh, Wilburta Q. *Therapeutic Communications for Allied Health Professions.* Albany, NY: Delmar Publishers Inc., 1992. "Abraham Maslow, Humanist," pp. 113–115.

Sources of Additional Information

American Sleep Disorders Association National Office, 1610 14th St. NW, Suite 300, Rochester, MN 55901

National Sleep Foundation, 122 S. Robertson Blvd., Los Angeles, CA 90048

REVIEW AND SELF-CHECK

Fill in the blanks to complete each statement below.

1. The levels of need in Maslow's Hierarchy of Needs are:

   _____

   _____

   _____

   _____

   _____

2. Dr. Maslow stated these needs as a hierarchy because _____ _____ .

3. In Maslow's Hierarchy, physical needs fit into the level concerned with _____ .

4. Some influences on the behavior patterns a person develops to satisfy physical needs are:

   a. _____

   b. _____

   c. _____

   d. _____

5. Five physical needs that are essential to survival are:

   a. _____   d. _____

   b. _____   e. _____

   c. _____

6. Two phases of the sleep cycle are _____ and _____.

7. Three effects of sleep deprivation for twenty-four hours or more are:

   a. _____   c. _____

   b. _____

ASSIGNMENT

1. In your mind, review some early influences in your life that shaped the patterns of behavior you now use to meet your physical needs. Do your patterns reflect dependence on others? Or self-reliance? How would these patterns be affected if you should become disabled? Visualize yourself in such a situation. How might your reaction to this enforced change be reflected in your behavior?

2. List five differences between two socioeconomic levels (lower class and middle class, or middle class and upper class).

3. State one aspect of a health care provider's philosophy that would ensure the same quality of care for a patient who is "different."

4. List five facts or beliefs to guide your behavior when you find that your clinical assignment is a young woman with a bullet wound inflicted during an attempted robbery of a convenience store.

5. List five facts or beliefs to guide your behavior when your assignment includes a young manic depressive male who was shot by a policeman when the young man was threatening to commit suicide.

6. You have learned about several influences on behavior patterns. List some possible differences in the behavior of people from three socioeconomic levels in each of the situations listed in the following chart.

SITUATION	EXTREME POVERTY	LOWER SOCIO-ECONOMIC CLASS	MIDDLE CLASS
Example: A severe "flu" epidemic	Resignation to sickness and death as a part of life; little tendency to assume personal responsibility to take action to control the uncertainties of life	Some tendency toward resignation; perhaps seeking medical assistance from a clinic; possible reliance on home remedies, hearsay, or superstitions	Seeking of "flu shots" from private physicians; medical help for victims from private physicians; perhaps criticism of medical profession for lack of precise methods for prevention and cure
Passage of a local ordinance requiring certain types of garbage containers, and a fine of $25.00 for not abiding by this regulation			
Serious illness in the "provider" of a family			
A public health campaign on the importance of obtaining a new type of immunization			
Hospitalization for the first time: Adult patient Child patient			

Unit 6

The Need for Self-Approval

OBJECTIVES

Upon completion of this unit, you should be able to:

- Explain social needs.
- Define compensation, autonomy, and self-esteem.
- Explain self-concept.
- Describe three important influences on one's self-concept.
- Compare self-concept and self-esteem.
- Explain the influence of success and failure experiences on self-concept and self-esteem.
- Describe the relationship between "success expectation" and "performance."
- List two essential steps for modifying a habit.
- List and explain six steps of the problem-solving process.
- Use systematic problem-solving to resolve life problems.
- Develop written goals for modifying personal traits and/or behavioral patterns.

KEY TERMS

Autonomy	Appraisal	Aptitudes
Hindrance	Competent	Derogatory
Potent	Socializing	Persistence

In the previous unit, you learned about influences on the ways people strive to meet their physical needs. There are other human needs that are just as important to comfort and happiness as physical needs. These other needs are also **potent** influences on behavior, but they are less obvious than the physical needs. This unit will help you learn about social and psychological needs as they relate to you and your self-concept.

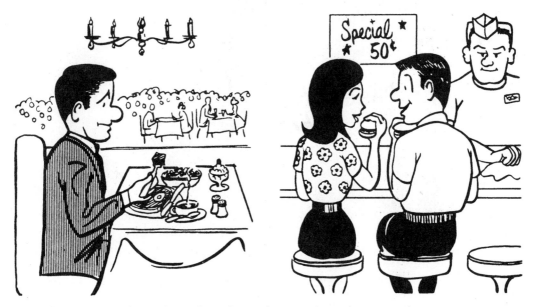

Basic physical needs can be met alone. Basic social
needs require satisfying interpersonal relationships.

SOCIAL NEEDS OF PEOPLE

For the most part, physical needs can be met either alone or in the company of
others. However, sharing with others is more satisfying than meeting these
needs alone. You enjoy your dinner much more if you have pleasant companionship than if you eat alone or in the company of someone you dislike. When
physical needs and social needs are met simultaneously, enjoyment is greater
and there is more likely to be a sense of well-being.

A social need involves relationships with other people. As used here,
"social" does not mean "socializing." **Socializing** is participating in recreational activities with other people.

Types of Social Needs

There are many different kinds of social needs: psychological, emotional, intellectual, spiritual, diversional, and recreational. These terms overlap, since each
term refers to groups of needs that are closely related.

Some social needs can be partially met alone, but relationships with other
people are necessary for full satisfaction. For example, the person who enjoys
studying a subject can partially meet intellectual needs alone. Greater satisfaction might be experienced, however, if there are opportunities to discuss the

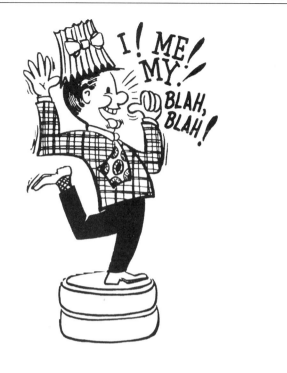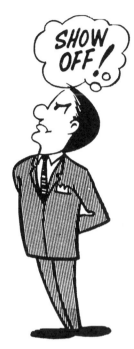

Compensation provides temporary relief when a basic social need is not being met.

subject with others who share the same interest. *Satisfying relationships with other people lead to full satisfaction of the social needs.*

Some social needs are related to the self; other needs are related to contact with other people. Each of us needs to feel important as a person, to have a sense of achievement, and to feel worthy. We also need to feel that we are important to others, that other people approve of us, and that we are accepted as a member of the group. These two sets of needs are closely tied together, for feelings and beliefs about oneself affect acceptance by others.

Compensation

You have learned that each of the physical needs can be met only in a specific way. With the social needs, a type of substitution known as **compensation** is possible. *Compensation does not satisfy a basic need.* It is a device that provides temporary relief from the discomfort felt when a basic social need is not being met.

Do you know a person who habitually talks loudly, tends to brag, is a showoff, or dresses in loud clothes? Is this person popular? Is this person accepted by the group? Probably not, for these are attention-seeking behaviors. For some people it is better to be noticed, even disapprovingly, than to be ignored. Behavior that gets attention can relieve the inner discomfort resulting from being ignored. Attention-seeking behavior is an example of compensation. This behavior temporarily relieves inner discomfort and effectively but temporarily gains attention from the group. Obtaining approval meets a basic need; getting attention compensates for not gaining approval. People who compensate are usually unaware that they are getting temporary relief from inner discomfort instead of the full satisfaction that comes only from meeting basic social needs. Now that you have a general understanding of social needs and their importance, let us turn our attention to self-approval and its relationship to social needs.

THE SELF-CONCEPT

Each of us has our own image of "self." We think of ourselves as a certain kind of person, possessing specific characteristics. Self-concept may be thought of as all the things a person thinks are true about the self. It is a mental image of "me."

A particular person's self-concept may be realistic or unrealistic. Suppose Joe thinks of himself as an honest person, yet he takes advantage of any situation in which he can gain something, regardless of whether it is honest or dishonest. Joe's concept of "Honest Joe" is not in agreement with his behavior when he is acting like "Joe the Cheat." Jim, on the other hand, thinks of himself as just an average guy, whereas his teachers see him as a person with exceptional ability. Neither Joe nor Jim has a realistic self-concept.

Behavior as an Indicator of the Self-Concept

The person with a realistic self-concept thinks of the self in terms that are consistent with behavior. Usually, behavior is an accurate indicator of a person's self-concept. Joe's behavior indicates that he is not honest, but if Joe's self-concept includes honesty as an attribute, then his behavior and his self-concept are not consistent. Which reflects the real Joe?

Behavior is not always an accurate indicator of a person's true characteristics. Behavior may not be consistent with a person's beliefs and values. Suppose a person in the health field talks about the philosophy of individual worth and treats all patients courteously and with impartial efficiency, yet actually has strong prejudice against members of certain groups. This prejudice may not be revealed in day-to-day behavior but would be reflected in an important decision. Such a person's public self—the self revealed to others—is inconsistent with the private self, the self known only to the individual.

A Realistic Self-Concept

The person who has a realistic self-concept is able to be honest about the real self. Such a person's behavior accurately reflects the person's own beliefs, values, and standards.

The person whose self-concept is unrealistic is not ready to set goals for personal growth until the self-concept has been revised. "What is" must be acknowledged before considering "what can be." An unrealistic self-concept may be either idealized or self-derogatory.

For example, Patsy has great difficulty with high school subjects, but thinks of herself as a person who can do anything she attempts. Her ambition is to be a scientist. Patsy's *idealized self-concept* may trap her into setting goals that she cannot achieve. In contrast, Patsy's friend Phyllis is an excellent student but lacks self-confidence. Phyllis has an older sister who is a good student, is very pretty, and sings extremely well. Phyllis does not seem to have any artistic talent. She is average in appearance. Because she has always compared herself unfavorably with her sister, Phyllis thinks of herself as a second-rate person, yet she has tremendous potential and can probably succeed in any field of study she undertakes. Phyllis has a **derogatory** *self-concept*, which may influence her to settle for goals less challenging than those she could achieve.

Formation of the Self-Concept

The self-concept begins to form at a very early age and is well established by about age six. It can be modified later in life, but only with conscious effort over a period of time. The self-concept is greatly affected by all life experiences, but it is most susceptible to the influence of other people *during the early formative years and during adolescence.* The young child's relationships with other people establish the early pattern. Is the child considered a person with rights and feelings? Many adults demand expressions of courtesy from a child, yet fail to use courteous behavior toward the child. The old saying, "Children are to be seen and not heard," reflects an attitude that children are not really worthy as persons, that what a child thinks and says is not important enough for an adult to hear.

A positive self-concept develops if the young child has positive experiences and positive verbal interactions with the important adults of his or her social environment:

"You are sweet."
"I love you."
"You are so strong."
"You are special."
"It's fun being with you."
"I like for you to ask questions."

A busy adult may forget to tell a child that he or she is loved and is important. But, a child needs to hear such positive statements in order to think of "me" as one who is loved and is important to other people. Children also need positive nonverbal messages: hugs and kisses, a squeeze of the hand, a pat on the shoulder, and other appropriate forms of touch. The most important message is conveyed through time spent with the child, time in which the child is the primary focus of a parent's attention. Working parents should plan for quality time with the child each day—reading, playing, walking, and talking. The amount of time is less important than the quality.

The form of discipline used with a child also has an extensive influence on the child's self-concept. If Greg is repeatedly told that he is a bad boy, he will begin to think of himself as being bad. Why should Greg try to be good if he has learned to think of himself as "bad" and believes that "everyone expects me to be bad"?

During adolescence, the peer group exerts a powerful influence on self-concept. There is pressure to conform to the group's standards and values. There is a tendency to label those who do not conform. It requires a rather strong self-concept for a teenager to resist those pressures, to stand up for personal beliefs and values, and at the same time gain acceptance from the peer group.

In these and many other ways, the people around a young child mold the developing child's self-concept. Throughout childhood many different aspects of one's personality develop and each aspect influences the self-concept. In the following sections, we will explore two aspects of personality development: self reliance (a strong, capable person) or dependence (a weak, incompetent person, who relies on others). Obviously, the tendency to remain dependent on others, versus the tendency to become progressively more self-reliant, has extensive implications for one's self-concept.

Learning Independence

One of the most important aspects of development during childhood and adolescence is a gradual increase in independence, with less and less dependence on others. The need for self-reliance is an inborn force. Many infant behaviors reflect the need for this type of development: efforts at self-feeding, attempts to help with dressing and undressing, and attempts to "do it myself!" A child's angry reaction when an adult interferes in something the child is trying to do reflects this need for independence.

Autonomy Versus Dependence

The struggle between self-reliance and dependence on others continues throughout life. Each of us has a need for *autonomy,* the ability to function independently without outside control. Yet, no one ever achieves complete autonomy. We are social beings, and in many ways our welfare depends upon our being able to function as a member of the group. The mature person has learned to live harmoniously with his fellow man, functioning autonomously in many ways and accepting that dependence on others for some things is a matter of necessity.

Autonomy must be achieved over a period of time, by gradually learning to be self-reliant in the simple tasks of daily living (e.g., dressing and eating) and then progressing to self-reliance in more complex situations. It is impossible to be dependent on others throughout childhood and adolescence and then suddenly, at age 18 or 21, become a self-directing, autonomous adult. Effective parenting provides for the gradual development of independence throughout childhood by encouraging the child to do simple tasks. It also requires being available when help is requested or frustration becomes more than the child can handle.

This struggle for a compromise between autonomy and dependence reaches its peak during adolescence. The young person struggling for autonomy rebels against dependence on others. The parents may resent the young person's insistence on greater independence than they believe the child can handle. Young people who do not successfully resolve this conflict may carry the struggle for autonomy into adulthood, usually as rebellion toward any form of authority, such as the teacher or the "boss." You may find it interesting to study examples of rebellious behavior in terms of the struggle for autonomy.

The self-concept can be modified in adulthood, either by experiences that change one's perception of self or by a conscious approach to self-study. A realistic self-concept is based on thinking of oneself as a worthy person with a high level of capability for some activities, but not for others. The concept of *self as a worthy person* must be accepted and believed before a constructive appraisal of strengths and weaknesses can be made.

SELF-ESTEEM

Self-esteem refers to one's *feelings about self at a given moment* or period of time. Self-esteem is closely related to self-concept, but is not the same. Whereas self-concept is established during the early years and is relatively permanent, self-esteem is quite changeable and is affected by life experiences. A person's self-esteem may be high in the morning; then, some negative experience may plunge that person's self-esteem to a very low point. For most people, a period of low self-esteem is short-lived. If a negative experience, such as being unemployed, extends over a period of weeks, then self-esteem may remain low throughout that period. Effectively dealing with a life problem usually restores self-esteem to a high level. Good life experiences tend to maintain self-esteem

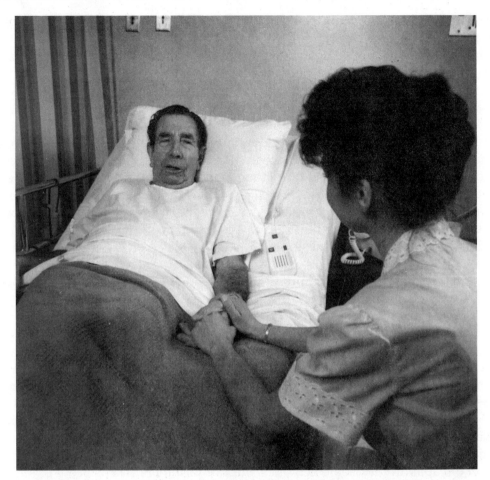

Illness and dependency are serious threats to an adult patient's self-esteem.

at a high level. But, self-esteem is always at risk—threatened by those negative experiences that are a part of life. The success/failure ratio of a person's life influences the frequency of low self-esteem. Someone with a positive self-concept has greater tolerance for periods of low self-esteem than one whose self-concept is relatively negative. Success and failure experiences, then, are critical influences on self-esteem.

INFLUENCE OF OTHERS ON ONE'S SENSE OF SELF

Other people have a strong influence on one's sense of self, beginning with the interactions of adults and the newborn baby. A sense of self-and-others begins to develop during infancy. The struggle for autonomy, "self" as separate from others, begins during the toddler stage, continues throughout childhood, and becomes intense during adolescence. During the infant and toddler periods, family members and care-takers influence the early sense of self. The child's exposure to the world widens with entry into preschool programs and school itself; from that time on, teachers and others make significant contributions to the formative sense of self. These early interactions help to establish the child's self-concept, which then acts as a sort of filter for the effects of later experiences and relationships.

The struggle for self-identity, a clarification of "Who am I?" intensifies during adolescence and early adulthood. Courtship and marriage introduce another influence, so powerful that it may lead to modification of some aspect of the self-concept. Any intimate relationship can have a powerful effect on one's self-concept, as well as day-by-day effects on self-esteem.

New social contacts and relationships influence one's feelings about self, and one's feelings about self affect relationships and social interactions. Communication style, a major component of one's behavior patterns, is so important that Section V consists of two units devoted to practicing effective communication, both verbal and nonverbal.

You should now become more aware of the role other persons play in determining how you feel about yourself at any given time. Your interactions with some people almost always make you feel good. Some people say and do things that make you feel good about yourself. Other people tend to have the opposite effect: they make put-down statements, are often critical, play the one-upmanship game, or otherwise have a diminishing effect on your sense of self. If there are many such people in your daily life, you are probably struggling to maintain a positive level of self-esteem. In order to correct the situation, you have certain choices:

1. Avoid such people.

2. Be assertive about not accepting negative statements.

3. Refuse to participate in their games.

4. Learn ways to respond to communications that have a negative effect on you.

Obviously, the first choice is not available to you if members of your family or your co-workers have a negative effect on you. In that case, you can begin to learn how to deal with such people through various activities, such as reading about effective relationships and participating in assertiveness training and communication skills workshops.

During the 1980s, some psychologists began to focus on differences in the way men and women communicate, the different values and expectations of the two sexes, and different emotional needs of men and women. As a result, many workshops and seminars on human relationships and family dynamics emphasize the need for men to understand the emotional needs and communication styles of women, and for women to understand that the emotional needs and communication styles of men differ from their own. By learning to relate to the other sex effectively, a person can not only be more effective in meeting the other's needs, but also achieve greater satisfaction of one's own needs.

Patricia Evans, who works with abused women, describes in *The Verbally Abusive Relationship* the destructive effects derogatory statements can have on self-concept, gradually undermining self-confidence and fostering a growing belief in one's incompetence. In most cases, derogatory statements are made only in private; the abuser does not reveal to others the use of put-downs and criticism. When the woman begins to realize that she is being abused verbally, she cannot find understanding from friends or relatives because the abuser has not revealed this tendency to them. Not finding emotional support, and hearing from others that she should be thankful for such a wonderful relationship, simply increases her self-doubt and further erodes her self-concept.

Evans emphasizes that most verbally abused women *believe what the abuser says,* without considering that there is no real basis for the criticism, accusations, and put-downs. Any woman who suspects that she is being verbally abused should consult a professional counselor, rather than seek understanding from friends and relatives. A counselor can help restore her belief in herself and also help her learn ways to cope with the verbal abuse. Verbal abuse usually accelerates and eventually includes physical abuse, which the abuser always explains as being the woman's fault. Abusers are not likely to agree to marital counseling. Most abusers derive satisfaction from *having power over another person* and are not willing to work toward establishing a mutually fulfilling relationship.

In summary, positive relationships can help one to develop a strong self-concept and maintain high self-esteem most of the time. Negative relationships can have a destructive effect on self-concept and may result in a chronic state of low self-esteem.

EFFECTS OF SUCCESS AND FAILURE

Have you ever had a task so difficult that you did not believe you could complete it? Perhaps it was a reading assignment that just did not make sense when you read it. Perhaps it was a written assignment, and you did not know how to proceed.

What was your approach to this task that appeared so hopeless? Did you pitch in, try your best, and find that you could do it, after all? How did you feel about your accomplishment? You should have felt good, for you overcame obstacles and successfully completed a difficult task. Each successful

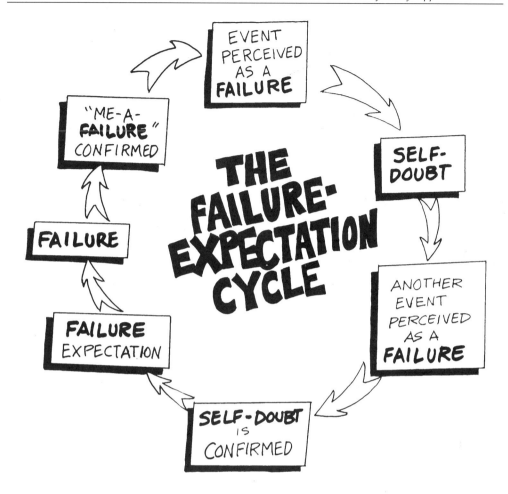

experience should be consciously recognized as a success. And, each success should help you believe in *yourself as a person who can overcome obstacles.*

On the other hand, you may have found a particular task just as hard as you expected and were unable to complete it. No doubt you still have some negative feelings about this experience. Perhaps you were angry at yourself for not finishing it. Perhaps you were angry with the person who assigned the task to you. In either case, your self-confidence was threatened. You were discouraged and probably approached the next difficult task with greater self-doubt.

Meaning of Failure Expectation

Discouragement and a sense of failure can be quite damaging to self-confidence, especially if experienced frequently. But this is only part of the problem. When failure occurs too frequently, there is a tendency to develop "failure expectation." Each failure adds to self-doubt; self-doubt creates failure

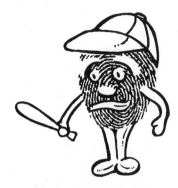

"What if I strike out?" (From Carol D. Tamparo & Wilburta Q. Lindh, *Therapeutic Communications for Allied Health Professions*. Albany, NY: Delmar Publishers Inc., 1992)

expectation; and, failure expectation interferes with performance. Thus, there is increased probability that the next task will result in another failure. If this cycle becomes well established, the individual may need professional help to break the pattern and believe in the possibility of future successful performances.

Success Expectation

For most people, however, the problem is lack of self-confidence rather than an established failure expectation. Self-confidence might be thought of as "success expectation." The key to building self-confidence is conscious recognition of each successful experience, with awareness that life includes both successful experiences and disappointing experiences.

Success expectation is an attitude that affects the way you attack a task. Your approach, to a great extent, will determine the outcome. Two personal traits that are helpful in the performance of any task are **persistence** and determination. Successful performance may be dependent upon time—some tasks require a slow, careful performance, while others should be performed quickly. A skill that is helpful in many situations is the problem-solving method. Successful performance as a health care provider requires that you choose the appropriate method of performance in a wide variety of situations.

Confidence comes from having a reasonable balance of successes and failures. Perhaps you have such a balance, but give undue attention to failure experiences and do not consciously acknowledge your successes.

Everyone has some failures and some disappointments in spite of a conscientious effort to do well. It is possible to make use of such experiences by viewing them as opportunities to identify factors that may have contributed to a poor outcome:

- Did I begin the task without proper preparation?

- Did I attempt to do the task too rapidly? Did I give enough attention to details (or technique)?

- Did I allow too little time for the task?

- Did I use efficient work habits? If not, what work habits might have been more effective?

- Did I use the appropriate method for this task? If not, what method would have been better?

- Did I give up too soon?

- Did I have control over the outcome or was the outcome controlled by someone else? If the outcome was controlled by someone else, then the failure is not yours. Habitually blaming others, however, can prevent you from taking responsibility for your actions and, therefore, inhibit learning from experience.

- If you used the problem-solving approach, which alternative solution might have resulted in a better outcome?

Successful experiences in life make it easier to accept the occasional failures that all of us have. If a reasonable balance can be maintained between successes and failures, if satisfaction is consciously experienced after each success, and if the attitudes and habits that facilitate successful experiences are progressively developed, then self-esteem will be high most of the time and any periods of low self-esteem will be brief.

SUCCESS

Do you think of "success" as making a lot of money, gaining power, having a late model car, perhaps even becoming a movie star? Only a few people get to the top, and some of those who do get to the top in their field find that their "success" does not provide happiness.

Influence of Success

Each of us has many opportunities for success if we recognize daily accomplishments and grant ourselves the right to feel good about them. Each time a job is done well, you should feel inner satisfaction. If others notice and express approval, this should add to your enjoyment. But even in the absence of expressed approval from others, you should feel good when you know, deep inside, that you did a job well.

If you recognize and acknowledge daily successes, each one will build your self-confidence and prepare you for succeeding in the next task you undertake. Each success diminishes the probability that self-doubt will interfere with success in future undertakings.

As a Student

As a student, you will have many opportunities to experience success. New information, new insights, new understandings, and new skills can give you a sense of accomplishment. Take pride in each achievement, seeing it as another step toward becoming a health care provider. Remember, however, that none of us can experience success in every task. There are times when we do not do as well as we would like. From the disappointments, however, we can learn what to avoid in the next similar situation. Thus "failures" can be used constructively as learning experiences, instead of being allowed to create destructive self-doubt.

As a Health Care Provider

When you have become a full-fledged health care provider, recognize your successes each day and gain a sense of satisfaction from them. Regard your "nonsuccesses" as learning experiences that will help you perform more effectively in the future. Set goals for developing those traits that are fundamental to self-confidence: persistence, determination, and adaptability. Learn to use a systematic, problem-solving approach. Develop efficient work habits. As successes increase, disappointments will be less damaging to your self-esteem. Thus, you can build belief in yourself as a **competent** person.

STRIVING FOR SELF-APPROVAL

Modifying Habits

In striving to build self-confidence, you must be realistic. You have many, many personal traits. Some are so highly developed that they characterize you as a person; in trying to describe you, someone would mention those traits. Other traits are not so prominent, but can be developed if you give your attention to them. Some traits are favorable; others are unfavorable. Try to identify the traits that will help you as a person and as a health care provider and strive to develop those traits to a high degree. Also, identify those traits that are a **hindrance** to you; strive to minimize or eliminate those traits from your behavior patterns.

You cannot overhaul yourself on a moment's notice. In fact, revising habits is a somewhat slow process. It takes effort and persistence to replace an undesirable habit with a more desirable one. You must practice the new habit at every opportunity. Do not let an exception occur; each time you lapse into the old habit, it becomes harder to establish the new habit. For example, if you tend to procrastinate, it will take much effort to overcome this one habit. Resist the temptation to put things off. Gradually, the habit of "do it now" will replace the habit of thinking "I'll do that later."

Developing Problem-Solving Skills

You can deal with problems more effectively by using a systematic method. The following steps to choosing successful behavior can be applied to a variety of situations:

1. Identify the problem. Think it through. Discuss it with someone who might help you to understand it or to see the problem in a new light. Write out a statement of the problem.

2. Collect information and/or ideas that might help you to understand the problem better.

3. Consider all available information, then look at your statement of the problem. Reconsider what the problem is and rewrite the statement if necessary.

   NOTE: At this point, your perception of the problem may have changed completely. You may eventually see the problem as being entirely different from what you initially thought.

4. Write down every imaginable solution. In a second column beside each possible solution, write out the possible consequences of trying that solution.

5. Select the solution that seems most likely to lead to the desired outcome and carry out the actions required.

6. Evaluate the outcome. If the result was not satisfactory, try another solution that appears likely to succeed.

It requires practice to become skillful in using a problem-solving approach, but if you apply it to daily problems, you will soon become skillful in thinking through these steps. In other words, thinking through a problem may become a work habit. Skill in problem-solving enables a person to choose a specific behavior for a desired result.

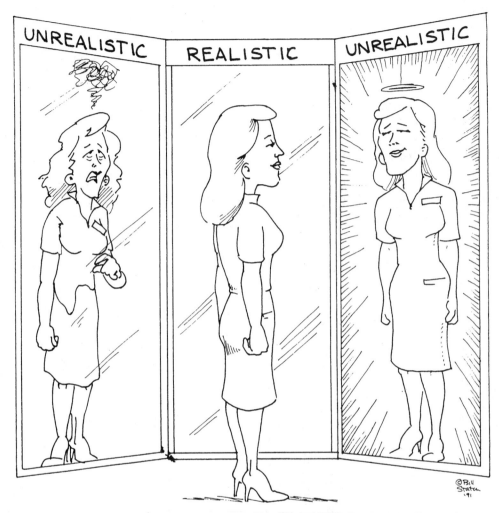

Strive to develop a realistic self-concept—neither derogatory nor idealized.

Building a Realistic Self-Concept

A realistic self-concept requires conscious and thoughtful consideration of "what is." By honestly appraising your strengths and weaknesses, identifying your interests, and clarifying your values, you will get in touch with the "real you." This is the starting point for planning ways to develop your potential and gaining greater satisfaction from living.

Setting Goals

Your true interests and **aptitudes** influence the success you are likely to experience and the satisfaction you are likely to gain from certain types of activities.

Each of us tends to do best those things that we enjoy doing. Also, we learn more easily and perform best those activities for which we have an aptitude. A realistic **appraisal** of "what is" provides the foundation for setting goals, "what may be."

Goals that are in accordance with your true interests and aptitudes are more likely to be achieved than goals set for you by someone else. If your goals offer a challenge, then reaching them will provide much satisfaction—the feeling of having overcome obstacles and of being a person who can achieve goals. This is self-approval. When goals are too high for your aptitudes or readiness, then you may experience disappointment, failure, and self-doubt. Goals that are too low are easily reached, do not challenge you to develop your potential, and provide only limited satisfaction.

It is desirable to have both short-range and long-range goals. Short-range goals are the stepping stones that lead to long-range goals. If JoAnn wants to study medicine and is qualified to do so, her high school curriculum and college courses will be a series of short-range goals leading to the long-range goal of becoming a physician. If there are financial problems, JoAnn may use a health occupations course as a short-term goal, obtaining job skills that enable her to work part-time while attending college. Thus, JoAnn may eventually reach her long-range goal through a series of intermediate goals. Intermediate goals provide inner satisfaction and a sense of achievement that help one persist in striving for the long-range goal.

References and Suggested Readings

Branden, Nathaniel. *The Six Pillars of Self-Esteem.* New York, NY: Bantam Books, 1995.

———. *The Power of Self-Esteem.* Deerfield Beach, FL: Health Communications Inc., 1992.

Evans, Patricia. *The Verbally Abusive Relationship: How to Recognize It and How to Respond.* Holbrook, MA: Adams Publishing, 1992.

Glass, Lillian. *Toxic People: 10 Ways of Dealing with People who Make Your Life Miserable.* New York, NY: Simon & Schuster, 1995. "You can't please everyone, so you've got to please yourself" pp. 51–52; Chapter 8, "Choosing a Technique Based on the Toxic Person's Role in Your Life," pp. 176–194.

Gray, John. *Men are from Mars, Women are from Venus.* New York, NY: HarperCollins Publishers, 1992.

McKay, Matthew & Fanning, Patrick. *Self-Esteem.* New York: Fine Communications, 1994.

Tannen, Deborah. *You Just Don't Understand.* New York, NY: Ballentine Books, 1990.

REVIEW AND SELF-CHECK

Complete the following statements, based on information in Unit 6.

1. The expression "social need" refers to such needs as _____ , and

   _____ .

2. Compensation refers to behavior that _____ .

3. "Self-concept" is _____ .

4. Three important influences on self-concept are _____ ,

   _____ , and_____ .

5. "Need for autonomy" refers to _____ .

6. The struggle for autonomy reaches its peak during _____ .

7. A realistic self-concept is based on thinking of oneself as a worthy person

   with _____

   but _____ .

8. Self-esteem refers to _____ .

9. Use the chart below to compare self-concept and self-esteem.

Self-Concept	Self-Esteem
_____	_____
_____	_____
_____	_____

10. The effect of a successful experience on self-esteem is strengthened belief

    in oneself as a person who _____ .

11. The effect of too many failure experiences is _____ .

12. Two personal traits that affect performance, and therefore one's success

    rate, are _____

    and _____ .

13. Two essential steps for modifying a habit are: _____

    and _____ .

14. The problem-solving method consists of the following steps:

    a. _____

    b. _____

    c. _____

    d. _____

    e. _____

    f. _____

15. You are more likely to achieve your goals if they are _____ .

ASSIGNMENT

1. Briefly describe one experience you have had in regard to each of the following:
   a. You attempted a task but gave up without completing it.
   b. You attempted a difficult task and finished it.
   c. You expected someone to praise your performance, but no one commented.
   d. Someone complimented you on how well you did something. It was a routine job that you do regularly without giving it much thought.

2. Review each of the above situations. Describe how each experience made you feel.

3. Consider how you feel when you complete a task satisfactorily, in your opinion, but your boss (or your teacher) criticizes the result. What does your reaction indicate in terms of your need for self-approval? What does it mean in terms of your need for approval from authority figures?

4. Select a problem you have had recently in your role as a student. The problem may involve a disagreement with a classmate, daily adjustments necessary in becoming a full-time student, a task you found difficult, or a patient situation in which there was a misunderstanding. Briefly describe the situation. Now use the problem-solving method to study the situation, including your own behavior and the outcome. Identify an action that probably would have had a better result.

5. Select a problem you now have and apply the problem-solving method. Write out several possible solutions; beside each, list the probable results. Select the solution you think will have the most desirable outcome. Try this solution. After one week, review the problem, your action, and the outcome. Evaluate your use of the problem-solving method. Did you select the best action? Do you now think another action would have had a better result?

Unit 7

The Need for Acceptance

OBJECTIVES

Upon completion of this unit, you should be able to:

- Explain the relationship of social needs to one's sense of worth.
- List four specific needs that are related to the need for acceptance.
- List three behaviors required for effective use of approval.
- Define conformity.
- State two components of caring.
- Differentiate sympathy and empathy.
- List three interpretations of appreciation.
- Explain the relationship of social needs to effective caregiver/patient relationships.
- Recognize behaviors that may represent someone's effort to meet the need for approval, acceptance, or appreciation.
- Help others to satisfy social needs by expressing approval, caring, or appreciation appropriately.
- Plan effective ways to satisfy one's own social needs.

KEY TERMS

Conformity   Mutual   Martyr complex

You have learned that social needs can be met fully only through satisfying relationships with other people. Satisfaction of social needs requires both self-approval and approval of and acceptance by the group. The person who has achieved self-approval finds it easier to gain approval and acceptance by others. On the other hand, acceptance by others makes us feel more comfortable with ourselves. So, these two needs are closely tied together; the person who can grow in self-approval can become increasingly acceptable to others and vice versa.

Two psychologists at the Menninger Institute have studied the relationship between "belonging" and motivation. They indicate that the need to belong "is more than just an urge. It's a fundamental human need—as essential and basic as the need for food or *the drive for self-preservation*." (Italics added) The need to belong can be satisfied through (1) frequent, positive interactions with the same people and (2) a life situation (framework) that provides a long-term, stable climate of caring and concern. A person who has established a relationship that fulfills some of these belonging needs is reluctant to end the relationship, even when it includes destructive elements such as abuse. It is interesting that feelings of belonging experienced occasionally are so powerful that they may outweigh the need to escape abuse. (The Menninger Letter, 3:8).

THE IMPORTANCE OF ACCEPTANCE

Each of us needs to believe that others accept us as a worthwhile person. To satisfy this need, we must see and hear expressions of approval from time to time, in order to remain convinced of this acceptance. We also need to believe that others understand our viewpoint, our feelings, and our problems. Obviously, satisfying the need for acceptance requires receiving indications of approval and caring from other people.

Friendships develop and are maintained on the basis of whether or not two people meet each other's needs. You may find it difficult to understand why your friend Melanie seeks Helen's companionship in preference to your company. Perhaps you do not care for Helen at all. In reality, the Melanie/Helen relationship continues because it provides **mutual** satisfaction of needs. Perhaps Helen is very ready to express approval or admiration of Melanie, whereas you assume that Melanie knows you approve of her. Friendships grow stronger or they weaken on the basis of the extent to which the relationship satisfies social needs of those involved.

Ideally, a relationship between two people involves a balance of give-and-take. This ideal can be met only if the behavior of each person helps the other to satisfy basic social needs.

In some relationships, the balance of give-and-take appears to be one-sided. One person exerts much effort to please the other and seems to get little in return. If the relationship continues over a long period without change in this balance, both parties are satisfying certain needs. Self-sacrificing behavior is sometimes referred to as the **"martyr complex,"** meaning that the individual actually derives satisfaction from being taken advantage of by another person.

To a great extent, we can understand our behavior and that of others in terms of basic needs—behaviors that satisfy a basic need, and behaviors that compensate for not being able to satisfy a basic need. Usually, a person puts up with certain circumstances or with the behavior of others because some need is

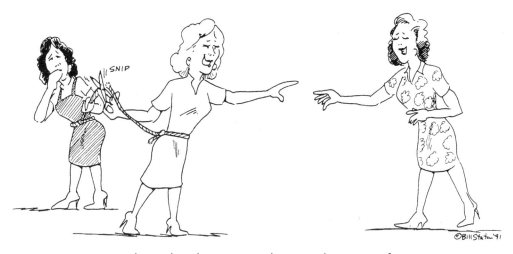

A relationship deteriorates when it no longer satisfies
the social needs of one or both parties.

being met. Perhaps compensation is taking place. Perhaps the need is a "sick" one, as illustrated by the martyr type of behavior. If no need is being met, the individual will usually engage in behavior that changes the situation or provides escape. Now let us turn our attention to some specific needs that are related to the overall need for acceptance.

APPROVAL FROM OTHERS

Have you ever expected to be praised for something you did, but instead you were criticized? How did it make you feel? How did you behave? How did you feel about the person who was critical instead of approving? This person, in failing to give approval, deprived you of a basic need. Each of us has had such experiences. The one who failed to give us our earned approval may have been a parent, friend, classmate, teacher, or boss. The hurt associated with such experiences is proportional to the importance we attach to the other person.

Let us look at the other side of the coin. Have you ever had a friend show you something new, yet you failed to express approval? Has a friend ever won an honor, but for some reason you could not bring yourself to offer congratulations? If so, you were depriving this person of approval. Why did you withhold your approval?

Hunger for Approval

Being deprived of approval early in life can create a hunger for approval that never seems satisfied. Do you know someone who "looks for compliments?"

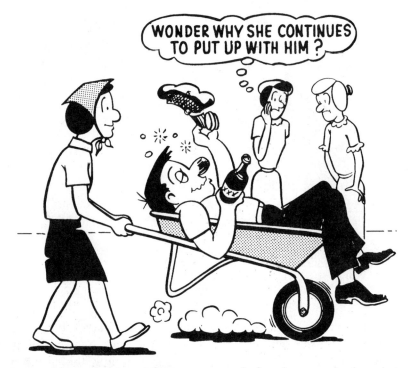

A continuing relationship is satisfying some need of each person in the relationship.

How do you feel about this person? Seeking compliments usually indicates a strong need for expressions of approval. The next time you observe such behavior, will you recognize the need for approval? Assuming it is deserved, will you express your approval freely and sincerely? If so, you will be helping that person meet an important need. You will be contributing to that person's inner comfort, but the cost to you is only the effort it takes to state your sincere approval.

Failure to Offer Approval

Some people fail to notice others. Some are indifferent to a job well done, but very ready to react to a job or a person who does not meet their approval. Some people may notice that a job has been well done, but make no comment. Some, for reasons of their own, deliberately avoid saying nice things to others. The habit of not expressing approval can be easily overcome, once you are aware that approval is a need we all have. Deliberately withholding approval is another matter, however. To understand this trait may be more difficult, for it indicates negative feelings toward others and, probably, toward oneself.

Appropriate Use of Approval

Approval should be given freely for the everyday tasks—not just for the big tasks that come only occasionally. The child who voluntarily does a task at home deserves expressions of approval. The student who does an assignment well deserves approval. The person who serves a tasty meal deserves approval. Each of us has opportunities throughout the day to express sincere approval to others. It only requires that we form the habit of noticing others and expressing approval when it has been earned.

When will you have your next opportunity to express approval to someone? Perhaps your young son washes his hands for dinner without being told. Perhaps a patient shows the first interest in grooming since an operation. Perhaps the teacher presents an especially interesting class. All these people need approval, too!

This is not a recommendation that you rush around paying compliments freely. Insincerity is worse than silence. The desirable behavior is *noticing others and unselfishly expressing approval when it has been earned.* This is an easy way to meet your own needs while also helping someone else satisfy a basic need. Giving approval to others can be quite enjoyable.

CONFORMITY

Have you ever arrived at a party and found you were dressed differently from most of those present? Perhaps you dressed casually and the others "dressed up." If among friends, you were probably not overly uncomfortable. But if you were trying to gain acceptance by the members of this group, discovering that you dressed inappropriately may have made you very uncomfortable.

Importance of Acceptance During Adolescence

During adolescence the need for acceptance by the peer group is very strong, and **conformity** is almost necessary to gain acceptance. Parents are often distressed to find that their teenager is more concerned about the opinions of friends than about their parents' beliefs. Some people never outgrow depending on conformity to win the acceptance of the group to which they wish to belong.

Group Standards and Conformity

Some of the policies of your school may seem unreasonable to you, but they are probably based on sound reasons and intended to benefit the entire student body. The ethics of the health professions are based on high principles and establish what is "appropriate" behavior for health care providers.

If you find yourself in a group whose standards are not acceptable, you must either change your beliefs, convince the group that their standards should change, or find another group whose standards reflect your own. In other words, use good judgment in deciding when to conform to a group's standards and when to go by your own standards, even at the risk of disapproval.

THE NEED TO BELIEVE THAT OTHERS CARE

Another social need that requires appropriate responses from other people is the need to believe that other people care. The extent to which we believe that a particular person does care about us has an influence on how we feel about that person. To put it another way, the more *important* a particular person is to us, the more strongly we need to believe that person cares about our feelings. Expressions of caring promote strong ties between people.

Sympathy

As a health care provider, you will be hearing the terms *sympathy* and *empathy.* Perhaps you think of sympathy as "feeling sorry for someone." Actually, sympathy is closely tied in with the need to believe that others care. It does not, as a basic social need, imply pity. Instead, it implies *caring and understanding* as an aspect of a relationship between two people.

Empathy

Empathy is similar to *some* of the meanings of sympathy, but it is not the same. Empathy means identifying with another person in such a way that we see things somewhat as that person sees them. Do you remember the previously mentioned farm wife who was extremely upset about her husband's accident? Another farm wife would probably have no difficulty in feeling empathy; she would understand this threat to the family's livelihood. On the other hand, a person without empathy may think, "Instead of being so upset, that woman ought to be thankful her husband didn't die."

As a health care provider you will be exposed to many situations in which an effort to feel empathy for the patient and the family—*to see the situation as they see it*—will help you to understand their behavior. Most patients do not want others to feel sorry for them. They *do* want others to care about them, to understand what they are experiencing, and to care about their feelings and beliefs.

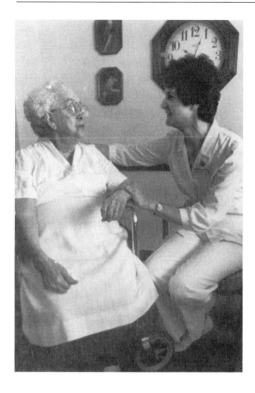

Patients want to feel that others care about them and understand what they are experiencing. (From Carolyn Anderson, *Patient Teaching and Communicating in an Information Age.* Albany, NY: Delmar Publishers Inc., 1990.)

NEED FOR APPRECIATION

Each of us needs to believe that someone appreciates us. We especially need to feel appreciated by those who are important to us. Appreciation may mean "to be grateful" as shown by saying "thank you" or "to have respect" as shown by the statement, "She has great appreciation for modern art."

Expressing appreciation might indicate either of these meanings and might even imply approval or caring as well. For example, a child's first attempt to help with a household task will be unsuccessful by adult standards, yet the child may be proud of the effort. The adult reaction will affect future efforts. For a positive effect, the parent could show gratitude for the attempt to be helpful, could show respect for the child's effort, or could show caring and pleasure with the child's intent to help. All of these should be shown sincerely, even though the result of the child's performance may not meet adult standards.

Expressions of approval, appreciation, and caring provide a sense of satisfaction. The absence of any such expressions can be as negative in effect as open criticism or disapproval. If a task has been attempted but not performed well, sincere *approval* cannot be given; yet it is quite likely that an expression of *appreciation* would be appropriate. If suggestions for improvement are needed, these suggestions are less likely to appear as criticism if they are preceded by an expression of appreciation, caring, and understanding. Thus, there are some situations where approval should be expressed, but indications of appreciation or caring are not necessary. At other times, approval is not needed or has not been earned, but appreciation could be shown. Sometimes neither approval nor appreciation can be expressed, yet an expression of caring would be appropriate.

Some of our highly commercialized holidays are built around the idea of showing appreciation: Mother's Day, Father's Day, and St. Valentine's Day. Gifts, however, are superficial ways of showing appreciation. Our words and actions toward another person reflect our true feelings more accurately than the gifts we buy for special occasions.

Obviously, the social needs are interrelated. The person who is aware of social needs and their importance in interpersonal relations will recognize opportunities to contribute to the satisfaction of another's needs. The person who is unaware may blunder through life, contributing little to the needs of others and lacking personal satisfaction from meeting social needs.

SEX DIFFERENCES IN EMOTIONAL NEEDS

In *Men are from Mars, Women are from Venus,* Dr. John Gray states, "Most of our complex emotional needs can be summarized as the need for love." (Gray, 1992) Believing the behaviors that satisfy emotional needs of men and women are different, Dr. Gray enumerates twelve *primary love needs*—six for men and a different six for women. Men need to receive expressions of *trust, acceptance, appreciation, admiration, approval,* and *encouragement* in order to feel loved. Women, on the other hand, feel loved when they receive expressions of *caring, understanding, respect, devotion, validation,* and *reassurance.*

If a person expresses love to a partner using only the behaviors he or she wants to receive from the partner, then the partner may feel unloved. Actually, everyone needs to have all twelve of these emotional needs met. The *difference* between men and women is the importance of the six primary needs. These six needs must be met "before one is able fully to receive and appreciate the other kinds of love." Dr. Gray maintains that understanding these differences in the primary needs of men and women can result in improved interpersonal relations, especially with one's partner.

SOCIAL NEEDS AND BEHAVIOR

Perhaps you are now more aware of the complexity of human behavior. One person seeks approval by strict conformity to a group's standards of behavior, another by getting good grades, another by acquiring symbols of success, another by doing favors for people, still another by being the life of the party. Some people find effective patterns of behavior that lead to self-approval and acceptance by others. Some people compensate with behavior that temporarily relieves their inner discomfort but fails to satisfy basic social needs.

Behavior and Causation

All behavior is caused; it does not just happen. However, it is seldom possible to pinpoint one particular cause of a specific action. The causes of behavior are numerous and complex. Some of these causes lie in the situation in which the behavior occurs; other causes are within the individual, as a result of past learnings and their continuing influence on behavior. Many behaviors are goal-oriented; that is, they represent an individual's efforts to achieve some goal, such as satisfying the need for acceptance. We can increase our understanding and tolerance for behavior of others by being more aware of possible contributing causes, some apparent and others hidden. It is also helpful to study behavior in terms of its effectiveness—the degree to which it satisfies some basic need.

BEHAVIOR AND THE HEALTH CARE PROVIDER

For health care providers, being aware of the social needs of others can mean the difference between effective and ineffective relations with patients and their families. People under the physical and psychological stress of illness are more likely to cope with their illness successfully if care-givers help them meet social and emotional needs, as well as physical needs.

As a health care provider, you can be more effective if you are also a student of human behavior. You know that there is no ready answer to the "why" of any one person's behavior. You know that basic needs, both physical and social, continue during illness. However, the need for relieving distress and releasing emotions such as fear may temporarily push the need for approval or acceptance into the background. On the other hand, some patients try to cover up their own emotional distress to win acceptance from health care providers by being pleasant and cooperative.

As you observe people in apparently similar situations reacting in very different ways, you are seeing evidence of individual differences. Patients differ in their behavior used to cope with stress, in the strength of different needs, in relative importance given to specific needs, and in the capacity to find behavior patterns to meet their needs in a particular situation.

The human scene provides a never-ending variety of situations for thoughtful study. You will become less critical of others, more accepting of behavior that you do not understand, and more tolerant of human weakness as you apply your learnings about human behavior to people around you.

References and Suggested Readings

Brassell, William R. *Belonging: A Guide to Overcoming Loneliness.* Oakland, CA: New Harbinger, 1994.

Burley-Allen, Madelyn. *Listening: The Forgotten Skill.* New York, NY: John Wiley & Sons, Inc., 1995. "Three Levels of Listening," p. 14; "Strokes," pp. 25–27; "Empathetic Listening," pp. 125–132; "The Accomplishments that Can Be Gained through Empathetic Listening," pp. 183–184.

Gray, John. *Men are from Mars, Women are from Venus.* New York, NY: Harper-Collins, 1992. Chapter 8, "Discovering our Different Emotional Needs," pp. 132–149.

The Menninger Clinic. *The Menninger Letter,* August, 1995 (3:8), p. 6.

Simon, Sidney B. *In Search of Values.* New York, NY: Warner Books, 1993.

Thoele, Sue Patton. *The Courage to be Yourself Journal: A Woman's Guide to Growing Beyond Emotional Dependence.* Berkeley, CA: Conari Press, 1996.

Whitfield, Charles L. *Boundaries and Relationships: Knowing, Protecting, and Enjoying the Self.* Deerfield Beach, FL: Health Communications, Inc., 1993.

REVIEW AND SELF-CHECK

Complete the following statements, using information in Unit 7.

1. Full satisfaction of one's social needs requires both _____ and _____ .

2. Each of us needs to hear and see expressions of approval from time to time in order to believe _____ .

3. Friendships develop and are maintained on the basis of _____ _____ .

4. The need for acceptance by others is related to four very specific needs:

   _____ , _____

   _____ , and _____ .

5. Effective use of approval involves _____

    _____ , and _____ .

6. Conformity refers to behaving according to _____ .

7. Caring may include _____ , _____ , or both.

8. Sympathy means _____ .

9. Empathy means _____ .

10. Two different meanings of "appreciation" include _____

    _____ , and _____ .

ASSIGNMENT

1. Consult a dictionary and list all meanings given for "sympathy."

2. Describe how you could use each meaning of sympathy in
    a. your relations with patients and their families
    b. your relations with co-workers, and
    c. your personal life.

3. Consult a dictionary and list all meanings given for "empathy." List ways you can convey empathy to another person.

4. Consult a dictionary for all meanings of "appreciation." Select those that relate to social needs and explain briefly how you could use each meaning as a basis for improving your relations with others.

5. Observe yourself and others for one week. Describe, in writing, examples of behaviors that illustrate the following:
    a. need for acceptance by others
    b. need for conformity
    c. need for believing that others care
    d. need for appreciation

6. We can express approval, appreciation, or caring to others through both verbal and nonverbal behavior. For each situation that follows, indicate with a checkmark the type of verbal expression(s) that would be appropriate:

SITUATION	INDICATIONS OF		
	APPROVAL	CARING	APPRECIATION
Your good friend and co-worker has just been fired.			
Your 5-year-old has made his own bed; the covers are lumpy and sagging on one side.			
Your sister has just become engaged to a boy you dislike.			
Your classmate is elated over getting an A on a test. You usually make much better grades than this friend, but on this test you made a C.			
According to rumor, your supervisor's husband has just left her. Your relationship with the supervisor is entirely professional, but you have found her very helpful when you seek assistance.			
A patient has been quite dependent since surgery. Today he voluntarily walks out into the hall.			
You are having dinner with a good friend. She proudly serves you a casserole that she has made from a new recipe. You do not like it.			

7. Refer to the examples you collected for activity #5. List ways you could have helped each individual meet a social need.

8. Engage in a small group discussion to identify various ways to satisfy one's social needs.

9. Develop a plan for meeting your own social needs more effectively.

10. In a class discussion, evaluate Dr. Gray's description of differences in the primary emotional needs of men and women.
    a. Male members of the class should express agreement or disagreement, then list six expressions or behaviors from a woman that would meet a male's primary emotional needs.
    b. Female members of the class should express agreement or disagreement, then list six expressions or behaviors from a man that would meet a woman's primary emotional needs.

Unit 8

Emotions and Behavior

OBJECTIVES

Upon completion of this unit, you should be able to:

- Define emotion.
- Explain the importance of emotions by listing five effects on the quality of life.
- Describe the physiological effects of emotional arousal.
- State the purpose of the body's adaptive response.
- Define stress, dis-stress, and stressor.
- List two positive emotions.
- List three negative emotions.
- Name one essential characteristic of unconditional love.
- State five influences on the formation of emotional patterns.
- State five differences in patterns for the expression of emotions.
- Define temperament.
- State five guidelines for using emotions constructively.
- Define self-control.
- State five guidelines for increasing one's self-control.
- State five ways a health care provider can use knowledge about emotions to foster effective relationships with patients.
- Modify communication habits to include "I talk" and eliminate accusative statements.

KEY TERMS

Adrenalin	Altruism	Hostility
Eruption	Homeostasis	Noradrenalin
Inevitably	Mind-talk	Psychosomatic
Physiological	Resentment	Stress
Repressed	Suppressed	TLC
Stressors	Cynicism	

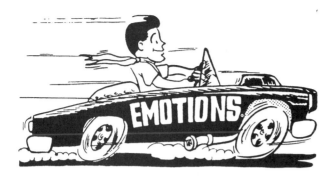

To use emotions constructively, one must be in control.

MEANING OF EMOTIONS

Emotions are the inner feelings that all of us have. They are responses to life situations, varying in type and intensity according to the experience of the moment. Many different terms are used to describe emotions. Some of these terms describe the *type* of feeling; other terms imply *intensity* of the feeling.

Emotions are neither good nor bad. We all experience these inner feelings according to what is happening to us and how we perceive the experience. To think of any emotion as good or bad, in a moral sense, is as pointless as considering hunger to be morally good or bad. Both positive and negative emotions are natural reactions to life experiences. The effects of negative emotions are unpleasant, but they are natural reactions to displeasing or threatening experiences.

IMPORTANCE OF EMOTIONS

Emotions have physical and mental effects. Indirectly, emotions determine the amount of satisfaction one gets from life, the degree of success in solving life problems, the satisfaction found in relations with other people, and ultimately, the degree of *physical* and *mental* well-being throughout life.

The relationship between negative emotions and physical health is now well-established, both by research and clinical findings. Anger, when experienced frequently, tends to evolve into resentment (chronic, low-level anger), hostility (an angry attitude toward a specific person or group), or **cynicism** (an attitude of contempt or distrust of others). Thus, anger can become incorporated into the personality.

The Type A personality has long been recognized as a risk factor for heart attack. Descriptions of the Type A personality include such behaviors as always being in a hurry, often doing two or more things at the same time, being driven by ambition (for achievement, success, recognition), displaying intolerance for the shortcomings of others, tending to become frustrated quickly when obstructed, and frequently manifesting anger or hostility.

Dr. Redford Williams, Director of the Behavioral Medicine Research Center at Duke University, studied cardiac patients and concluded that only the anger and hostility components of Type A personality are "toxic." Some aspects of this personality type are positive. For example, behaviors related to striving for achievement were found to be related to good health, provided they were not associated with anger. So it is now known that the risk factor for coronary disease is not Type A personality itself, but the anger and hostility component.

Another emotion that is known to have significant effects on physical health is grief. Ever since the days of Hippocrates, physicians have recognized the correlation between significant loss and serious physical illness. Today we know that grief suppresses the immune system, thereby rendering a person more susceptible to infections, cancer and other disorders for which the immune system normally provides adequate protection. Grief also affects mental processes significantly. Advice often given to a newly widowed person is, "Don't make any important decisions for at least a year." If you have ever experienced a significant loss, you may remember that it was difficult to concentrate or think clearly; even your memory was affected. The duration of these effects depends on the significance of the loss and the intensity of the grief reaction.

Since our emotions have powerful mental and physical effects, it is important that we learn to use emotions effectively, rather than allow emotions to control our behavior. The person who has learned to express feelings in socially acceptable ways is competent in dealing with life situations—both good and bad. A person who has not learned to use emotions constructively is likely to lose control when feelings become strong. The sudden **eruption** of powerful feelings may result in behavior that is ineffective in dealing with a situation.

PHYSIOLOGICAL EFFECTS OF EMOTIONS

Emotions influence physical functioning, with particular effect on the autonomic nervous system. The autonomic nervous system, in turn, influences the functioning of internal organs. Through this indirect influence, the emotional state can stimulate certain organs and inhibit the activity of others. If the emotion is strong, the effect is of short duration. If the emotion is long-term, as in chronic anxiety, internal processes are kept in a state of "semi-emergency alert." Over a period of time, this long-term **physiological** situation can lead to actual physical changes.

The human body is an organized system that carries out numerous life-sustaining processes. The body makes certain adaptations in response to a variety of life situations so that **homeostasis** is maintained. Homeostasis is the

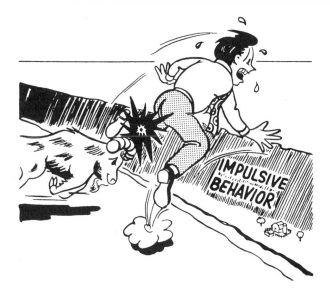

Suppressed emotions can erupt suddenly and propel an individual into undesirable behavior.

balance of chemicals and hormones necessary for ideal physiological functioning. When the body is unable to make this adaptation (i.e., homeostasis does not exist), there is serious threat to physical health until homeostasis is reestablished.

Studies of body reactions to situations that arouse fear or anger show that the adrenal glands discharge large amounts of **adrenalin** and the sympathetic nervous system produces **noradrenalin.** These two hormones speed up the circulation of blood, accelerate blood clotting, dilate the blood vessels that serve the skeletal muscles, and increase the respiratory rate. The purpose of these changes is to prepare the body for unusual activity, that is, a "fight or flight" state to deal with the emergency situation. While the body's resources are being mobilized to strengthen the musculoskeletal system, other areas of the body have a diminished supply of blood. These physiological changes are adaptive, meaning that they enable the individual to deal physically with a threatening situation.

✓STRESS

Dr. Hans Selye studied the physiological effects of unusual life situations for over thirty years. Dr. Selye noted that there is a *generalized* body reaction in addition to the alarm ("fight or flight") reaction. He labeled this pattern of response **stress.** Dr. Selye labeled the generalized reaction "General Adaptation Syndrome" or GAS. It is the sum total of physiological changes that occur in a state of stress. The stress response is essential to survival; it occurs in response to either a positive or a negative emotional state. Thus, a happy event such as marriage or the birth of a baby, as well as an unhappy experience, can trigger the generalized stress reaction.

Extreme emotional states are generally of short duration; they can be measured in terms of minutes or hours. The "fight or flight" arousal generally subsides as soon as the emergency has passed, although the aftereffects, such as sweaty palms and trembling, may continue for several hours, until the amount of adrenalin and noradrenalin in the bloodstream has returned to normal. On the other hand, stress (the generalized response) does not subside quickly; when this aroused state exists for a long period, then the body is in a state of dis-stress. The physiological arousal is not serving a useful purpose and is, in fact, interfering with normal body functions. Stress over a period of years can lead to depletion of the adrenal glands.

The term stress refers to the adaptive response itself. The outside influences that create a state of arousal are **stressors.** The word "stress" should be reserved to refer to the psychological state of emotional arousal and/or the physiological adaptive response.

Dr. Selye's research led to the discovery that the stress reaction includes increased body resistance to outside agents such as infectious organisms. This is the basis for immunity to specific diseases (i.e., production of antibodies). During a period of increased resistance to a specific stressor, resistance to other stressors is decreased. For example, working long hours, eating improperly, and not getting sufficient sleep and recreation add up to stress. A person with such a lifestyle is likely to have lowered resistance and therefore be more susceptible to infection.

The person whose stress reaction is due to invasion by a specific infectious agent, such as the measles virus, has the physiological response specific to that infectious agent (e.g., in case of measles, fever, rash, runny nose). At that time, the measles victim has lowered resistance to other organisms, such as the bacteria or viruses that cause pneumonia. While the body mobilizes its resources to deal with the measles virus, only limited resources are available to deal with other threats to health.

Unfortunately, resistance to psychological stressors does not automatically develop, as is the case with immunity to some infectious organisms. Nor does the stress reaction subside as quickly or as completely after a psychological threat is no longer a part of the immediate life situation. Because of mental/emotional/physiological interactions, we can experience stress by remembering a past event, by anticipating some undesirable future event, or even by imagining that something has happened or is happening.

One of the advantages man has over other forms of animal life is the mental ability to deal with the future by planning, setting goals, or preparing for

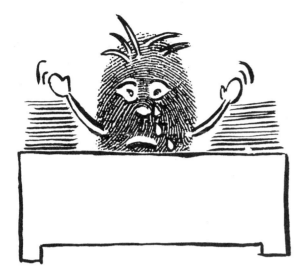

"I'll never finish on time." A heavy workload can be a major source of stress. (From Carol D. Tamparo & Wilburta Q. Lindh, *Therapeutic Communications for Allied Health Professions.* Albany, NY: Delmar Publishers Inc. 1992.)

specific future events. When one's thoughts are directed to an undesirable event (e.g., failing a course, being fired, being deserted by one's spouse), the emotional reaction to this *mental activity* triggers the adaptive response.

Another major source of stress for many people is **"mind-talk."** This almost continuous stream of thoughts and memories is most likely to occur when an individual is performing routine tasks (i.e., ironing, raking leaves) that do not require concentrated thought or during quiet times when trying to relax. Mind-talk contributes to insomnia, since the physiological reaction to thoughts can lead to increasing wakefulness, rather than increasing sleepiness. Mind-talk, as used in this discussion, is ongoing, not fully under conscious control, and not purposeful. It is different from conscious use of mental processes for thinking, planning, evaluating, analyzing, and remembering.

Mind-talk that deals with past events may include an embarrassing situation, a failure or an unsatisfactory performance, a disappointment, a lost opportunity for a smart response, or an extensive review of a conversation. Many people carry a heavy load of resentment (i.e., anger) or anxiety (i.e., fear) regarding past events. But—past events cannot be changed; only the present and the future can be altered. This habit of frequently recalling past events that aroused a negative emotion results in a state of chronic stress that can lead to permanent physiological changes—the basis for **psychosomatic** (psycho—mind; soma—body) illness.

Mind-talk can also deal with future possible events, rather than memories of past events that did occur. These thoughts may involve rehearsal of an expected conversation, something "bad" that could happen to oneself or to a loved one, a loss, or the possibility of abandonment. If worrying about possible future events is habitual, the individual maintains a state of anxiety. The resulting physiological response is continuous—a state of stress exists.

Obviously, mind-talk can include remembering good things that happened, or anticipating some type of good experience. Mind-talk concerned with "good" things is satisfying, however, rather than stress-inducing. Mind-talk can arouse any of the emotions—positive or negative. Everyone experiences mind-talk, but people vary in the extent to which they react emotionally. Stress management requires learning to control mind-talk so that it does not arouse negative emotions or interfere with sleep. While *planning* and mind-talk are similar, *planning* is a specific thought process. Its purpose is to prepare to deal with a future event effectively.

The importance of learning to use your emotional responses constructively and to deal with stress effectively cannot be emphasized too strongly. Your physical and emotional health in the future will ***inevitably*** be affected, for better or worse, by the behavior patterns you are using to express emotions throughout each day.

√POSITIVE EMOTIONS

The positive emotions, primarily joy and love, contribute to our feeling good. Words such as elation and ecstasy describe extremely high states of joy, whereas pleasure and satisfaction imply a less intense state of joy. Love is a complex emotion; there are various types of love and the intensity varies according to type, the object of the love, and circumstances of the moment.

These two emotions are essential to the state we call "happiness." Some degree of joy is experienced whenever good things happen, when our life is relatively free of trials and tribulations, and when we are aware of loving others and being loved. Yet happiness is possible even when our life situation includes problems, some degree of stress, and times of negative feelings. The experience of happiness is dependent upon one's ability to focus on positive aspects of life—the sources of pleasure and satisfaction—and minimize negative feelings by dealing competently with the problems and challenges that are a part of daily living. Because it is so important to happiness and health, love is discussed in greater detail below.

√Love

Love is an important positive emotion. Strong feelings of warmth for another person might be thought of as *love,* with milder feelings of the same type being termed *friendliness. Affection* implies a feeling less intense than love, but stronger than friendliness. Love implies caring about someone else, being concerned enough to help, understand, and respect the person loved. Love and our patterns for expressing it affect the relationships we have with others. The capacity for feeling love influences one's outlook on life and attitudes toward people. The ability to love and to receive love also has a powerful effect on physical and mental health.

Kinds of Love

There are many kinds of love: the love of a mother for her child; the child's love, at first self-centered and then extended to others; love for one's playmates; love for material things associated with pleasant memories; love for friends with whom life experiences have been shared; love for unfortunate ones wherever they might be; and love for a patient and his family who are all struggling with their stressful situation. Sexual love should involve both self-love and selfless love, the desire for oneness with the loved one including a desire to please that exceeds the desire to be pleased. Spiritual love is different still and varies according to one's concept of the Divine. Needless to say, each kind of love is expressed in specific ways. Newspaper accounts of some family's misfortune often result in a flood of contributions from strangers, illustrating the capacity of many people to express love for strangers who are less fortunate than themselves.

Learning to Love

Love is essential to an infant's normal development. Babies who must remain in an institution tend to waste away and die, unless the staff makes certain that the baby is frequently touched or held. The importance of tender loving care **(TLC)** for institutionalized infants has only been recognized in the past few decades. If you ever work in a nursery or neonatal unit, you may see "TLC" orders for certain infants who have been there for some time. The infant who receives the love of parents and other caretakers also learns trust and develops a sense of security.

Throughout childhood, one gradually learns to extend love to others: parents, siblings, other family members, caretakers, and eventually a widening circle of friends and associates. This learning is basic to the development of such traits as generosity, **altruism,** respect, and courtesy toward others. During adolescence, romantic love becomes a primary concern, which may extend throughout adulthood. Mature love is a special type of love that evolves through a long-term adult relationship. Each of these types of love can flourish only if the individual's early experiences fostered the development of self-love.

Learning to Love

*The place above all others
where children should receive love
and thereby learn to love
is in the family.
One of the curses of our world
is selfishness,
and probably the only effective way
to be rid of it
is to begin with our children.
They have to learn to love at an early stage,
which means within the family.*

*William C. Menninger, MD, 1899–1966
Reprinted courtesy of The Menninger Foundation*

Self-Love

Self-love is basic to the experience of love. Without self-love, a person is not able to truly love others. Self-love is not selfish, nor is it egotistic. It is an awareness of "self" as a worthwhile, lovable being who deserves to be cared for. A religious person may experience self-love through the belief, "I am a child of God." Loving oneself and believing oneself to be lovable are fundamental to a positive self-concept, the best protection one can have against threats to self-esteem as various difficulties of life are experienced.

Self-love enables a person to experience joy and happiness. It also contributes to health and well-being, in part because those who have self-love care enough about themselves to practice habits of safety and health maintenance. They do not abuse their bodies with toxic substances, such as alcohol, nicotine, or other addictive drugs. They eat right, exercise appropriately, get enough sleep, wear seat belts in the car, do not drive recklessly, or otherwise place themselves at needless risk. In other words, a person who has self-love takes responsibility for "self" in all aspects of living.

Unconditional Love

Love should be *unconditional*, which means that it is not subject to being withheld whenever one is displeased. Conditional love has an "if/then" basis: *if* you do (or do not do) such and so, *then* I will love you. All too often, conditional love is used as a manipulative tool to control another person. This is destructive to a relationship, but is especially damaging when used by parents to control a child. Conditional love teaches, "You're not lovable as a person; you're only lovable when I consider that you are being 'good.' " This style of parenting can lead to a negative self-concept, the belief that one is only lovable when meeting the demands of another. Dr. Bernie Siegel, a surgeon who devotes much time to working with cancer patients, states in his book, *Love, Medicine and Miracles:*

> *"Many people, especially cancer patients, grow up believing there is some terrible flaw at the center of their being, a defect they must hide if they are to have any chance for love. Feeling unlovable and condemned to loneliness if their true selves become known, such individuals set up defenses against sharing their innermost feelings with anyone."*

Dr. Siegel believes that all disease can be traced to lack of love or to experiencing only conditional love during significant periods of their lives. Noting that the majority of his patients did not experience unconditional love, Dr. Siegel states, ". . . 80 percent of my patients were unwanted or treated indifferently as children." Feeling unloved and unlovable depresses the immune system, making the individual more susceptible to disease.

Unconditional love, then, not only provides a growing child with a strong, positive self-concept, it also prepares the individual for a more healthful future life. Unconditional love does not mean that one must put up with undesirable behavior from others. It is important to differentiate between the person and that person's behavior. It is also important to realize that you can love someone even when you do not like them. Unconditional love is available at all times; it survives the ups and downs of a relationship. Liking, on the other hand, is quite variable, depending upon behavior, the quality of interaction, even personality traits.

Insofar as behavior is concerned, love for a child includes teaching appropriate behaviors at each stage of development; boundaries must be set in terms of what is acceptable behavior and what is not. Setting boundaries—making it clear that one will not tolerate a specific behavior—is a way of clarifying a relationship; it is not a matter of withholding love.

Unconditional love can be learned (and received) at any stage of life, in sickness or in health. Dr. Siegel believes that helping cancer patients learn to love themselves unconditionally, and then extend their unconditional love to others, is a powerful tool that influences the course of illness. Even seriously ill patients can achieve this goal and find new joy in living. How much better it would be if everyone could learn early in life to give and receive unconditional love and then reap the benefits, including improved health and better relationships, throughout life.

NEGATIVE EMOTIONS

The negative emotions make us feel uncomfortable. The intensity of each emotion can range from mild to very strong, with various degrees of feeling in between these two extremes. The effects on the individual may be a vague restlessness, a feeling of dissatisfaction, or a state of intense agitation.

The arousal of negative emotions may occur as a response to the behavior of another person, a specific event or piece of information, or mind-talk. The emotional arousal may be anger, fear, guilt, or sadness. Regardless of which emotion is being experienced, it results in stress and the physiological changes described by Dr. Selye. The intensity of the emotional response is based on how the individual perceives the precipitating events/thoughts. The effects occur regardless of whether the emotional response is to actual events or mind-talk.

√Anger

Anger is an emotion aroused by obstacles, threats, or otherwise offensive situations. It is usually short-term and directed at a specific object or person, but can be generalized as anger at the world or society. *Hate* may be thought of as intense anger felt toward a specific person or persons. *Annoyance* is used to describe a mild form of anger. *Rage* describes intense anger and implies that the anger is expressed through violent physical activity. ***Hostility*** is a mild form of anger/hate directed to a specific person or group; often it is unintentionally conveyed to others either verbally or nonverbally. ***Resentment*** is chronic anger that may be entirely subjective—it is not conveyed verbally or nonverbally—and can be a powerful influence on one's behavior.

Anger is the emotional response to one's perception of a situation. The perception usually involves feeling wronged, neglected, cheated, deprived, ignored, or exploited. If the anger is not resolved, it becomes resentment and may be harbored for a lifetime. Many resentments have their origins in childhood, with a parent or sibling as the object of the resentment. Both anger and resentment can arise from feeling powerless to change a situation or to fight back. Anger may be aroused by an unsuccessful effort to control another person, or by awareness of being controlled or manipulated by another person. When anger is shared by a large number of people and control is held by a faceless group ("administration" or "the owners" or "government"), the anger of powerlessness can erupt as rebellion.

As individuals, we may generate our own anger. Dr. Thomas Gordon, a psychologist who works with parents to help them improve family relationships, believes that anger is often secondary to some other emotion. A parent feels fear when a child cannot be found; once the child's safety is assured, anger is directed at the child for having "caused" the situation. Anger may be secondary to other primary feelings, such as embarrassment or disappointment. When one experiences anger toward a friend or family member, it is advisable to consider whether or not the anger is due to some need of our own not being met. If the anger is due to some type of problem/situation, it is better to state that one is experiencing anger, and then suggest that an effort to solve the problem situation be undertaken by all parties involved. If the anger is not used constructively, it may develop into smoldering resentment, hostility, or even hatred. **Suppression** of these feelings is likely to result eventually in an explosive verbal outpouring or even destructive physical actions.

One unfortunate example of destructive anger is domestic violence, now recognized as a growing problem in American society. (Perhaps it is a long-standing problem that is only now being acknowledged.) Violence against another person is an inappropriate expression of anger. Domestic violence involves directing anger toward one's spouse or child, usually through physical assault; it also includes verbal assault and any menacing actions that arouse fear in the victim.

The problem of child abuse has received increasing attention over the past two decades. Studies of child abusers reveal that many were themselves abused as children. This is a tragic example of how inappropriate adult behavior influences the child's future patterns for emotional expression. The child who grows up in a home where violent behavior occurs regularly perceives this pattern of family interaction as "normal." That perception must change, either through education or counseling, before that person can adopt a different standard of values in which violent behavior is unacceptable.

Fear

Fear is an emotion aroused primarily by threat. The threat may be related to physical harm or it may be related to one's sense of security. Fear of physical harm is usually of short duration; the danger passes or the person is able to cope with the dangerous situation. *Terror* and *panic* are terms for describing intense fear; the person who is in a state of terror or panic may flee the situation or may be immobilized by the intensity of the emotional reaction.

Fear is a natural reaction to a situation that is perceived as dangerous or life-threatening. It serves a useful purpose by mobilizing the body for action—for fighting or fleeing a threatening situation. The body's response is an outpouring of adrenalin, which increases the flow of blood through the body, raises the rate of respiration, and stimulates muscle tone. Under these circumstances, the body is literally mobilized for action. If physical activity does not occur, this readiness for action may be released through "the shakes." Perhaps you have been involved in a dangerous situation, remaining calm until the danger was over and then finding yourself shaking all over or "weak in the knees." Many examples of heroic action involve physical exertion that the individual could not repeat after the excitement had subsided. The outpouring of adrenalin resulted in physical strength far beyond the person's usual abilities.

Fear can also be a natural reaction to mind-talk. *Worry* is fear based on thoughts about a *possible* event, such as losing one's job, losing a loved one, losing some type of property, or displeasing someone. *Anxiety* involves a higher intensity of fear than worry; it is likely to be a chronic pattern of emotional response to mind-talk. *Apprehension* and *dread* describe fear based on thoughts about some pending event that one perceives as threatening.

Fear is healthful when it is a reaction to a threatening event or situation. When self-generated through mind-talk, fear is pointless and destructive, unless it is used to plan ways to deal effectively with an expected situation. If one is apprehensive about a speech to be delivered on Monday, the best way to deal with the fear is to prepare well, practice the speech until completely comfortable with it, mentally picture oneself delivering the speech effectively, then remember to take several deep breaths before starting to deliver the speech. In the process of preparing for an effective delivery, self-confidence will replace apprehension.

Grief

Grief is the emotional response to loss. It can range in intensity from momentary disappointment to deep sorrow that completely absorbs the individual. *Grief* is used to describe intense feelings; *sorrow* implies grief without indicating intensity; *sadness* implies grieving of moderate intensity; *disappointment* implies a mild form of grief. Whereas fear and anger tend to arouse one physically, grief has the opposite effect. A person who is grieving may find it difficult to perform simple tasks. The body seems to reserve energy at this time for the individual to work through the grief. It is highly desirable, even healthful, to consciously grant oneself time to grieve when loss of any type has been experienced.

Guilt

Guilt as discussed here refers to self-blaming, rather than to any legal/criminal aspects. A clinical psychology professor once referred to guilt as the "most useless emotion there is." We can feel guilty about many things: things we did or said in the past, things we now wish we had done but did not do at the proper time, words we could have spoken but didn't. These are sometimes referred to as the "sins of commission and omission." Painful regrets, with or without feelings of guilt, are experienced by almost everyone who has lost a loved one through death.

It is impossible to change the past, so it is pointless to wallow in guilt about what cannot be changed. Some things can be remedied by doing "now" what should have been done in the past. Another remedy is forgiveness—of self and others. But forgiveness is not easy; self-forgiveness is especially difficult for people who have been controlled by guilt. Those who try to control others, especially family members or lovers, tend to use guilt as a manipulative tool.

Striving for self-understanding and learning effective interpersonal skills are one's best protection against the damaging effects of guilt. Anyone who realizes his or her behavior is strongly influenced by guilt feelings, or that someone is controlling him or her through guilt, may find professional counseling helpful.

FORMATION OF EMOTIONAL PATTERNS

Emotional patterns are learned through experience and according to the satisfaction or distress that accompanies various life experiences. Each person's capacity to feel specific emotions may be hereditary, as indicated by the fact that newborn infants show marked differences in their responses to distress. In spite of this hereditary factor, the great differences in adult emotional patterns are primarily the result of learning.

The people of a baby's world—the social environment—determine to a great degree whether the baby's experiences are pleasing or distressing. Throughout infancy, childhood, and adolescence the formation of emotional patterns is influenced by the emotional expressions and behaviors of others, especially primary care-givers and family members. Later in life, the balance of successes and failures in daily living has great influence on emotional expression. Also, the reactions of other people to one's expressions of emotion influence the tendency to show one's feelings or attempt to hide them. The development of patterns for expressing feelings, then, occurs within a framework of various influences on behavior: heredity, environment, basic needs, the consequences of behavior that follow specific life experiences, and interactions with other people.

Family patterns of emotional expression influence the formation of a child's emotional patterns. Ideally, the child receives loving care from both parents and other family members, thereby learning love and trust. In these days of single-parent and two-wage-earner homes, the primary care-givers may be the staff of a child-care facility, rather than a parent. The demands of a full-time job plus homemaking responsibilities limit the amount of time and energy a parent has to invest in parenting. And so, the child may be exposed to a hectic schedule, rushed to the child-care center in the morning and picked up later in the day by a parent exhausted from the demands of the workplace. At times, the balance of emotional expression may be more negative than positive. The behaviors of the adults, especially those behaviors that express an emotional state, are the behaviors the child will learn. In addition, the behaviors of child-care personnel and their beliefs about the expression of feelings are important influences on the child's developing emotional patterns.

Dr. Harriett Lerner, a psychotherapist at the Menninger Institute, has studied the emotional patterns of women for several decades. In her book

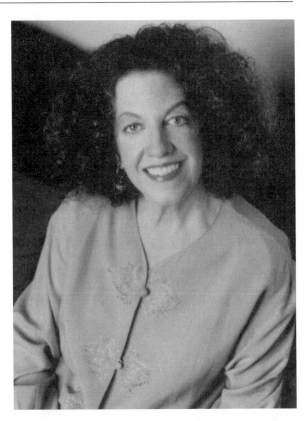

Dr. Harriett Lerner has written extensively on the subject of anger, especially as it affects women. (Photo by Penni Gladstone, courtesy of Jo-Lynne Worley.)

The Dance of Anger, she describes patterns for expression of anger as a legacy handed down from generation to generation. A young woman who tends to suppress her anger probably has a mother who suppressed anger, and her mother was reared by a woman who probably suppressed anger. Thus, a particular pattern of emotional expression may characterize a family, extending through several generations as the children of each generation learn, through imitation, the emotional patterns of the adults. The formation of these behavioral patterns will change only if some members of the family learn a *different* pattern of behavior for expressing emotions. This relearning may mean a rejection of parental influence; some people, therefore may find it difficult to modify long-standing patterns for expressing one's feelings.

Although these patterns are learned early in life, they are influenced later through exposure to widening circles of relatives, friends, schoolmates, co-workers, and various peer groups. These patterns extend to all the emotions, positive as well as negative. As you study the remainder of this unit, be aware of your own patterns for expressing each emotion. As you remember specific behaviors you saw in your home as a child, speculate about the emotions that were being expressed. Also, consider (1) whether or not you, as a child, adopted that pattern of behavior and (2) what modifications you have made in expressing feelings during adolescence and adulthood.

INDIVIDUAL DIFFERENCES IN EMOTIONAL PATTERNS

Everyone has both negative and positive feelings. The tendency to respond to a certain type of situation with a specific emotion, the intensity of our emotional responses, ways in which we express our feelings, the balance between positive and negative feelings, and the duration of a particular emotion are all characteristic of each person as an individual. People differ, then, in regard to the inner experience (feeling) and in the outward manifestation (behavior) of that inner experience.

The behavior that results from a specific feeling state is a person's *expression* of that particular emotion. Another person may use a very different behavior for expressing the same emotion. If one is experiencing a particular emotion but chooses not to express it, then the emotion is being **suppressed.** Some times we suppress an emotion while in the situation that arouses it, then express it later; this is especially common with anger. If an emotion is extremely intense, and/or the situation that aroused the feeling is painful or unacceptable, then the emotion may be *repressed.* The memory of a traumatic event and the feelings associated with that event may both be repressed, meaning that they are not available to conscious memory. Several therapeutic approaches can help a person access repressed memories/feelings. In addition to differences in behavioral expressions of feelings, people differ in their tendencies to feel various emotions.

Intensity and Frequency

Some people have the capacity for very strong feelings, whereas others seem to feel less intensely. Some people react frequently with strong emotion, even to daily annoyances such as traffic slowdowns. Other people react with strong emotion only to unusual situations in which an intense emotional reaction is justified. Some people hide their feelings, which can result in a chronic state of stress.

Temperament

The type of emotion (positive or negative) that a person feels most of the time is known as *temperament.* An optimistic person is one whose feelings are primarily positive; a pessimistic person is one whose feelings are primarily negative. Temperament is indicated by the way emotions are expressed: words and tone of voice, facial expression and other nonverbal behavior, and actions.

Most of us prefer the company of people who usually reflect positive emotions. Sometimes people with a pessimistic outlook find mutual satisfaction in each other, which brings to mind the saying, "Misery loves company." And then there are those who do not show their feelings readily; their appearance is somewhat the same whether they are feeling good or bad inside. This lack of expressiveness may indicate suppression of emotion, rather than lack of feeling. It is difficult to know how such people feel and, therefore, difficult to adapt your own behavior appropriately.

Some people overreact to difficulties in life, thereby having many negative emotional responses. This is similar to the person we previously described as giving great attention to each of life's disappointments and hardly noticing the things that go smoothly. Some people allow a negative state to persist longer than the situation warrants. A disappointment is cause for a relatively short period of unhappiness. Persons who allow disappointments to dominate their emotional state are overreacting to normal life events.

Mood Swings

Another difference in individual emotional reactions is the tendency to have mood swings. Each of us has times when we are "blue"; each of us has times when we feel especially good for no apparent reason. This swing from up to down is normal. Some people, however, swing from one extreme to another or remain "down" for long periods and "up" for long periods. Extreme mood swings and/or a prolonged mood at one extreme or the other may indicate a need for professional counsel. Those whose mood swings are within normal range can learn to make full use of the times when they feel good and develop techniques for coping with periods when they feel "low."

The tendency to have long "down" periods can indicate that a person is clinically depressed, a condition now referred to as "unipolar." Extreme mood swings, down periods alternating with periods of high energy and productivity, may indicate that a person has bipolar disorder (formerly known as manic depressive illness). The line between "normal" mood swings and those indicative of a mood disorder is not clearcut. Many unipolar and bipolar people function relatively well at jobs and within the family, especially if they are under psychiatric care. In fact, bipolars tend to be highly productive when they are in the "hypomanic" state; this is especially true of creative people, such as writers, poets, composers, musicians and others in the performing arts.

If the mood swings are serious enough to interfere with work, study, or family relations, then the individual should seek medical evaluation. If destructive or threatening behavior accompanies the "up" cycle, the individual should have a psychiatric evaluation as soon as possible. Dr. Kay Jamison, an authority on Bipolar Disorder, states that only two out of five persons with this illness have been diagnosed and are under treatment. This means that many

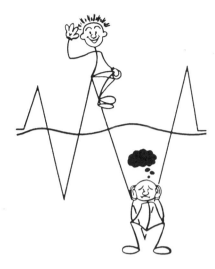

Everyone has "ups" and "downs."

people who are perceived by friends and family as "moody" or "unpredictable" may in fact be bipolar and in need of medical evaluation.

USING EMOTIONS CONSTRUCTIVELY

Accentuating the Positive

Many people who appear happy much of the time actually have had more than their share of unhappy experiences. Happiness is determined by how we react to both pleasant and unpleasant experiences in life. Some people use their unhappy experiences for endless conversational material. Others give only short notice to unhappy experiences, rapidly turning their attention to activities that give them satisfaction.

Each of us is free to choose between a negative and a positive outlook. We cannot eliminate all of life's disappointments, but we can refuse to let negative emotions dominate our lives. We can cut short the time and attention we give to negative feelings aroused by unpleasant experiences and give greater attention to pleasant experiences and the good feelings that result. It is important, however, to consider each negative experience in terms of any lesson that can be learned. By using negative experiences as opportunities for learning, we become more competent for coping with life events.

Open and Honest Communication

Dr. Gordon recommends a number of techniques for handling situations effectively. Owning your feelings involves stating how a situation is affecting you. For example, a health care provider may have a supervisor who frequently changes the schedule, for no apparent reason. Some people may rearrange their personal plans in order to work the changed hours, but criticize the supervisor to co-workers and the family. Another person might confront the supervisor in anger and possibly even refuse to accept the changed hours. Still another worker might say nothing about the change, but take sick leave on the day for which the hours were changed. Each of these three approaches has disadvantages. None is likely to alter the supervisor's habit of changing hours on short notice. A cooperative approach is preferable; but first, the supervisor must become aware that there is a problem.

Suppose the health care provider approaches the supervisor at an appropriate time and calmly states, "I have a problem when my hours are changed. I have to make different arrangements for care of my children." The health care provider has made statements of fact, using "I" to describe the effect of the schedule changes. This is "open and honest" communication. No accusation has been made; no blame has been laid on the supervisor. The climate is right for a discussion of the problem and a cooperative approach to finding a solution.

Perhaps there is a good reason for the change in hours. It is easier to accept an undesirable situation if you know that it exists because of unavoidable circumstances, rather than because of someone's poor planning. Perhaps the supervisor was not aware of the health care provider's child care problems and, therefore, was unaware of the inconvenience created by a change in schedule. Regardless of how the supervisor responds, the health care provider has diffused any anger that was felt; it will not erupt later in an uncontrolled outburst of feeling. Even more important, the anger will not be displaced onto patients, co-workers, or members of the family who did nothing to cause the anger.

This approach is called, "I talk," meaning that *feelings* are expressed in a statement beginning with "I" rather than a "you" statement that accuses or blames the other person. Compare the suggested "I" statement of the health care provider with an accusative statement: "You are always changing the hours! You are forcing me to change my babysitting arrangement! Why can't you make up a schedule and stick to it?" These statements would result in an angry supervisor. Certainly being on the defensive would not put the supervisor in a problem-solving frame of mind.

"I talk" is valuable as a means of expressing both positive and negative feelings. If substituted for suppression of feelings (holding them in) and for accusations ("you talk"), this technique can lead to improved interpersonal relations. Dr. Gordon warns, however, that when an "I" statement is used to express anger, it may be perceived as an accusation ("you made me angry"). Consider the possible effect of the following statements:

- "You always keep me waiting."
- "I really get angry when I have to wait."

- "I was disappointed when I arrived and you were not here yet."

- "You are fifteen minutes late."

Obviously, the "you" statements put the other person on the defensive, may create angry feelings toward you, or may arouse feelings of guilt. Any of these feelings will interfere with your enjoyment of each other's company now that you are together. On the other hand, the "I" statements simply state how you feel (although #2 may be perceived as an accusation). The other person cannot deny you your feelings. There is no basis for argument. And, you have discharged the feeling verbally and are no longer burdened with anger.

Open and honest communication of positive feelings will greatly improve relations with others. All of us like to hear good things. Our needs do not get satisfied when others withhold their positive feelings on the assumption that we know how they feel. But open and honest communication is especially important as a means of dealing with negative emotions. The following sections deal with approaches to handling specific negative emotional states.

Dealing With Anger

Negative emotions must be dealt with constructively, or they will have destructive effects. When inner tension builds up from anger, this tension needs release. If a patient makes you angry, you cannot throw a bedpan or physically attack the patient. It is not desirable to "blow up" at your supervisor; not is it fair for you to bottle up your anger until you get home, and then let it loose on your family. (This is called "displaced anger.") Perhaps the tension built up from your anger can help you mow the grass, repair that broken gate, or whip up a cake. In other words, use energy generated by anger in some type of constructive physical activity. Do not "blow up" in a way that will harm relations with other people. Do not hold the feeling in or deny its existence.

While you are in the situation, use "I" statements as appropriate or ask questions that will help you understand the other person's views or the circumstances. As you gain understanding, your anger may subside.

Once you are out of the situation in which you became angry, try to understand the reason for your anger. Is the reaction related to old resentments? In other words, do you have a "response set" for becoming angry with this person or in this type of situation? Were you frustrated in your efforts to meet some need? Did you have expectations that the other person failed to meet? Were you treated unfairly (in your opinion)?

If you still feel anger, there are several techniques for safely diffusing the feelings. Talk with someone who knows how to listen. Just talking about the situation—the facts and also your feelings—can provide effective release. If you cannot talk to someone about it, set up a tape recorder, visualize it as the person at whom you are angry, and tell it exactly how you feel. Then, listen to a playback of the tape. Continue until your anger has been released. (Don't forget to erase the tape!)

Another technique for working off feelings is to "punch out" a pillow, preferably a large, firm one. The physical activity provides for release of energy generated by the anger.

Dr. O. Carl Simonton is an oncologist who encourages cancer patients to deal with whatever anger and resentment they may have. He teaches patients to use mental imagery to visualize good things happening to a person who is the object of the anger or resentment. Although it does not seem appropriate, the technique is quite effective, according to Dr. Simonton. The positive thoughts seem to dissipate negative feelings.

Many therapists consider that the most effective technique for dealing with anger is forgiveness. It is difficult to forgive someone who has hurt you or cheated you. Yet, the anger you carry with you is actually harming *you*—your health and well-being—rather than the one who is the object of your anger. Learning to forgive may be one of life's most difficult lessons. But the power of another person to harm you psychologically is diminished when you are able to forgive. The forgiveness must be genuine; it must be at the emotional, rather than mental level. Forgiveness of those who are deceased is just as important as forgiveness of those who are still living.

Self-forgiveness is especially important. It is only human to make mistakes. We all have regrets about things we did or didn't do, about what we said or didn't say. Some matters can be corrected by taking action, sometimes referred to as "mending fences." If the other person is deceased, then the only recourse is self-forgiveness. It is desirable that we learn from the past, however, so that new regrets do not accumulate.

Dealing With Fear

To deal with fear effectively, we must first acknowledge the fear. We all encounter situations that arouse mild fear: a test, an oral report, returning to care for the patient who was critical of you yesterday, reporting to the supervisor that you broke a piece of equipment. In some situations the fear is justified, and the only recourse is to deal with the situation as effectively as possible. Sometimes mentally rehearsing the event as a successful experience prepares you to deal with the situation with less fear.

Sometimes a person's fear is out of proportion to the expected event; fear tends to magnify the dreaded aspects of the situation. Sometimes one's fear is based on a faulty assumption or expectation. Fear can interfere with realistic thinking about a problem, but the problem-solving approach often reveals that there is an acceptable solution. Once a solution is apparent, fear tends to decrease.

Some people have intense fear, known as a phobia, regarding something that most people do not find fearful (i.e., heights, being closed up in a small space such as an elevator, flying in an airplane). These fears are "abnormal" when they interfere with daily activities or cause the individual to take extreme measures to avoid the feared experience. Psychotherapy often results in the identification of some past traumatic event that the person had repressed, so that it was not available to conscious memory. In severe cases, the phobia requires a process of systematic desensitization, which may be done by various licensed mental health practitioners.

A more serious example of fear-related memory is known as Post-Traumatic Stress Disorder (PTSD). This is manifested by panic attacks, in which the individual relives a traumatic experience through sudden flashbacks or nightmares. This disorder came to the attention of the public after many Vietnam veterans had difficulty adapting to civilian life following discharge from military service. PTSD can have a severe disabling effect if left untreated.

A less severe, but quite distressful, reaction is experienced by most people who are involved in a serious accident or experience a frightening event such as a flood, hurricane, or tornado. For several weeks or months after such an experience, the individual may relive the experience when trying to go to sleep, or wake up suddenly in a cold sweat with rapid heartbeat, clammy skin, and uncontrollable shaking—a panic attack. Usually this tendency passes after several weeks, as physical healing occurs. If not, the individual should have professional counseling; it requires skilled professional intervention to desensitize survivors of traumatic events and free them from recurrent panic attacks. These examples illustrate again that there is a thin line between "normal human behavior" and the deviations from normal that indicate the need for therapeutic intervention.

Dealing With Grief

Grief is an emotion that lasts over a period of time. It may take weeks or months to work through the intense feelings and readjust one's life pattern. Whenever a loss occurs, permit yourself to grieve. When feelings of guilt are associated with grief, professional counseling may be needed to work through both emotions; such a combination is very difficult to handle alone. Unit 21 is devoted to a full discussion of the grief process.

EMOTIONS AND BEHAVIOR

Self

In striving to understand yourself and your behavior, you must give attention to your emotional patterns. Do you usually react to unpleasant situations with fear or anger? If you tend to overreact, you may need help in understanding reasons for your strong feelings. Some situations call for intense feelings, but most life situations do not justify a strong emotional reaction.

Do you give too much attention to negative feelings, perhaps even "enjoying" them? Enjoyment of misfortune is manifested through conversation, pessimism, self-pity, and other attention-getting behavior. You have only to think of one person who manifests such behavior to recognize the unfavorable effect on others. Obviously, such behavior is not appropriate for health care providers.

Emotions do exist, and they do affect us physically, psychologically, and mentally. To deny these feelings is a form of suppression. Suppressed emotions will have their effects sooner or later, through "blowing up" in an uncontrolled display of emotion, illness, poor coping mechanisms, or poor interpersonal relations.

Self-control is a constructive way of *using emotions,* rather than *not showing emotions.* Self control is a *learned behavioral pattern for expressing feelings in socially acceptable ways while dealing with a situation intelligently.* The following guidelines can be used to increase self-control.

- Express your feelings at the time they are experienced; if for some reason that is not appropriate, express the feelings as soon as possible in a "safe" setting.

- Own your feelings; use "I" statements rather than accusative "you" statements in your interactions with other people.

- Acknowledge (do not deny to yourself or others) that you experienced a particular emotion in a specific situation.

- Ask yourself, "Is this situation important enough to me to justify these feelings?" If the answer is "No," turn your attention to other matters. If "Yes," then deal with the situation effectively, perhaps using some of the guidelines below.

- Be assertive in getting others to work with you to clarify the problem and find a solution acceptable to all—a "win-win" situation; constructive efforts may dissipate any anger associated with the problem/situation.

- As you begin to experience anger, ask questions about the situation, then *listen* to the answers; better understanding of the other person's point of view may dissipate your anger.

- When you become aware of fear or apprehension, ask yourself whether or not you are in *real* danger. If the answer is "Yes," take appropriate

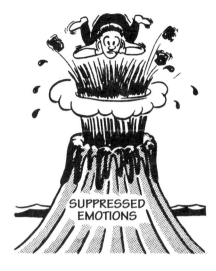

Suppressed emotions eventually lead to a blow-up.

action; if "no," analyze the basis for your feelings and take preventive action if needed.

- Use problem-solving to deal with a situation, present or future, so that you feel competent to find a solution and no longer need to feel apprehensive.

- Take responsibility for your feelings and your behavior; avoid blaming others for "causing" your feelings.

- Try to control mind-talk. If your thoughts involve future possible events and you become anxious, realize that mind-talk, not a real event, is the source of your anxiety.

- If you have a particular phobia, seek professional help so you can free yourself from this unrealistic fear. If you succeed in exposing the basis for your phobia, it no longer has the power to control your behavior.

- Use and enjoy humor; be willing to laugh at yourself for getting upset over something trivial. Diffuse a tense situation, as appropriate, with a humorous comment or anecdote.

- If you are still "worked up" after a situation that aroused strong emotions, use the energy for some type of constructive physical activity, such as mowing the grass, working out, running, or walking.

- Allow yourself to grieve for any loss you have experienced; if the loss arouses feelings of sadness, it is important enough to justify a period of grieving.

- Become aware of the events of your daily life that give you pleasure; be conscious of your pleasurable feelings as they occur and allow time at the end of the day to enjoy thoughts of these good experiences.

- Love yourself. Take credit for your strengths, your competence, your willingness to grow; forgive yourself for being less-than-perfect.

The foregoing suggestions are intended to help you understand yourself and your emotions better. As you become more open and honest with yourself and others about your feelings, you will have a favorable effect on others. As you learn to replace impulsive emotional behavior with actions based on reasoning, you will be free to control situations more effectively. As you develop greater sensitivity to the feelings of others, you are more likely to react appropriately to their behavior.

Others

Emotions are somewhat like a chain reaction. Hostile behavior by one person tends to bring out hostility in others. Aggressive behavior by one person brings about defensive behavior in others. When a person's behavior indicates that he or she may be experiencing some type of negative emotion, do not allow that behavior to arouse a negative emotion in you. Instead, maintain a positive feeling and show your concern with such statements as, "I sense that you are angry" or "I sense that you are really feeling down today." This approach is called "reflecting," meaning that you act as a mirror for the person's feelings. Reflecting indicates that you are "tuned in" to what that person is experiencing, that you care, and that you are giving that person your full attention. On the other hand, if you are not sensitive to the feelings behind that person's behavior, your response may provoke more negative behavior from the other person.

It requires practice to develop sensitivity to the feelings of others. Yet we can best adapt our own behavior and respond effectively to another person only if we are aware of the other person's emotional state.

As you work with patients and their families, strive to understand their feelings. Become observant of behavior that may indicate fear, anger, or grief. Avoid adding to such feelings by your own behavior. Take a little more time with the fearful patient, giving effective reassurances as best you can. Grant the grieving person the right to sorrow, recognizing that this emotion needs expression and cannot be worked through quickly. Grant your patient the right to be angry in certain situations; instead of becoming defensive, listen. Then, try to resolve the problem that aroused the patient's anger.

Through continuing effort, you can become a health care provider who practices the *art of human relations* along with the technical skills of your field.

References and Suggested Readings

Borysenko, Joan. *Guilt is the Teacher, Love is the Lesson.* New York, NY: Warner Books, 1991.

Bradshaw, John. *Creating Love.* New York, NY: Bantam Books, 1994.

Dacher, Elliott. *Psychoneuroimmunology: The New Mind/Body Healing Program.* New York, NY: Paragon House, 1993. Chapter 3, "Mindfulness," pp. 33–56.

Frankel, Lois P. *Women, Anger & Depression.* Deerfield Beach, FL: Health Communications, 1991.

Gordon, Thomas. *Parent Effectiveness Training.* New York, NY: New American Library, 1975.

Jampolsky, Gerald G., M.D. *Good-Bye to Guilt.* New York, NY: Bantam Books, 1988.

Lerner, Harriett, Ph.D. *The Dance of Anger.* New York, NY: Harper & Row Publishers, 1985. Chapter 5, "Using Anger as a Guide," pp. 88–107; Chapter 6, "Up and Down the Generations," pp. 108–121; Chapter 7, "Who's Responsible for What," pp. 122–153.

Siegel, Bernie S., M.D. *Love, Medicine and Miracles.* New York, NY: Harper & Row Publishers, 1990.

Simonton, O. Carl, Matthews-Simonton, Stephanie and Creighton, James. *Getting Well Again.* New York: St. Martin's Press, 1978. Chapter 4, "The Link between Stress and Illness," pp. 43–51; Chapter 13, "Overcoming Resentment," pp. 164–172.

Wegscheider-Cruse, Sharon. *Learning to Love Yourself.* Deerfield Beach, FL: Health Communications, 1987.

Williams, Redford, M.D. & Williams, Virginia, Ph.D. *Anger Kills: Seven Strategies for Controlling the Hostilities That Can Harm Your Health.* New York, NY: Harper-Collins, 1994.

REVIEW AND SELF-CHECK

Complete the following statements, using information from Unit 8.

1. Emotions are _____ .

2. Emotions are important because they affect us _____

    _____ and _____ .

3. If one does not learn to use emotions constructively, there is danger of

    _____ .

4. The purpose of the body's adaptive response to strong emotion (the "fight or flight" reaction) is _____ .

5. Stress, described by Dr. Selye, is _____ .

6. Dis-stress, according to Dr. Selye, is _____ .

7. Stressor refers to _____ .

8. Words that describe positive emotional states include _____ , _____ , _____ , _____ , _____ , and _____ .

9. The overall effect of experiencing one of the positive emotions is _____ _____ _____ .

10. The overall effect of experiencing one of the negative emotions may be _____ , _____ , _____ , or _____ .

11. Words that describe some degree of anger include _____ , _____ , _____ , or _____ .

12. Words that describe some degree of fear include _____ , _____ , and _____ .

13. Grief is an emotional response to _____ .

14. Words that express various degrees of grief include _____ , _____ , and _____ .

15. People differ in their emotional patterns, especially in regard to _____ , _____ , _____ , _____ , and _____ .

16. Temperament refers to the type of emotion (negative or positive) that characterizes a person; temperament is indicated by _____ , _____ , and _____ .

17. In order to use emotions constructively, one must learn to _____ ,

    _____ , _____ ,

    _____ , and _____ .

18. Self-control may be defined as _____ .

19. Guidelines for increasing one's self-control include _____ ,

    _____ , _____ ,

    _____ , and _____ .

20. Some ways a health care provider can use knowledge of emotions to foster effective patient relationships include _____ ,

    _____ , _____ ,

    _____ , and _____ .

ASSIGNMENT

1. Consider how you are affected by anger and how you usually express it:
   a. Can you think clearly when you are angry?
   b. Do you usually express your anger *verbally* by:
      saying something you later regret?
      calling the other person a "dirty name"?
      raising your voice? shouting or screaming?
      threatening to do something the other person would not like?
   c. Do you usually express your anger *physically* by:
      throwing things or kicking something?
      slamming a door?
      attacking the other person with your fists?
      slapping the other person?
   d. Do you try to express your anger, but burst into tears?
   e. Do you usually leave a situation when you become angry?
   f. Do you manage to appear completely calm even though you are seething with anger inside?
   g. Do you express your anger later, "taking it out" on someone other than the person at whom you are angry?
   h. Do you believe that other people or events *cause* your anger?

2. Consider how you are affected by sadness and how you usually express it:
    a. Can you think clearly when you are unhappy?
    b. Can you concentrate when you are unhappy?
    c. Is it difficult to do things you know you should do?
    d. Is it difficult to make decisions?
    e. Have you ever made a decision while feeling sad, then later realized you did not use good judgment?
    f. Do you believe another person or some situation is the cause of your unhappiness?

3. Do you tend to feel anger toward those you believe caused your unhappiness? What are some alternatives to holding this anger?

4. Your husband has just come home and states that he and a colleague "really got into it today." You sense his anger and want him to talk about what happened. Instead, he changes clothes and goes out for a five-mile jog. What do you think of this behavior?

5. Mary Ann is 17 years old. Her mother died the day before her seventeenth birthday. Mary Ann occasionally states, somewhat proudly, "I didn't even cry." You know that she and her mother were very close. What do you think of Mary Ann's behavior?

6. Your sister has a son who is four years old. Each time you visit in their home, you notice that your sister frequently says to the child, in an alarmed tone of voice "Don't do that. You will get hurt." Consider some possible effects of these repeated warnings on the child's emotional patterns.

7. You are assigned to Mr. J. today. You enter his room and say "Good morning" in your most cheerful voice. Mr. J. answers in an angry tone, "What's good about it?" What would be an effective response? What are some possible reasons for Mr. J. responding in such a way? How would you feel about Mr. J.?

8. Mrs. K. is scheduled for heart surgery. She is cheerful, never has a complaint, and tries to be helpful to the other patients. Your co-worker says, "Mrs. K. is certainly unusual. She is not at all worried about her surgery." Do you agree with your co-worker? Explain your answer.

9. Your supervisor calls you to the office and angrily says, "I'm changing the hours. You will have to work Saturday and Sunday." You have no plans, but it is your turn to have a weekend off. You become angry and say you will not work, even if it means being fired. Later that day you learn that two members of the staff are sick and one has been called out of town because of family problems. Describe the supervisor's probable emotional state when she called you into the office. List five ways you could have responded that might have prevented the unpleasant scene.

10. Consider each of the following statements. Be prepared to discuss each in terms of possible effects on the listener's emotional patterns:
    a. "You must not cry. You're a big boy now!"
    b. "If you do that again, I'll shut you in the closet."
    c. "You're a bad boy!"
    d. "It's wicked to hate someone. You must love everyone."
    e. "My friend had that same operation you're going to have. She had a terrible time and hasn't been the same since the operation."
    f. "Oh, you don't have a thing to worry about" (to a patient scheduled for surgery).
    g. "Shame on you! I expect you to get all As."
    h. "How dare you stomp your foot! You're a little girl; you must be sweet."

11. During the remainder of this course, collect examples of the following:
    a. "Innocent" statements that could arouse fear or anger in the listener, especially a child
    b. Ineffective reassurance offered to a patient or member of the family
    c. Effective reassurance, either verbal or nonverbal
    d. "You" statements in which the speaker projects blame instead of using open and honest communication
    e. Failure to express anger in a situation where anger is justified
    f. Denial of grief when there has been a great loss from one's life
    g. Statements that discourage the honest expression of feelings
    h. Statements that imply *conditional* love

12. Your child usually goes to his room whenever his older brother teases him. What does this mean, in terms of his pattern for expressing feelings? Now that you've noted his behavior, what should you do?

Unit 9

Adjustment and Patterns of Behavior

OBJECTIVES

Upon completion of this unit, you should be able to:

- Define adjustment.
- List five characteristics of a person who is well adjusted.
- List three characteristics of a person who is poorly adjusted.
- Explain why poor adjustment is a vicious cycle.
- State one reason change may affect adjustment.
- State five guidelines for improving adjustment.
- State four steps for adapting to a new situation.
- State two requirements for adapting to the role of health care provider.
- Name four ways one's emotional patterns influence adjustment.
- List five examples of daily hassles that affect adjustment.
- List five examples of satisfying daily experiences that affect adjustment.

KEY TERMS

Adjustment	Disruption	Vicious cycle
Hassle	Burnout	

Adjustment means the degree of success an individual has achieved in dealing with life situations. Each person's adjustment is variable, depending upon circumstances. A person may be well adjusted most of the time, but poorly adjusted during a period when there is a serious problem. Some people are poorly adjusted most of the time. They have not learned to deal with ordinary life situations effectively.

GOOD ADJUSTMENT

A person who is "well adjusted" deals effectively with problems and finds much satisfaction in living. Such a person has developed the habits and skills needed to solve common problems and has developed patterns of behavior that satisfy basic needs. Such a person is well prepared to weather a crisis and reestablish good adjustment within a reasonable period of time.

POOR ADJUSTMENT

A person who is poorly adjusted is not living a full life. Such a person feels restless and dissatisfied much of the time. Actually, the poorly adjusted person may not have any more problems than a well-adjusted person. The difference is that the poorly adjusted person has not learned to cope with obstacles or effectively deal with everyday problems of living.

The biggest obstacle for the poorly adjusted person is the poor adjustment itself. The habits, attitudes, emotional reactions, and behavior patterns that are a part of poor adjustment create additional problems for the individual. Poor adjustment is a **vicious cycle.** Ineffective behavior often creates additional problems that the individual handles with more ineffective behavior. For that reason, poor adjustment is a vicious cycle that can be broken only if the individual learns to deal with life situations more effectively.

EFFECTIVE BEHAVIOR VERSUS INEFFECTIVE BEHAVIOR

The key to adjustment is learning to recognize ineffective behavior and replacing it with another behavior that gets better results. The person who is willing to change can improve adjustment. The person who is unwilling or unable to change behavior patterns will not improve adjustment.

Transitions

Life is transitions
professional and personal.
Transitions help us to grow
and force us to change.
It is our choice—
to make these transitions or not.
Listen for cues,
follow the signs.
Life is transitions!

L. Robert Hudson
e-mail: lrhudson@magicnet.net

Any change is a test of one's ability to adjust. If familiar habits are used in new situations, the results may be quite different from results in the old situation. A change calls for conscious evaluation of habitual behavior. Ineffective habits should be discarded and new, more effective ones, established. To acquire new friends, to fit into a new community, to succeed in a new job, and to do well in a course of study all require that some old habits be discarded and that some new, more appropriate ones be developed.

Change is always a threat to adjustment. It is easy to continue using familiar habits; it requires effort to form new habits. It is distressing to find that established patterns of behavior do not bring the familiar result. Such inner discomfort may lead to snacking, criticizing the new situation, telling new companions about the old situation, or even trying to change the new situation to make it more like the old one. These types of behavior indicate poor adjustment.

Linda and Kay are two high school juniors enrolled in the health occupations course. Both are new in the school, faced with a new and unfamiliar setting. Kay wants desperately to be popular; when her new classmates ignore her, she feels resentment. She becomes critical of the class leaders, looking for opportunities to make uncomplimentary remarks about them. Her classmates soon tire of her negativity. They do not understand that Kay gets some relief from her inner discomfort by criticizing those she envies. Instead of becoming popular, Kay soon has fewer friends than ever.

Kay is using ineffective behavior. Criticizing others makes her feel better momentarily, but it interferes with her forming new friendships. Unless Kay gains insight into her own behavior, she is likely to continue to use a behavior that provides only temporary satisfaction. After a period of time, she may become so dependent on this habit that she will be unable to change.

In the meantime, Linda decides to broaden her interests. She becomes more active in school affairs, helping with the newspaper and joining several clubs. Each new activity leads to new friends for Linda. People who were once just acquaintances become friends with whom she has common interests. Linda is learning new skills and acquiring new outlooks through these various activities. Also, she is becoming an important person in her class because of her interest and enthusiasm.

Linda is using effective behavior to improve her adjustment. She took action to adapt to her new situation and that action proved to be effective. Do not conclude, however, that her sole motive was "to become popular." Goals that are superficial often do not provide satisfaction. Linda's real goal was to become comfortable in the new situation and broaden her range of interests; gaining many new friends was only one of several benefits.

Julie is a student in the surgical technician program. She knows the procedures must be performed correctly, but her performance often includes errors. The instructor has talked with Julie about her performance. Every error and every problem, according to Julie, was the fault of someone else: the circulating nurse, another student, whoever set up the tray or pack, some member of the surgical team. Julie does not learn from her mistakes or from the

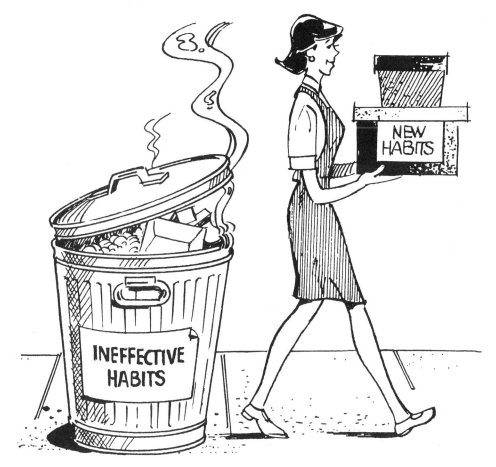

Improving your adjustment requires giving up ineffective habits.

instructor/student conference, because she is unable or unwilling to admit that she can make a mistake. She has not learned to take responsibility for her actions, and she denies the consequences of her errors by claiming "it wasn't my fault." Unless Julie changes this pattern of behavior, she will have problems throughout life. She will not be acceptable as a health care provider, because she would not be a safe practitioner.

EMOTIONS AND ADJUSTMENT

Emotions are a major influence on one's adjustment. A person who experiences positive emotions several times a day is likely to have better adjustment than one who frequently experiences negative emotions. Sometimes the emotion one experiences is a matter of choice. For example, you drop your keys as you try to unlock the car door. You feel somewhat annoyed as you pick them up and try again to fit the key into the lock. Somehow the keys slip out of your fingers and fall to the ground a second time. At this point, you can utter a string of four-letter words to express your anger and exasperation. Or, you could pick the keys up again, laughingly comment that you seem to have butterfingers today, then pay close attention to getting the key into the lock successfully.

Everyone has daily experiences that represent some type of difficulty. Everyone has daily experiences that proceed smoothly, without any problems. At the end of the day, one person remembers a number of these "good experiences" and gives little thought to the things that did not go well. Another person may finish the day feeling angry about several problem situations that occurred, and have little or no conscious awareness of any good experiences. Each of us may *choose* the type of experience to which we give most of our attention. In most situations, we may either choose to be angry or to deal with a situation unemotionally, working toward a resolution of the difficulty. Dr. Norman Shealy, whose work is discussed in Unit 23, stated in a workshop that he regards anger to be a destructive emotion that serves no useful purpose; by this, he means that it is better to deal *effectively* with an anger-arousing situation, than to indulge in angry feelings and ineffective behavior. Another workshop leader commented that when he begins to feel angry, he goes for a walk and thinks about *why* he is angry; often, the answer involves a way to resolve the situation and his anger simply dissipates.

Hassle denotes "any event that causes you to feel irritated, annoyed, frustrated, fearful or angry." How one copes with "daily hassles" is a reflection of one's adjustment. However, one's usual state of adjustment is also a factor in how well one copes with the "daily hassles." A current expression can serve as a guide to decreasing your tendency to become angry, or even just annoyed, in dealing with daily events:

"Don't sweat the small stuff; remember, most things are small stuff."

Fear is also a powerful influence on adjustment. A person who lives in fear of what "might happen" is expecting bad things to happen. Such expectations influence behavior and also affect how that person perceives events. It is normal to experience fear when faced with a real threat; the well-adjusted person reacts appropriately to such threat. A person who is chronically anxious, however, is living with fear that arises from negative thinking, rather than any real threat. Habitual negative thinking represents a state of poor adjustment.

Sadness also may be experienced appropriately or inappropriately. Each of us has life experiences that arouse sad feelings. Each of us is exposed to world news revealing the terrible things are happening, events that we are powerless to change. Someone who is truly grieved by conditions in a third world country might join the Peace Corps and devote two or more years to try to improve

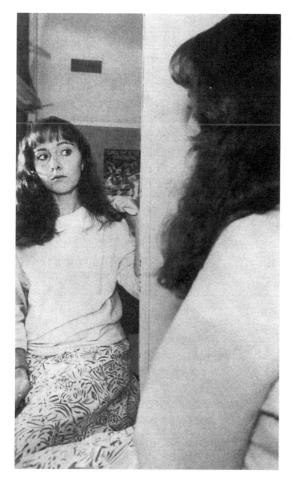

When you look in the mirror, do you see a person who finds much satisfaction in life, or someone who focuses on negative experiences? (From Carolyn Anderson, *Patient Teaching and Communicating in an Information Age.* Albany, NY: Delmar Publishers Inc., 1990.)

those conditions. Others might feel real empathy for the victims of some distant tragedy and send a contribution to an organization that is providing help. Others may feel a brief period of sadness and then shift their attention to their own affairs. These reactions indicate healthful use of sadness.

A person who chooses to focus on such events may remain in a sad state, indulge in "Ain't it awful" talk, yet take no action to correct the situation. This focus of attention on tragic events allows sadness to interfere with adjustment. As with anger and fear, a person can *choose* the extent to which a particular emotion is allowed to affect one's overall feeling state.

Table 9–1 on the following page is designed to help you identify hassles in your life. Table 9–2 permits you to identify the "good" things that occur. You choose which type of events receive most of your attention, and therefore which type of emotions dominate your daily life.

TABLE 9–1
Hassles in My Life

Instructions: In the following list circle (1) for each event you experienced yesterday and (2) for each event you experienced during the past week or month. Substitute appropriate words (i.e., "my glasses" for "keys") to adapt a statement to your situation. If a statement just does not apply to you, leave it blank.

1. I couldn't find my keys.	1	2
2. My neighbor's dog barked all night.	1	2
3. My sister called to talk about her problems.	1	2
4. There's no way I can pay all my bills this month.	1	2
5. My spouse is thrilled with our new sound system; I'm not, because our charge card is now "maxed out."	1	2
6. I had to make a difficult decision.	1	2
7. My co-workers take extended breaks and I end up doing more than my share of the work.	1	2
8. One of my clients was especially unpleasant, even though I had given him or her extra time.	1	2
9. I am having a plumbing problem (again!).	1	2
10. My job is just the same old routine day after day.	1	2
11. I am really bored with my life: work, problems at home, bills, never enough time or money for fun.	1	2
12. The children need new shoes (again!); last time I bought shoes for them, I expected to be next.	1	2
13. I'm having a really bad hair day.	1	2
14. I tossed and turned all night. (I went to bed really sleepy, then couldn't go to sleep; or, I woke up at 2 a.m. and couldn't get back to sleep.)	1	2
15. My car wouldn't start.	1	2
16. I locked my keys in the car.	1	2
17. Traffic was terrible this morning.	1	2
18. I've gained another three pounds.	1	2
19. The news is full of crime reports; I just don't feel safe any more.	1	2
20. There's a rumor that administration plans to "downsize" the patient care staff.	1	2
21. Even on my day off, I just couldn't relax.	1	2
22. Someone (insert name or title) is taking unfair advantage of me; I'm afraid to confront him or her.	1	2
23. Someone (insert name) smokes too much; I'm afraid he or she will develop lung cancer.	1	2
24. It's harder and harder to please my spouse; I'm afraid he or she is planning to leave me.	1	2

Total your score for each column. Note that items 1–18 deal primarily with anger and frustration; items 19–24 are more closely related to fear and anxiety. Now follow the same procedure with Table 9–2 to identify some "good" experiences in your life.

TABLE 9–2
Satisfactions in My Life

Instructions: In the following list circle (1) for each event you experienced yesterday and (2) for those you experienced during the past week or month. Substitute appropriate words to adapt statements to your situation. If a statement does not apply to you, leave it blank.

1. I had a good night's sleep.	1	2
2. My supervisor complimented me on my work.	1	2
3. I am scheduled to be off on my birthday.	1	2
4. I found a good buy on my family's favorite food.	1	2
5. I enjoyed talking with a new co-worker during break.	1	2
6. One of my patients said, "You are the best!"	1	2
7. When I reconciled my checkbook with my bank statement, I "found" a $50 deposit I had failed to enter.	1	2
8. My energy level has been up lately.	1	2
9. I stopped smoking.	1	2
10. I ate less fat (sugar, snacks, caffeine).	1	2
11. I exercised for twenty minutes.	1	2
12. I am learning to manage my time better.	1	2
13. I included some recreation in my schedule.	1	2
14. I spent time with friends and really enjoyed it.	1	2
15. I confronted (insert name) about (insert issue) and, to my surprise, we had a very satisfying discussion.	1	2
16. I lost three pounds.	1	2
17. I was able to relax and enjoy my day off.	1	2
18. My neighbor got rid of his barking dog.	1	2
19. My sister liked the birthday present I gave her.	1	2
20. My child's grades have improved and he or she likes the new teacher.	1	2
21. I was able to get the lavatory unstopped, so I saved the cost of a plumber.	1	2
22. While eating lunch, I realized the handsome/pretty person at the next table was showing interest in me.	1	2
23. I didn't think I could handle an assignment, but I did and was complimented on my work.	1	2
24. I received a favorable work review (grade).	1	2

Total the two columns. Now, compare your "Hassles" scores with your "Satisfaction" scores. Which score is higher? Was it easier to recognize hassles than satisfactions? Or, were the satisfactions more recognizable? Do you tend to focus more on your satisfactions or hassles?

IMPROVING ADJUSTMENT

How does one go about trying to improve adjustment? It is easier to make the effort while in a familiar situation. The following guidelines apply to improving adjustment:

- Find patterns of behavior that satisfy basic needs and solve problems effectively.

- Assume conscious control of your behavior.

- Use problem-solving to find the best possible solution for a problem situation instead of acting impulsively.

- Use emotions constructively. When appropriate, express feelings at the time they are experienced.

- Evaluate your behavior in a specific situation. Was the outcome favorable for you? What other possible behavior on your part would have been appropriate? Is it likely that another behavior would have been more effective?

- Self-evaluate in a constructive sense. Look for ways to improve but avoid feelings of guilt or inadequacy.

- Select appropriate goals in terms of "all that I can be" and plan how you will reach these goals.

If you can achieve reasonably good adjustment in your usual life situation, then you will be prepared for the challenge of adapting to new situations and dealing with the occasional crisis situations that are an unavoidable part of life.

Maintaining a Healthful Lifestyle

The above suggestions for improving your state of adjustment are somewhat broad and require conscious effort over a period of time. But, steps for improving your daily habits can be taken immediately, and these daily habits definitely contribute to one's state of adjustment. A diet that consists largely of junk foods eaten "on the run," the use of substances detrimental to wellness, lack of balance in work and play, sedentary habits, and inadequate sleep can all interfere with good adjustment. Your diet should include generous amounts of fresh vegetables and fruit, some eaten raw. Drink at least eight glasses of pure water each day. Exercise regularly. Avoid harmful and addictive substances. Participate regularly in recreational activities that help you release stress and regenerate your energies. Allow adequate time for sleep. Most of these habits are discussed elsewhere, and some you are probably learning about in other courses.

One daily habit that is essential to good adjustment, yet is seldom included in a course of study, is sleep. You learned about the physical need for sleep in Unit 5. The purpose here is to re-emphasize that 7 to 8 hours of sleep are necessary in order to get the full benefit of REM sleep, which tends to occur most often during hours 6 to 8. So be aware that an important first-line defense against stress overload is getting your full quota of sleep. When you start your day well-rested, it is easier to work toward other aspects of achieving good adjustment.

Avoiding Burnout

Every health care provider is at risk for developing burnout syndrome. **Burnout** is a state of deterioration that affects an individual physically, mentally, and emotionally. It develops gradually over a period of weeks, months, or years of living or working in a high-stress situation, during which the individual may not eat properly, gets minimal rest, has few opportunities for recreation and self-renewal, experiences much frustration, receives little emotional support from others, and/or ignores signs of illness in order to keep going. Anyone with a tendency to be a "workaholic" is risking eventual burnout.

A conscientious worker who begins to make errors, take longer to perform tasks, or fail to complete assigned work may be in the early stages of burnout. Other early signs include increasing frustration and loss of interest. The worker may believe that his or her efforts are unappreciated and develop a negative attitude about the job. As the condition worsens, it becomes increasingly difficult to fulfill job responsibilities. Co-workers may notice increased irritability or complaining. Physical symptoms include fatigue, frequent minor illnesses, gastrointestinal disorders, headaches, or various aches and pains. There may be increased consumption of caffeine, tobacco, alcohol or a tendency to seek relief through drugs, either legal or illegal.

The causes of burnout may lie within the individual—unhealthful life habits, failure to take responsibility for one's own well-being, a dedication to the job that results in too much work and not enough self-care, and failure to use effective stress-management strategies. Often the causes of burnout are within the work environment—stressors such as uncomfortable physical conditions, unpleasant working relations, supervisor or management behavior, lack of encouragement and emotional support, and lack of recognition or reward for work done well.

In any individual case, the contributing causes of burnout syndrome are probably a combination of personal habits and working conditions. The period of service in a high-stress area (i.e., air traffic controllers, intensive care personnel) should be limited, with periodic rotations to less stressful work assignments. Supervisors in high stress occupations should be alert for early signs of burnout. Early intervention can protect the worker and prevent errors and accidents by a person whose functional capacity is diminished. In the final analysis, it is the individual worker who has responsibility for preventing burnout.

The best protection is a lifestyle that includes all of the above suggestions for improving adjustment plus the regular use of effective stress management techniques (discussed further in Unit 25). If the stressors of the work setting affect numerous workers, management should be made aware so that steps can be taken to eliminate as many stressful conditions as possible. If work conditions cannot be improved and the worker is not able to deal effectively with the resulting stress, then it is time to seek employment elsewhere!

Adapting to New Situations

When a change occurs in your life situation—for better or worse—modify some of your patterns of behavior in order to achieve a state of good adjustment in the new situation. If the change is rather minor, you may adapt with little awareness of stress. If the change is great, however, you may go through a stressful period before you achieve adjustment. You may even be very unhappy at first, wishing that you could return to the old situation. As you successfully adapt, you will gradually begin to feel as comfortable in the new situation as in the preceding one.

The degree of **disruption** a change causes in one's usual pattern of living is dependent upon the type of change. Some changes you are likely to encounter from time to time include job changes, moving to a new neighborhood, a change of supervisors, a new administration in your place of employment, and changes in operational procedures and policies. A major change all of us have to face at some time is the loss of relatives and friends.

In general, adapting to change requires acceptance of the new situation and a conscious effort to adapt. If the change involves new tasks and new people:

1. Study the situation carefully.

2. Observe the behavior of others.

3. Learn the policies and regulations of the new situation and abide by them.

4. Consciously adopt behaviors that are appropriate for that situation.

If you find that the new situation requires you to follow procedures that are unsafe (for your or your patients) or are unethical, you have a conflict: you can lower your standards and console yourself with the thought, "I'm just doing what everybody else is doing"; you can use appropriate procedures to try to change practices, a risky approach for a new employee; or, you can leave the situation. Conflicts are discussed in detail in Unit 12.

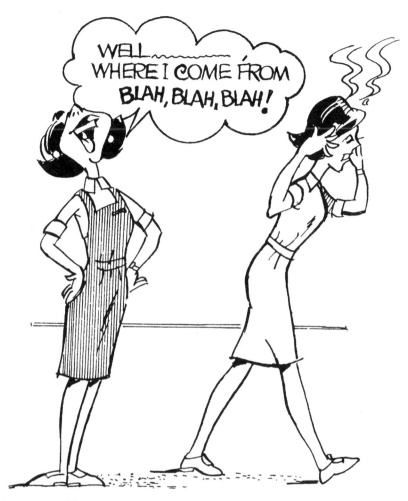

Clinging to old situations indicates poor adjustment to the present situation.

There is also the possibility that the new situation has more rigorous standards than your previous position. In that case, you have a challenge: to improve your performance in order to be acceptable to your new co-workers and supervisors. Willingness to learn and to improve performance will earn favorable evaluations for you; rebelling against the higher standards will mark you as an unsatisfactory employee.

A type of behavior that interferes with adapting to a new situation is clinging to the old situation. Comparing the old situation to the new, especially in terms that indicate your preference for the old, reveals that you do not yet accept the present situation. One sure way to antagonize new co-workers is to tell them repeatedly how you did things on your previous job. This behavior indicates poor adjustment to one's present job situation.

Adapting to the Role of Health Care Provider

You are already aware that becoming a health care provider requires certain modifications in behavior. Perhaps your previous job permitted smoking at any time while you worked; this is not appropriate in your new role. Perhaps you have had a job in which you were allowed to do many different tasks and accept as much responsibility as you were able to handle. As a health care provider you will have a well-defined role. You may find it annoying to have limitations placed on your role, especially if others perform tasks you believe you can do. Performance within one's defined role is necessary within the health field; to exceed that role may endanger a patient and also may have legal implications. You are already aware of the change you must make in giving health care suggestions to your friends. Refrain from any advice or actions that appear to be efforts to diagnose or prescribe. Essentially, adjustment to being a health care provider requires knowing one's role and performing within it, while also accepting and abiding by the code of ethics appropriate to that role.

References and Suggested Readings

Casargian, Robin. *Forgiveness: A Bold Choice for a Peaceful Heart.* New York, NY: Bantam Books, 1992.

Kaufman, Barry Neil. *Happiness is a Choice.* New York, NY: Fawcett Books, 1991.

Luban, Ruth. *Keeping the Fire: From Burnout to Balance.* Laguna Beach, CA: ChoicePoints, 1995. A two-hour audiocassette program and book. Available from the publisher at 412 North Coast Hwy, Ste 197, Laguna Beach, CA 92651.

Taubman, Stan. *Ending the Struggle Against Yourself: A Workbook for Developing Deep Confidence and Self-Acceptance.* New York, NY: Putnam, 1994.

REVIEW AND SELF-CHECK

Complete each of the following statements, using information in Unit 9.

1. Adjustment means _____ .

2. A person who is "well-adjusted" could be described as someone who

   _____

   _____

   _____

   _____ .

3. A person who is poorly adjusted may be described as one who

    _____

    _____

    _____.

4. Poor adjustment is a vicious cycle because _____.

5. The key to improving one's adjustment is to _____.

6. To improve adjustment, a person must be willing to _____.

7. Change in one's life situation is a threat to _____.

8. Indications of poor adjustment to a new situation include

    _____

    _____

    _____.

9. State five guidelines for improving one's adjustment.

    _____

    _____

    _____

    _____

    _____.

10. State four steps for adapting to a new situation.

    _____

    _____

    _____

    _____.

11. Two requirements for successfully adapting to the role of health care
    provider are

    _____

    _____.

ASSIGNMENT

1. Consider anxiety to be a state of chronic fear, the cause of which is vague or unknown. Write a brief paragraph explaining how anxiety affects a person's adjustment.

2. List ten observable behaviors that may indicate poor adjustment.

3. List ten observable behaviors that indicate a person is relatively well adjusted.

4. Using the above lists, place an X beside each behavior that is characteristic of you. Count the number of Xs beside "poor adjustment" behavior; count the Xs beside "good adjustment" behavior. Subtract the "poor" score from the "good" score. If the remainder is less than 5, begin *now* to plan ways to improve your adjustment.

5. Select one behavior listed under "poor adjustment" and plan how you will modify or eliminate that behavior. Set a time limit (for example, 3 months) at which time you will evaluate your success in modifying, or eliminating, this behavior.

6. Your classmate says, "I think all this study about understanding yourself is a waste of time." Write a brief response to this statement. Use the following as a basis for your reasoning: (a) the importance of adjustment to living a full life and (b) the importance of self-understanding to an effective health care provider.

7. Refer to your scores for Tables 9–1 and 9–2 and review the items that you marked. Tonight before going to bed, list the hassles you experienced today; select one particularly annoying event and consider ways you could prevent that particular hassle from recurring.

   Now, list the satisfying events of the day and consciously experience "good feelings." As you drift off to sleep, feel a sense of gratitude for the good experiences you had today.

8. List five behaviors you will modify in order to improve your adjustment to the role of health care provider.

9. List four behaviors that could help you adapt to a new situation.

10. During the next week, observe yourself and others for behavior that indicates poor adjustment. List five examples.

11. Observe those around you for behaviors that do not solve the immediate problem and/or create additional problems. Write a brief paragraph describing a situation you observed in which someone used an ineffective behavior. Suggest two other behaviors that might have been more effective. Be prepared to lead a group of your classmates in discussing this situation and brainstorming possible effective behaviors and the probable outcome of each.

Section III

Behavior and Problems
in Living

Life does not always flow smoothly. There are many problems in daily living. The goals we set for ourselves can be reached only through continual striving, and progress is often blocked by some type of difficulty. Behavior in the face of threat, blocking, failure, and other unsatisfying experiences can resolve the difficulty or create additional problems. This is especially true if a defensive reaction or aggression occurs.

Anyone with a health deviation has new problems in addition to those of the usual life situation. Health care providers must be aware that many of their patients are reacting to threat and, possibly, overwhelming problems. The patient needs acceptance, understanding, and caring from those who provide health care.

Section III is designed to help the health occupations student understand some types of behavior likely to result from threat. By learning to cope effectively with personal threat and its effects, the health care provider prepares to understand and accept the behavior of others who are reacting in their own way to threats in their life situations.

Unit 10

Threats to Adjustment

OBJECTIVES

Upon completion of this unit, you should be able to:

- List six milestones in life that can threaten adjustment.
- Name one significant change that occurs in each of six life stages.
- Name three types of experience that represent a major life change.
- State four guidelines for dealing with threats to adjustment.
- Name three reasons a victim of a traumatic experience may need psychological counseling, in addition to treatment for physical injuries.
- State two reasons a health care provider should be aware of the various effects of traumatic experiences.
- List five examples of traumatic experiences that may occur during childhood.
- Name three serious, long-term effects of child abuse.
- List three examples of traumatic experiences that may occur during adolescence.
- Explain the significance of peer pressure on an adolescent.
- List five examples of traumatic experiences that may occur during adulthood.
- List three examples of sexism.
- List three traumatic effects of each of the following: discrimination, sexism, rape, domestic violence.
- Explain the phrase, "blaming the victim."

KEY TERMS

Abuse	Bereaved	Crisis
Desensitize	Deviant	Discrimination
Heterosexual	Homosexual	Immature

152

Incest	Milestones	Paraphilia
Pedophilia	Peer	Perpetrators
Perversion	Prepubescent	Ritual
Senescent	Sexism	Sexual deviation
Sexual variation	STD	

The adjustment of any one person can be very poor, very good, or anywhere in between. Each person has a relative state of adjustment that characterizes that person most of the time. Adjustment, however, is always subject to change. Life experiences require changes in behavior to adapt to new situations and cope with new problems. No one achieves a state of adjustment that cannot be threatened by difficult situations.

A state of good adjustment *most of the time* is the best protection a person can have against the difficulties of life. As a goal, each of us should develop skills that will help us deal effectively with our usual life problems. These skills are our most valuable resource for coping with unusual situations. In other words, we prepare ourselves for dealing with big problems by learning to deal effectively with our daily problems.

CHANGE AS A THREAT TO ADJUSTMENT

Most people are reasonably well adjusted to their usual life situation. They are able to deal with familiar problems, and they get along fairly well with family and friends. Then a change occurs. Perhaps the change appears rather ordinary—a move to a new neighborhood, a change of schools, even a change of jobs. We adapt to "ordinary" changes with slight modifications in our behavior. Perhaps the change is major, such as going away to college or leaving a protective home to enter military service. When major changes occur, many of our usual patterns of behavior are no longer appropriate.

Any type of change is a threat to one's adjustment. Many changes that occur during specific periods of life require the learning and acquiring of new behaviors, which most people accomplish with relative ease. Other changes require major adaptations in behavior and may be a serious threat to adjustment. Certain significant events can occur at any period throughout life; some of these are traumatic events that are serious threats, not only to adjustment, but also to physical, mental, and emotional health.

LIFE STAGES AND CHANGE

Certain **milestones** in life require changes in behavior or the formation of entirely new patterns. Each of these milestones represents a threat to adjustment.

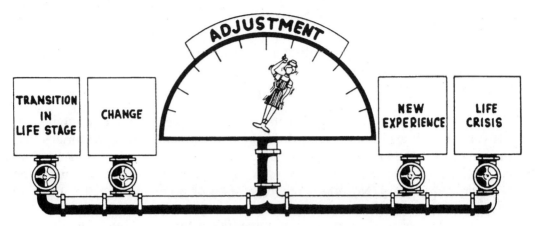

Adjustment is a relative state that shifts according to life experiences.

Early Childhood

Adults tend to forget how frightening new situations, places, and people can be to a young child. Much of a child's sense of security is derived from familiarity, from doing things the same way each time and from having a regular routine. Around the age of two or three, a child likes to follow a ritual for certain daily activities. The child even becomes upset if an attempt is made to vary the **ritual.** After this stage has passed, however, the child is better able to accept small changes in the daily routine. During the preschool period, the child should be introduced to changes in daily routine, to new experiences, and to new people in the presence of a familiar figure who can provide comfort and reassurance as the child faces each new situation.

The School Years

By kindergarten age, the child should be able to face a new situation without overwhelming fear. The child's sense of security and the variety of experiences as a young child influence readiness to accept the big step of entering kindergarten or first grade. Lack of readiness for this first big change in daily routine creates problems, not only for the child but also for parents and teachers.

After entering school, the child faces new situations with regularity. Each year there are new teachers, new classmates, new classrooms, and new learning experiences. Eventually the child enters a junior high school and, in a few more years, high school. Each of these steps represents change and therefore is a threat to adjustment: a minor threat for those who are relatively well adjusted, but a major threat for those who have not learned to adapt to new situations.

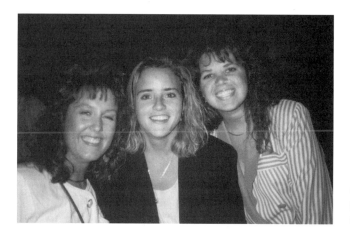

Acceptance by the peer group is especially important during adolescence.

Adolescence

Adolescence is a period of life when adjustment is quite variable. The adolescent is inclined to worry about appearance, self-worth as a person, the future, and—very important—the opinions of others. This is a period when it is important to feel accepted, approved, and a part of the group. Thus, the ability to form friendships, to communicate with others, and to share interests and activities influence acceptance by others. Any disappointment or rejection can threaten the adjustment of the adolescent. Likewise, special notice from schoolmates may produce elation. Mood swings and variable adjustment are typical of the adolescent period.

The teenager who has a positive self-concept and relatively good adjustment is likely to adapt to the challenges of the adolescent period. If one enters adolescence with a negative self-concept, poor interpersonal skills, ineffective behavior patterns, and/or inability to adapt to change, the problem may become more intense. If adolescence proceeds at a favorable pace, childhood patterns are gradually replaced by more mature patterns of behavior. If such growth does not occur, then childish patterns of behavior may continue into adulthood. We tend to label such people as **"immature,"** though immaturity actually involves more than childish behavior.

Young Adulthood

Change is the dominant characteristic of young adult life: new educational ventures, the first job, marriage, the challenges of setting up a home and starting a family. Each undertaking during the years immediately following high school is likely to be a new and challenging experience, requiring changes in habits and many new learnings. Failure to make such changes can lead to numerous problems, such as failing in an educational program, losing one job after another, or failing to establish a harmonious marriage.

Striving for good adjustment during early adulthood requires continuous effort. The experiences of this period will influence the remainder of one's life. The importance of education for a career, of succeeding in a new job, and of succeeding in marriage need not spelled out here. It is apparent that a failure in any one of these major life experiences has strong emotional effects, threatens one's adjustment, and may interfere with success in the next undertaking.

Middle Age

During middle age one becomes painfully aware of the passing of time. Perhaps early ambitions have not been realized. Early job experiences may not have been satisfactory, and one wonders whether it is "too late" to start again. Perhaps early goals have been achieved and, suddenly, life seems empty and lacking in challenge. Children are growing up and leaving the home. The mother who has devoted her young adult years to her children may now feel that no one needs her anymore. Physical changes, especially in women, may create strange feelings accompanied by negative emotional states. A man's physician may tell him to give up some activities, to "slow down." All of these add up to disappearing youth. For some people, loss of youth is difficult to accept. Middle age may be the greatest threat of all to the adjustment of those who place a high value on youth and a youthful lifestyle.

Senescence

The senescent period of life brings many frightening changes. The elderly person may attend funerals of friends and relatives at frequent intervals. The employer may encourage retirement long before the individual is ready to withdraw from work that has been a major part of life for many years. The widow or widower may find it necessary to change homes. Sometimes family and friends rush an elderly person, just **bereaved** of a life partner, into a decision to give up the home and move in with one of the children. Such radical changes should not be made until the widow or widower has worked through the grief process (one to three years).

Old age is accompanied by numerous fears: loss of independence, lack of sufficient money, dependence on others (financially or physically), illness, and death. The uncertainties of **senescence** are an ever-present threat that affects attitudes, feelings, relations with others, and total behavior. Many elderly persons view the future as dismal, offering only the prospect of increasing losses and eventually, death.

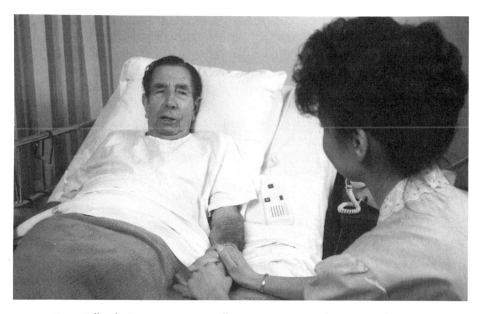

Especially during senescence, illness is a serious threat to adjustment.

MAJOR CHANGES

New experiences, crisis, an accident or serious illness may occur at any time during one's life and result in a major change in one's life situation that requires significant changes in behavior to cope with the new circumstances.

New Experiences

New experiences have been mentioned in relation to life stages. They are so important as threats to adjustment, however, that they deserve special mention. The well-adjusted person who enjoys new experiences does not perceive them as threatening. There may be a period of poorer-than-usual adjustment while new coping strategies are developed. But, for the poorly adjusted person, new experiences are a big threat. The poor adjustment is itself an obstacle to developing the coping skills needed in the new situation. Therefore, the poorly adjusted person is likely to react defensively to a new situation. Thus, the new situation pushes the poorly adjusted person toward still poorer adjustment.

Crisis

A **crisis** involves a major change, or the possibility of a major change, in one's life. Any crisis disturbs one's state of adjustment. Extreme changes may have to be made in one's patterns of behavior. Decisions with long-range influence may have to be made. Illness or death of the wage earner in the family changes an entire family's pattern of living. The offer of a new job may present exciting opportunities, yet require moving to a strange city. A job interview may be handled well and lead to a job, or be handled so poorly that the opportunity is lost. Failing to get a job or losing a job can threaten self-confidence and financial security.

Death, serious illness, divorce, and loss of a job are all crisis events for those involved. Other events in life may or may not assume the importance of a crisis, depending upon the individual involved. For the person who is not ready for a new experience, a major change can become a crisis. The bride who is not ready to assume the role of a wife may try to cling to her role as a daughter, or even transfer the daughter role to the relationship with her husband. For the new mother who is frightened by the responsibilities of motherhood, the birth of her baby is a real crisis. The person who is not ready for the responsibility of being a health care provider may find that the ethics and job requirements of the health field create a need for adjustments beyond those the individual is willing or able to make. Any crisis in regard to a vocational decision is a serious threat to adjustment. For people who have not learned to adapt to change, every life problem can add to poor adjustment. Any life event can become a crisis that creates anxiety and unhappiness for one who has not learned to deal with change.

Illness

Illness is always a threat to adjustment. It interferes with the usual pattern of living, is accompanied by discomfort, may involve doubt as to the outcome, and often creates financial problems. Patients and their families react to illness according to the degree of threat it represents. Adjustment is always poorer during illness. Sometimes behavior patterns that are not typical of a person appear during illness. Someone who is usually easy to please, for example, may be very difficult to please during an illness. A person who is usually quite well adjusted may show signs of poor adjustment during the period of illness. The patient may react with anger or fear to feelings of helplessness or to being dependent on others. Interestingly, the poorly adjusted person may react with positive feelings if the illness provides an escape from having to deal with daily problems.

The person who is self-reliant and has learned to deal with life problems usually finds illness frustrating. Familiar techniques for solving problems do not cure the illness. Perhaps the patient is accustomed to giving orders; now, the physician, nurse, laboratory assistant, radiology technician, and other personnel seem to be in charge. The shift from being independent to a state of

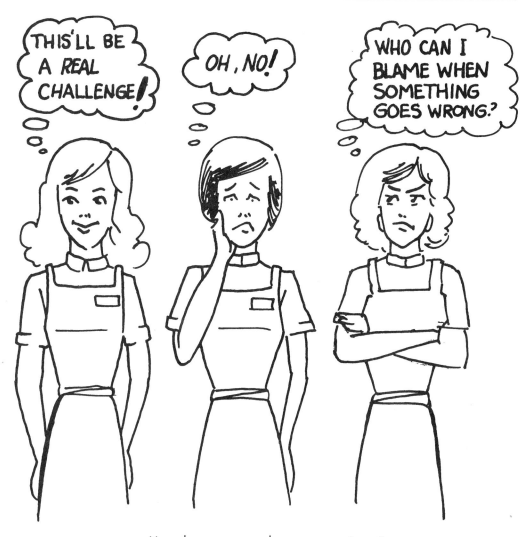

How do you approach a new experience?

dependency seriously threatens adjustment. The behavior of a patient may be markedly different from that person's usual behavior.

SOCIETAL AND CULTURAL ISSUES AS THREATS TO ADJUSTMENT

The preceding paragraphs describe threats to adjustment that are experienced by everyone. Some people are fortunate, in that they have never experienced *severe* trauma; but today more and more people, of all ages and from all walks of life, are having some type of traumatic experience. In addition, various types of abuse, once closely kept secrets, are now being exposed. **Discrimination** continues in schools, the workplace, and the community, in spite of federal laws that were intended to guarantee equal opportunities and protection for everyone. Health care providers need to be aware of these problems and issues that are serious threats to adjustment and have implications for the physical, mental, and emotional health of victims.

You, as a health care provider, are more likely to encounter victims than perpetrators. The purpose of the following section is to help you be fully aware of the effects of traumatic experiences on victims. You also need to have a high level of suspicion about the possibility that a patient is actually a victim, even if the patient does not volunteer information to that effect. Any suspicion that you have should be reported to your supervisor and/or the physician for further evaluation and possible legal action. *Follow the policies and procedures of your employing agency; do not attempt to handle such a matter yourself.* Just as important, *do not ignore the indications that aroused your suspicion.*

Reactions to Threat

Reactions to threatening situations vary from one person to another. Reactions to life situations are also highly individualistic. One person may perceive threat where another sees challenge and excitement.

The pattern for these reactions is established during childhood, yet as adults we *can* make changes. We can strive for self-understanding and consciously work for improved adjustment in our daily living. We can study our reactions to specific types of life experience and try to understand when and why we feel threatened. It is possible to **"desensitize"** ourselves to the common life situations that arouse our negative feelings by using the problem-solving method. This is an example of substituting controlled "thinking through" for relatively uncontrolled emotional reactions.

Each of us determines what events require big reactions. We then react to life situations with appropriate degrees of emotion. We are able to use intellectual skills instead of impulsive or emotional behavior to deal with problems. Over a period of time, these habits will lead to effectiveness in handling the challenges of daily life. Then, when a real crisis does arise, we can weather the experience and return to a state of adjustment within a reasonable period of time.

Reactions to Trauma

Each victim's reaction to a "bad experience" is influenced by all the factors discussed in Units 8 and 9 regarding emotions and adjustment. The type of experience also is a major influence on the intensity and duration of the victim's emotional reaction. Whether a person's emotional reaction to a traumatic event is normal or a deviation from normal must be determined on an individual basis; the line of demarcation is not always clear.

Victims of a single event, such as a mugging, experience intense emotional reactions in addition to their physical injuries. After the physical injuries have healed, professional counseling may be needed for processing the emotional trauma. Victims of recurrent trauma, such as long-standing **abuse,** need help in escaping their situation; these victims always benefit from professional counseling—develop new insights and resolve deeply rooted emotional trauma.

The Perpetrator

In reading the following paragraphs, remember that there are traumatic *events* (i.e., accidents), there are *perpetrators* (i.e., persons who inflict the trauma), and there are *victims* (persons suffering from the event). There are also various disorders that cause an individual to be misjudged and to experience difficulties, with traumatic effects, until a diagnosis is made. The behavior of a perpetrator may be the result of one or more of the following: early learnings in the home or on the street, cultural patterns, uncontrolled emotional expression, criminal tendencies, psychiatric disorder. The perpetrator's behavior may fall within the "normal" range of behavior (i.e., acceptable behavior within that particular culture) or may fall into the category of psychiatric disorder or criminal behavior. Discussion of the "causes" of a perpetrator's behavior is beyond the scope of this book; the study of such behavior falls within the disciplines of sociology, psychology, psychiatry, and criminology.

Traumatic Experiences

The following discussion of traumatic experiences focuses on the victim, with reference to the perpetrator only when especially relevant. Although many of these traumas can occur at any age, the sequence of topics below is based on the age at which each type of trauma is *most likely* to occur. Children may experience traumas such as divorce, death of a playmate or family member, an undiagnosed disorder that results in maladjustment, bullying by a family member or other children, mental/emotional or physical abuse. Adolescents may suffer the trauma of violence, including various types of accidents, and are subject to peer pressure that may result in some type of trauma. During adulthood, traumatic experiences may involve racism and/or **sexism** (taboos, discrimination, harassment), rape, domestic violence, crimes and accidents. Regardless of the age at which a traumatic experience occurs, the victim may experience additional trauma in the form of blaming. Also, survivors of traumatic experiences in which others did not survive may suffer the trauma of "survivor guilt."

Bullying

Many children experience teasing and bullying in the home, on the playground, and at school. The child who is noticeably different (i.e., has a physical handicap or a tendency to stutter) is especially at risk for teasing by the **peer** group or bullying by larger children. School policies regarding children with behavioral disorders or learning difficulties set these children apart, a practice that often results in a child being labeled and possibly rejected by classmates. Bullying, however, is a more serious problem.

Bullying consists of a person or group threatening, taunting, or physically assaulting someone who is smaller and weaker than the bully. The victim feels intimidated or humiliated and may suffer physical injuries. A bullying situation always has certain characteristics:

- The victim *is especially vulnerable*—smaller than the bully, physically weak or handicapped, female, or elderly.

- The bully selects a victim and a time when winning is certain.

- The bullying may occur at a time when there is an audience, but no one with the authority to intervene.

- If the bullying is done by a group, one member leads the initial taunting, but all members may participate in physically assaulting the victim.

A bully is a coward lacking courage, compassion, self-discipline, and a sense of responsibility. Jose' Chegui Torres was world light-heavyweight boxing champion in 1965–1966. As a former boxing champion, he expresses concern about the widespread tendency to glorify—and excuse—athletes who assault someone or batter their wives. According to Torres, "(Two prominent athletes) both established themselves as true champions. To do this, they had to be *experts at self-control. . . .*To say that boxers and football players *are primed by their sports to burst into fits of rage at the slightest provocation is absurd."* (Torres, 1995)

Torres deplores the cultural climate that glorifies and rewards violence by someone who has athletic superiority. Sports, especially the training regimen necessary to become a champion, are effective builders of character and self-control, according to Torres. If that is true, then the athlete who assaults others *chooses* to do so *in spite of* the self-discipline and self-control required by his sport. Today, cultural support for violent behavior is reflected in rap videos, TV programs, movies and much of the print media. Unfortunately, those most susceptible to these influences are children and adolescents, who may come to believe that violence is the method of choice for solving any dispute. Bullying as a pattern of behavior may manifest during adulthood as violence within the home—child or spouse abuse.

The child who has positive emotional support in the home may survive teasing and some degree of bullying without serious damage. The child who does not have opportunities for processing feelings about these experiences is likely to suppress anger and fear, develop a negative self-concept, and have problems with interpersonal relations. These experiences, though not as dramatic as some types of trauma, can have lifelong effects.

Undiagnosed Disorders

Some people are victims of a disorder that affects their ability to cope with daily life situations. Two relatively common neurological problems can cause rejection or humiliation by teachers and peers. Attention Deficit/Hyperactive Disorder (AD/HD) is especially distressing to teachers, because affected children have difficulty completing a task and may distract other children from doing so. This condition starts in childhood, usually by the age of seven, but a mild case may go undiagnosed throughout the school years and even into adulthood. Indications of this disorder include impulsivity, difficulty in concentrating, tendency not to finish a task, and restlessness. The behaviors of AD/HD cause many difficulties for the individual and are an annoyance to teachers, peers, and family members.

When hyperactivity is extreme, the child may experience frequent punishment for "being bad," when in actuality the child is unable to control the AD/HD behaviors. Some hyperactive children are eventually referred for psychological evaluation, at which time a diagnosis may be established and appropriate treatment planned. Except in cases where hyperactivity makes the child unmanageable at times, these characteristics may be perceived by others as simply part of a person's personality.

Adult Attention Deficit Disorder (AADD) has now been established as a diagnosis. This is another example of the fine line between behavior that is "normal" and behavior that indicates the need for medical evaluation and, possibly, therapy.

Dyslexia is a reading disorder in which the individual transposes letters or syllables; needless to say, this results in learning problems that distress both student and teacher. Many dyslexic children are not diagnosed, so the child may endure years of being regarded as a slow learner or, at best, a "poor student." Yet, many of these victims are highly intelligent; about 10% of left-handed people are dyslexic. Once a person has been diagnosed as dyslexic, special aids can be provided to facilitate learning. Until the diagnosis is made, the child may be wondering, "What is wrong with me?" The threat to self-esteem is obvious.

Divorce

Divorce is almost always a traumatic experience for everyone involved, especially the children. Even if both parents agree that divorce is preferable to continuing the marriage, children are affected emotionally as they see their home and family breaking apart. Their daily life changes in many significant ways. The adults are dealing with their own emotional reactions to the trauma of marital discord. They may be unaware of the child's reactions: anger toward one or both parents, belief that the parent who is moving out "doesn't love me any more," or possibly guilt, believing that he or she is the cause of the family breakup. If the divorce is hostile, there may be a custody battle. Then the child has a serious conflict of loyalties and may witness numerous hostile encounters between the parents. The child experiences emotional turmoil: a mixture of love and hate, anger and grief, guilt about divided loyalty, and negative feelings toward one or both parents.

When either parent remarries, a step-parent enters the picture, further complicating the child's emotional life. If the parent who remarries is the custodial parent, and the new step-parent also has children, the result is a "blended family." A period of turmoil may last for months, because each person must adapt to new family relationships and establish new patterns of interaction. Ideally, these adaptations occur with minimal trauma, and family dynamics eventually become positive. It is unrealistic to expect this to happen immediately after the wedding. Family counseling can assist blended families in making these adaptations.

Death

The death of a family member or friend can be very traumatic to a child. A child needs help in understanding death, accepting the permanence of death, dealing with feelings associated with the deceased, and coping with the sense of loss or abandonment. Effective grieving is very important to a child's development and future attitudes. If grief is not processed, the suppressed emotions can affect future attitudes, emotional expression, and behavior when another loss is experienced. Unit 19 discusses the effects of losses on children and adolescents in greater detail.

Child Abuse

The most tragic examples of child-as-victim are those in which the child is abused by an adult. This is the ultimate betrayal of the adult/child relationship. The role of an adult is to care for and protect a child. By violating this basic responsibility of the adult role, the abuser may destroy the child's trust in adults. Child abuse is a pervasive problem in American society. Approximately

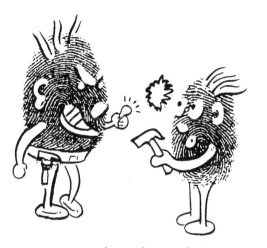

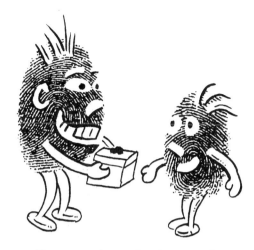

"Can't you do anything right?"

"I'm sorry about what happened.
It won't happen again."

(From Carol D. Tamparo & Wilburta Q. Lindh, *Therapeutic Communications for Allied Health Professions.* Albany, NY: Delmar Publishers Inc., 1992)

one child in 10 is subject to abuse by a parent or other caregiver; in 1993, there were over one million documented reports of child abuse or neglect. According to research findings, 20 to 45 percent of women and 10 to 18 percent of men in the United States and Canada experienced sexual abuse as a child. Among girls who are sexually abused, about 20 percent later develop a serious psychiatric disorder.

Child abuse may be physical, mental, or emotional. Physical abuse can be in the form of bullying, assault, corporal punishment, prolonged isolation, restraints, or sexual acts. The abuser may be angry or inebriated, or the abuse may be a manifestation of **perversion** or mental illness. Mental/emotional abuse does not receive as much publicity as physical assaults, but it is even more destructive. It may take the form of verbal put-downs, addressing the child with a derogatory term, using profanity, making unfavorable comments about the child in the child's presence, neglecting the child, or openly rejecting the child. Indifference, to the extent that the child's emotional needs are not met, is also a form of abuse.

Both boys and girls can be victims of sexual abuse, but two out of three victims are girls. The perpetrator is most often a close family member, but may be a family friend or authority figure. If the perpetrator is a parent or sibling, the sexual encounter is **incest.** If the child is under thirteen years old and the perpetrator is five to ten years older than the child, it is **pedophilia;** the abuser is a *pedophile.* Studies of pedophiles indicate that four out of five were themselves sexually abused as children. Sexual abuse of girls is almost always

heterosexual (i.e., male/female). Sexual abuse of males is most often **homosexual** (i.e., male/male). Because the majority of sexual abusers are male, the pronoun "he" is used for the remainder of this discussion. There are, however, cases of sexual abuse of a male by a female.

Traumatic Effects

The effects of sexual abuse on a child are profound and can affect adjustment throughout life. Sexual abuse is not limited to physical sexual acts; it includes mental and emotional abuse. The perpetrator uses various devices to keep the child from exposing him. The act may be presented as "our secret" and the child made to feel that she or he is being given very special attention. If the child reacts negatively, the perpetrator may use threats to keep the child from telling anyone. Some perpetrators convince their victims that they are to blame, thus using shame and guilt to control the child. This enforced silence results in suppression of intense feelings: anger, fear, grief, and guilt.

Unfortunately, many adults refuse to believe a child who does try to tell them about being sexually abused. It is very difficult for a mother to believe such a report, especially if a little girl is saying that the father, stepfather, brother, uncle, or grandfather committed such an act. For example, little five-year-old Edette told her mother repeatedly what the big brother was doing to her, and repeatedly she was punished for "telling lies." Even when she developed a recurrent bladder infection, neither the mother nor the urologist (male) believed her story.

It is especially difficult for a parent to believe that a respected authority figure, such as a teacher, coach, or member of the clergy, would sexually abuse their child. Yet, abuse is most likely to occur in a dominance/submissive relationship, in which the child is powerless. Many adult survivors of child sexual abuse tell of seeking help from an adult, only to encounter disbelief and accusations of lying. Parents, teachers, ministers, adult friends and neighbors, and especially health care providers must *listen* when a child tries to tell what some adult did to them. Although the child may not have the vocabulary to describe the event in adult terms, it is important to *let the child tell what happened in his or her own words.* Do not suggest words you think might help the child's description, since that could be construed legally as having "planted the idea in the child's mind."

The damage of sexual abuse is physical, mental and emotional. These victims grow up with low self-esteem, suppressed anger and fear, feelings of guilt, distrust, and perceptions of the world as a hostile place. They may contract a sexually transmitted disease **(STD)** or sustain other physical injuries. As adults, many survivors of childhood sexual abuse have difficulty forming an intimate relationship. Many have one relationship after another; others avoid intimacy altogether. Failed marriages are common. The life-long effects of child sexual abuse are now acknowledged by the mental health community. Through psychotherapy and techniques such as hypnosis, many adults have been able to bring repressed memories to the conscious level, a necessary step in order for therapy to proceed. Support groups for survivors of abuse and incest have been established in many communities.

Appropriate action depends on the situation. Criminal charges may be filed against the perpetrator, but adults should not let that possibility prevent them from protecting the child against further molestation. Pedophiles tend to repeat their behavior, so every child within range of a pedophile is at risk.

Societal Views

Every culture has *sexual mores,* meaning that the society draws the line between what is acceptable sexual behavior and what is not. Almost all cultures have a taboo against incest, and most cultures exclude **prepubescent** children as sexual partners. Terminology reflects to some extent the changes in societal attitudes about sexual behavior. Prior to this century, any type of atypical sexual behavior was labeled perversion. As psychological studies of sexual behavior proliferated during the mid 1900's, **sexual deviation** became the term of choice. Currently, **sexual variation** is used, indicating reluctance to label specific sexual behaviors as "**deviant.**" The diagnostic term used in psychology and psychiatry is **paraphilia,** a blanket term for a variety of atypical sexual behaviors. The legal system uses the simple term, sex offender.

The sexually abused child enters the adolescent period having already experienced some type of sexual activity. Some behaviors, emotional patterns, attitudes toward sex, trust in others, and interpersonal relations differ from those of their sexually inexperienced classmates. Some children try various forms of escape: alcohol, drugs, food, sleep, or withdrawal. Those who have strong guilt feelings may inflict physical pain on themselves by head banging, beating hard objects with the fists, cutting or mutilating themselves, or even attempting suicide. These behaviors may be exhibited during adolescence or adulthood, years after the sexual abuse stopped or the individual escaped from the abuser.

Stressors of Adolescence

All the sources of childhood stress continue through adolescence—accompanied by additional sources of stress: the pressure of competition (athletics, extracurricular activities, school politics), pressure to excel (especially if college-bound), the need to belong, the need to be attractive to members of the opposite sex, eagerness to finish Driver Education and get one's own car. These are the familiar pressures of adolescence.

There is also the threat of school violence. Gangs exist in many schools; by belonging, there is safety in numbers, but one must conform to the gang's practices and beliefs. Initiation rites may include having sex (or committing a rape), shoplifting, car theft, "beating up" someone of a different race or ethnic group, or mugging. The initiate who fulfills this assignment then "belongs" to the gang, but not just as a member; any attempt to leave the gang may result in blackmail—gang members could provide testimony about the crime, resulting in a prison sentence for the would-be defector. Thus, the gang leader has power and control over members of the gang.

Those who are not gang members may live in fear of gang activity or reprisals following any dispute with a gang member. Weapons, once unheard of in a public school, are now prevalent. Some schools have electronic devices to detect weapons; but weapons are present in the parking lot. Assaults do occur, with both teachers and students as victims.

Peer Pressure

Adolescence is a period when peer approval is extremely important. It is a time of life when family influence is challenged by the peer group because of the individual's need to belong. For that reason, each adolescent must choose between participating in certain practices that are widespread through the student body and the risk of being the outsider. Those who resist may experience pressure from their classmates to get involved, or "just try it."

Drugs

Drugs are a major problem, sometimes being sold and used in school restrooms and the parking lot. At social events there is peer pressure to use drugs such as marijuana, crack, cocaine, and now heroin. "Just say 'No!'" is not easy advice to follow; by saying, "No," the student risks disapproval of the peer group. By saying "No" to someone who wants to sell the drug, a student risks some type of reprisal by the disgruntled dealer, especially if the dealer is a gang member.

Sexual Activity

When the adolescent begins to date, there may be pressure almost immediately to engage in sexual activity. This may conflict with beliefs about morality the adolescent has learned in the home and at church. The adolescent experiences an internal conflict: the need for acceptance by the peer group and the need to uphold one's standards and maintain self-esteem. Today's trend toward becoming sexually active during the teens has serious health implications: pregnancy, sexually transmitted diseases, and the emotional effects of abandonment by a partner to whom one has become emotionally attached. In many communities, sex education remains a controversial subject. The provision of information on self-protection, and especially the provision of prophylactic materials, through a school program is emphatically opposed by many adults. A health care provider is very likely to be approached by a teenager who needs information or help in regard to sexual activity.

Fortunately, not every adolescent is exposed to some of these stressors, but many are exposed to all of them. Numerous stressors experienced by adolescents today did not exist, or were not prevalent, when their parents were in high school. Many parents, therefore, do not understand or believe the problems today's adolescents face at school. Every adolescent needs to be able to discuss these problems regularly with an adult who understands the problems, encourages the expression of feelings, and helps identify appropriate ways to deal with these difficult situations.

Stressors of Adulthood

Many of the stressors and serious traumas of childhood and adolescence continue into adulthood. Some that are discussed below also occur during childhood or adolescence. But certain stressors, such as discrimination, rape, and domestic violence seem more appropriate for discussion within the framework of adulthood.

Discrimination and Sexism

Members of minority groups in all cultures and throughout time have experienced discrimination. There seems to be an innate human need for perceiving people in "Us/Them" terms, favoring those who are members of the "Us" group. But this tendency does not excuse discrimination that violates the rights of others because of sex, race, nationality, ethnic group, age, or religion. It required many years of campaigning by a group of courageous women before American women finally gained the right to vote. Until about forty years ago, it was illegal in some states for a Caucasian to marry an Oriental. African Americans have gained many rights as a result of the Civil Rights Movement of the 1960s. Heightened awareness on the part of many Americans and a series of Congressional acts have brought about numerous changes.

Federal laws pertaining to equal employment opportunities and prohibiting discrimination on the basis of race, sex, and age have been passed only in the past thirty years. Such laws do make it illegal to continue certain long-standing policies and practices. But laws do not change attitudes or beliefs. It is relatively easy to find examples indicating that discriminatory practices still exist, in educational settings as well as in the marketplace. As a new generation that grew up with civil rights and feminist activities assumes decision-making positions in business and government, fairness and equal opportunities may prevail. In the meantime, discrimination continues as a serious stressor to those who are victimized by such practices.

Discrimination may be practiced against anyone because of a specific attribute, such as race, sex, religion, age, weight or other physical attribute. The most common basis for discrimination, however, is either race (racism) or sex (**sexism**). Other traumas related to sex include harassment, rape, and domestic violence.

Sexual Discrimination

As more and more women become part-time homemakers and full-time workers, there is increasing awareness of the extent to which discrimination against women is practiced. The male teacher is more likely to be encouraged to move into administration than a female teacher. A male health care provider is likely to be "promoted" to a supervisory position after a few years of work experience, while female colleagues with more experience are not considered for the position. In the business world, women who rise to relatively high positions in a corporation may encounter a "glass ceiling" in their organization; everyone above that ceiling is male. Until recently, women who experienced discrimination on the job had no recourse; now, because of federal legislation, there are procedures for protesting discriminatory practices. Those who protest are at risk of losing their jobs; but that, too, provides a basis for filing charges of discrimination.

Sexual Harassment

A more serious example of sexism is *sexual harassment,* which is the most frequently reported complaint in the workplace today. It may also occur in an educational setting. Usually the victim is someone with limited power (student, secretary); whereas, the perpetrator (teacher, supervisor, customer) has some degree of power over the victim. The victim of sexual harassment is usually female, but may be male. The harassment may be verbal, may consist of inappropriate touching, or may involve requests or demands for sexual acts. Sometimes the victim perceives the harassment as including the threat of being fired; sometimes the promise of favorable treatment (a good grade, a promotion, a "business" trip) is implied or stated directly. Some women enjoy the attention and use these "offers" as opportunities for self-advancement; some who make that choice later regret it when the male turns his attention to his next victim. The majority of women, however, consider these unwanted sexual advances as harassment and themselves as victims. The person who believes that he or she is being harassed should consider several questions:

- What can I do about this situation?

- How can I protect myself?

- What options are available to me?

- What is the best way to stop these unwanted advances?

Emotional reactions to sexual harassment include anger, fear, and guilt; the threat to self-esteem is obvious. The male who is accused of sexual harassment usually either denies that it occurred or blames the woman. At one time the female victim of sexual harassment had no recourse. If she reported the incident to a supervisor, she risked being fired, accused of lying, or worse. All-too-often, the perpetrator would be the supervisor. Today, however, it is possible to take legal action, since sexual harassment is covered by federal laws against discrimination. The woman who chooses to file a complaint should have some type of evidence, other victims who are willing to join the complaint, and/or witnesses who have heard or seen examples of harassment. The complaint probably will not be handled in the woman's favor if it becomes a matter of "her word against his."

The best approach is to stop harassment when the first incident occurs. Using "I" statements, the victim can express feelings and then in a matter-of-fact way establish limits on behavior. If this does not stop the harassment, then the employer's procedure for filing a complaint should be followed. A complaint can be filed with the proper federal agency if the employer does not take action to stop the harassment. If the victim does decide to file a complaint, she should be aware that there is risk of reprisal from the accused, from the employer, or even from colleagues who choose to side with the accused.

Sexism and Female Anger

A cultural aspect of sexism that is a threat to the mental and emotional health of women is the taboo against female anger. Women who express anger are judged differently than a man who expresses anger in the same situation. Dr. Harriet Lerner, in *The Dance of Anger*, notes that the English language contains eight derogatory terms commonly used to describe a woman who expresses anger. There are only two derogatory terms to describe an angry man, and both terms cast aspersions on the man's mother, rather than on the man himself! In fact, a man who expresses anger is likely to be described admiringly in terms referring to his genitalia or to his having a high level of testosterone. And so, any woman who expresses anger, even if she does so in a calm manner, risks being judged as "strident," a "nag" or worse. Her message about the situation that aroused her anger may go unnoticed, and therefore uncorrected! This means that women are much more likely than men to carry a burden of suppressed anger.

Rape

The use of threats or force in order to engage in a sexual act is *rape*. It is a crime and should be reported, even if the perpetrator is a relative, friend, date, or co-worker. *Rape is not a sexual act; it is an act of aggression that violates the victim physically and emotionally.* Rapists tend to have a hostile attitude toward women. They may also have an intense need to experience a feeling of power over others. Some rapists want to inflict pain and enjoy the woman's fear. Because the experience satisfies the rapist's need for power and control, he is likely to rape repeatedly and to have more than one victim. The rapist who does not feel powerful enough to force himself on an adult woman may choose a child as victim. Rape is one of a number of acts included in the legal term, "sex offender."

The rape victim often is victimized further by family members and/or "the system." If the rapist is a relative, family members may not believe the victim's report; some may actually side with the accused rapist. If the victim reports the rape to police, she may be subjected to dehumanizing procedures by officers who do not understand the significance of rape. Comments made about a rape or a rape victim often show total lack of understanding that *rape is a violent act of aggression.*

If the police take the victim to the Emergency Room, personnel busy with medical emergencies may keep the victim waiting for several hours. Once she does get attention, she may encounter a physician who is indifferent to her humiliation during examination of the genital area and collection of specimens. Possibly, no one attempts to help the victim deal with the emotional trauma of the rape. In many communities, the concerns of rape survivors, health care providers, and law enforcement personnel have led to educational efforts to sensitize officials to the needs of a rape victim. In one Georgia city, a house has been renovated to serve as the setting for care of a rape victim, sparing a traumatized woman the additional stress of the Emergency Room setting. In this private atmosphere, specially trained Registered Nurses perform the necessary physical examination to collect evidence. Other specially trained women provide emotional support to the victim. Women with special training for dealing with rape victims conduct an interview to obtain information for law enforcement officials. In addition, there is a community support group for rape victims.

Every rape victim should have professional counseling to help her deal with intense emotions and the serious threat to self-esteem. Counseling and a support group can help the victim regain confidence in her ability to go about her daily routine without fear.

Domestic Violence

Spousal abuse is now recognized as a public health problem in the United States. It affects about one-third of all marriages and is involved in about 12 percent of all homicides. Although male abuse of a female partner is more common, female abuse of a male partner occurs in about 10 percent of known cases. (*The Menninger Letter,* 1995) Domestic violence is the *leading cause of injury to women ages 15 to 44 in the United States*—more than auto accidents, muggings, and rapes combined. (FBI *Uniform Crime Reports,* 1991) Spousal abuse is found in all cultures, races, occupations, income levels, and ages. About one-third of the men counseled at one center were professional men, highly respected in their communities: doctors, lawyers, ministers, psychologists, business executives. (*For Shelter and Beyond,* 1992)

Spousal abuse can take various forms, including physical aggression (assault), emotional trauma, "mind games," deprivation of needs (including access to money), isolation from relatives and friends. Because the abuser is most often male, the term "battered wife syndrome" is commonly used. Battered women are often severely injured; between 22 and 35 percent of female patients in the emergency room are there because of injuries inflicted by their male partners.(Adams, 1989) Medical expenses from domestic violence total $3 to $5 billion dollars per year.(Colorado Domestic Violence Coalition, 1994) Women who attempt to leave an abusive spouse are at risk for being killed by the abuser; about half of the homicides of female partners by a male partner occurred *after separation.* (Hart, 1992)

Abusers have two personalities: the public personality, that of "a really nice guy" and the private personality, controlling and demanding. Few women would enter knowingly into an abusive relationship. The abuser initially is charming and shows care and concern, so the woman enters the relationship expecting romantic love and a "warm, cozy relationship." Gradually the abuser begins to make demands that lead up to isolating the victim from family and friends, getting control of the money (including the victim's paycheck), controlling the couple's activities (eliminating her activities and interests), requiring explanations for her behavior or comments, demanding a report on any time spent away from the abuser, making decisions that any adult woman should make for herself. These demands are first made within an acceptable, and possibly flattering, context:

- I can't stand to be away from you.

- I want you to spend more time with me.

- You spent all afternoon with your sister when I needed you to be with me.

- I want you to be here while I watch the ballgame.

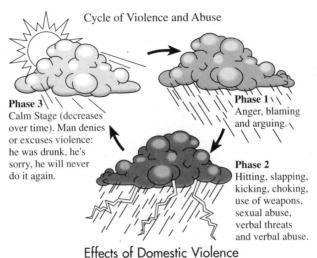

Cycle of Violence and Abuse

Phase 3
Calm Stage (decreases over time). Man denies or excuses violence: he was drunk, he's sorry, he will never do it again.

Phase 1
Anger, blaming and arguing.

Phase 2
Hitting, slapping, kicking, choking, use of weapons, sexual abuse, verbal threats and verbal abuse.

Effects of Domestic Violence

- I want you to be home when I get back from the ballgame.

- You know how important you are to me.

Initially the abuser makes the woman feel important and loved, but comments such as the above are leading up to controlling not only the relationship, but also all aspects of her life. The abuser's objective is *power*—total control over the other person.

The statements below illustrate the increasing degree of control:

- What did you and your sister talk about all afternoon?

- What did you do while I was at the ballgame?

- I'll take care of paying the bills; I handle money better than you do.

- Wear the red dress; you really look great in it.

- Don't wear slacks when we go out.

- Don't wear that short skirt to the party.

- What were you and Joe laughing about?

- Why did you stay in the kitchen with Amy so long?

- What did you mean when you said . . . ?

Next, the abuser begins to chip away at her self-esteem, then he works on making her feel guilty as well as inadequate:

- Why did you say (. . .)? That was stupid!

- Why can't you be more fun when we party?

- I don't like it when you dance with Jim.

- Why can't you be a better wife (mother, girlfriend)?

- You can't do anything right.

- You made me angry (jealous).

- You caused us to run out of money.

- You had me so upset I ran a red light; it's your fault I got this ticket.

- Yes, I drink too much, but it's because you make me so (. . .).

- I didn't get the promotion; you should have been nicer to my boss at the Christmas party.

Once the woman begins to believe that she really is the cause of his (and their) problems, he has tremendous power over her. With low self-esteem and overwhelming feelings of guilt, she is less able to evaluate the relationship and definitely less able to free herself from it. Once the man's power over her is established, he feels safe expressing his feelings through physical actions. Initially, it may be a slap; later there will be multiple blows, usually with the fists. After hitting the woman, the abuser points out that she is to blame: she didn't do as she was told, she didn't have dinner ready on time, she was late getting home from work, or whatever excuse he can think of at the moment. The physical abuse may escalate until the woman sustains serious injuries or is killed.

Women who grew up in a home where domestic violence was a way of life may simply accept abuse as part of a woman's role. At some point, a woman may realize she does not have to submit to abuse. She may seek escape, but if she has no money and no job skills, escape requires help from others. If her family is supportive, she may seek their protection. In some cases, the wife's family has been so charmed by the abuser that they side with him and refuse to help her escape the abuser. Sometimes religious beliefs are a factor: "You are his wife for better or worse."

Even well-educated women, some with positions that would enable them to support themselves, may find it difficult to leave an abusive relationship. The abuser maintains control by alternating periods of abuse with periods of proclaiming his love and promising "never to do it again." Survivors of abusive relationships refer to these periods as the "honeymoon" time; the woman, thinking each time that the abuse is a thing of the past, stays in the

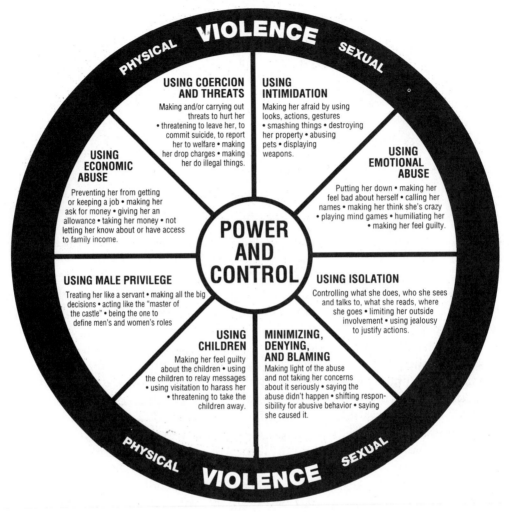

Abusers have a strong need for power and control. (From Domestic Abuse Intervention Project, 206 West Fourth Street, Duluth, MN 55806)

relationship. Sometimes a woman accepts the abuse in order to have the "honeymoon" periods, during which she is treated well. Any woman who has a negative self-concept and believes herself to be unlovable, may become dependent on an abuser for love and approval. ("He's the only one who'll put up with me.") Some women stay in an abusive relationship rather than risk the uncertainties of being alone or undertake the struggle to establish a fatherless home for her children.

Most victims of domestic violence need outside help to escape the abusive relationship. Since an abuser takes control of the family's finances, the woman

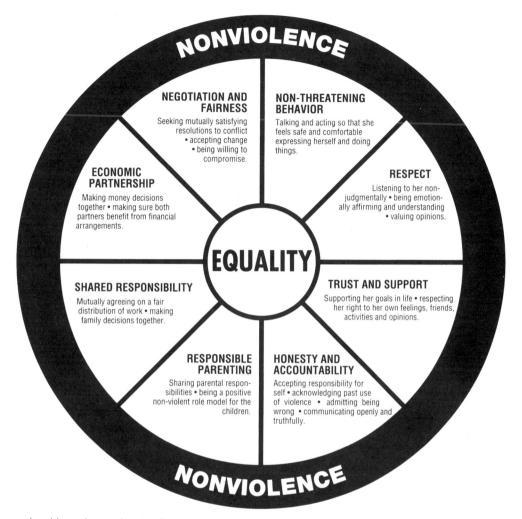

A healthy relationship is characterized by equality and an absence of violent behavior. (From Domestic Abuse Intervention Project, 206 West Fourth Street, Duluth, MN 55806)

has no financial resources to aid in her escape. Sometimes the abuser tries to ensure that she remain financially dependent on him by interfering with her efforts to keep or obtain a job. He may assault her just before a job interview or hide the clothes she planned to wear to the interview. If she has left him, he may stalk her at work or at a training site.

Personnel in women's shelters report that many women who appear ready to become self-reliant actually go back to the abuser. Sometimes it takes several attempts before the woman finally frees herself. Many of these victims need several types of help:

- Convincing that a woman does not have to submit to abuse

- Financial assistance

- A separate place to live

- Child care,

- Job and/or job-training,

- Child support

- Legal protection

As soon as arrangements are made for physical survival, it is important that the woman receive extensive counseling to counteract the destructive effects of the abusive relationship. The damage to self-esteem may take years to overcome. Processing her fear, anger, and guilt may require many months. Without effective counseling, the woman may not be able to trust other men or establish another intimate relationship.

Hopeful Signs

The problem of domestic violence in American society is finally gaining recognition. In April, 1995 the NOW Legal Defense and Education Fund (LDEF) sponsored a Leadership Summit on how domestic violence contributes to women's poverty and homelessness for women and children. The keynote speaker was U.S. Attorney General Janet Reno; participants were attorneys, policy-makers, researchers, and activists. Subsequently, in 1995 the U.S. Congress passed the Violence Against Women Act (VAWA). This is the first federal law that recognizes and attempts to stop violence against women. VAWA contains a civil rights remedy for victims of violence to file charges through a federal court and seek monetary compensation, court-ordered protection, and costs of legal expenses.

The effectiveness of VAWA will depend on changes in the attitudes and procedures of law enforcement agencies and the court system. LDEF has developed a curriculum for training judges on appropriate procedures for hearing and ruling on cases involving domestic violence, rape, and child abuse. There remains a need for widespread educational efforts to improve family relationships and parenting skills. Most important, there is need for change among those male groups who perceive women and children as "property" and believe a male is entitled to subject wives and children to any treatment he wishes.

The Menninger Institute, devoted to treatment and clinical research in the field of psychiatry and mental health for the past seventy years, has just established a Child and Family Center to focus on the problems of domestic violence and child abuse. According to Dr. W. Walter Menninger:

"America faces a crisis. Families are embattled, and violence is common. One-fourth of our children under age three—some 12 million youngsters—live in single-parent families. Social problems related to these family problems are reported in the daily news: Neglected and runaway children. Drugs. Gangs. Violence in our schools and on our streets." (Menninger Perspective #4, 1995)

This new unit at Menninger will address these social problems through projects to explore the cycle of violence in families, ways to increase involvement of fathers in effective parenting, methods to deal with bullying, and the effects of childhood abuse on adult behavior. Ideally, such projects will be replicated in many communities so that the trend toward violence can be reversed.

Crimes and Accidents

Muggings, carjackings, burglaries, gang beatings, and other types of violence are all-too-prevalent. Once considered to be dangers characteristic of big cities, these crimes are now commonplace in the suburbs and in small cities and towns. Even more common are automobile accidents, a leading cause of death, especially for males under the age of twenty-five. In addition, thousands of people each year sustain disabling injuries. Complete safety from crime or accidents does not exist.

Anyone who is the victim of a crime or who survives a serious accident has emotional trauma in addition to any physical injuries sustained. The health care system tends to focus on physical injuries, however. Once victims have been treated in the emergency room or discharged from the hospital, they usually receive follow-up treatment primarily for their physical injuries.

Fear and anger inevitably accompany the physical trauma of crimes and accidents. Some people can process these feelings over time; others need professional counseling to deal with the intensity of the feelings and any disabling effects, such as panic attacks or chronic anxiety. It is appropriate, within the role of some health care providers, to suggest to victims that they may benefit from counseling to deal with the emotional effects of their traumatic experience.

Blaming the Victim

The trauma experienced by the victim is magnified when others choose to blame the victim. Those who would defend a rapist are likely to claim the victim "was just asking for it," citing her manner of dress or her presence in a particular location. If the victim was a child, someone may comment that she was often "flirtatious" or note that she would sometimes climb into a male relative's lap. Thus, an innocent child's natural ways of seeking attention and affection may be used to imply that she was responsible for an adult's sexual behavior.

This tendency to blame the victim sometimes extends even to those who are the victim of a criminal act or are involved in an accident:

> *Why were you out at that time of night?*
> *Why did you go to that place? You should have known better!*
> *How many times have I told you not to drive so fast?*

Being blamed for what happened adds to a victim's emotional trauma. It is only natural to feel anger when being blamed at a time when one's need is for expressions of caring and emotional support. Although blaming may actually be a friend's or relative's expression of concern, it is inappropriate and not what a victim needs to hear. Also, blaming may be an example of displaced anger, from the cause of the event or the perpetrator, to the victim; this too is inappropriate. The health care provider sometimes has an opportunity to point out to relatives a victim's need for expressions of caring, emotional support, and protection from being blamed.

The Survivor Role

Each victim reacts to trauma in accordance with his or her established patterns of behavior. For some, the role of victim provides certain benefits that he or she does not want to give up, and so "I am a victim" becomes part of the self-concept. Some refuse to work through the emotional effects, choosing instead to hold onto their anger, fear or hatred. Others find valuable lessons in their traumatic experience and make significant lifestyle changes to improve the quality of their lives. And there are some who use the experience for a constructive purpose.

One woman who was the victim of sexual harassment filed complaints through appropriate channels, with no results. She later filed a lawsuit and eventually received a substantial financial settlement. Instead of simply enjoying her financial gain, she chose to set up a nonprofit organization to provide assistance to others in dealing with sexual harassment. She also serves as a consultant to businesses and provides on-site seminars to help employers establish safeguards against sexual harassment in the workplace. This is an example of how a person can learn from a bad experience and eventually use that learning for a constructive purpose.

THE CHALLENGE

Achieving a state of adjustment after having a traumatic experience is more difficult for some victims than others. When a victim finds it difficult to fulfill job or family responsibilities several weeks or months after a traumatic event, even though physical injuries have apparently healed, what sort of help is needed?

Is the person now in a state of clinical depression?

Has the victim developed a phobia?

Is the person having panic attacks? nightmares? flashbacks?

Is the person unable to resume daily activities because of a pervasive distrust of other people?

Or is the person's prolonged inability to resume his or her daily routine a severe, but still normal, reaction to trauma? It is difficult to differentiate a "normal" from "not normal" reaction in many such situations. Psychological trauma can be just as disabling as physical injuries.

The victim is usually discharged from health care once the physical injuries have healed. But members of the family, friends, and co-workers may notice that the victim "just isn't the same since . . ." or comment that "he just can't get his act together." The victim does not need criticism or judgmental attitudes. Rather, such a person needs understanding and emotional support. If improvement does not occur within a reasonable period of time, the victim should have the benefit of professional counseling.

Health care providers should encourage victims and relatives to understand the serious nature of psychological trauma and help them recognize the need for professional assistance. Although the disabling effects of physical trauma are obvious, psychological trauma is less likely to be understood or acknowledged. With encouragement from a health care provider, the victim may accept that he or she needs professional assistance in dealing with the psychological effects of the traumatic experience. With therapy, the victim may regain a healthy state of adjustment within a few weeks or months. Without therapy, the victim may remain in a state of poor adjustment for months or years.

References and Suggested Readings

Adams, David. "Identifying the Assaultive Husband in Court: You Be the Judge." *Boston Bar Journal,* July/August 1989, pp. 33–34.

Allen, Jon G. Ph.D. *Coping with Trauma: A Guide to Self-Understanding.* American Psychiatric Press, Washington, DC: 1995.

Bachman, Ronet, Ph.D. "Violence Against Women: A National Crime Victimization Survey Report." *Report of the Bureau of Justice Statistics,* U.S. Department of Justice, January, 1994.

Colorado Domestic Violence Coalition. *Domestic Violence for Health Care Providers;* Fifth Edition. Denver, CO: The Coalition, 1994. (Available from the Coalition, POB 18902, Denver, CO 80218).

Crawford, Christina. *No Safe Place: The Legacy of Family Violence.* Barrytown, NY: Station Hill Press, 1994.

Education Programs Associates (EPA). *No One Deserves to Be Abused: Help for You or Someone You Know.* Available from EPA, Distribution Dept., 1–408–374–3720.

Evans, Patricia. *The Verbally Abusive Relationship.* Holbrook, MA: Adams Media Corporation, 1992.

Glass, Lillian. *Toxic People: 10 Ways of Dealing with People Who Make Your Life Miserable.* New York: Simon & Schuster, 1995.

Hart, Barbara (Legal Director, PA Domestic Violence Coalition). *Remarks to the Task Force on Child Abuse and Neglect,* National Domestic Violence Coalition, April 1992.

Hunter, Mic. *Abused Boys: The Neglected Victims of Sexual Abuse.* New York: Fawcett Columbine, 1990.

Kalman, Natalie and Waughfield, Claire G. *Mental Health Concepts;* Third Edition. Albany, NY: Delmar Publishers Inc., 1993. Chapter 4, "Relieving Anxiety," pp. 80–90; Chapter 5, "Psychotherapies," pp. 99–116.

Lerner, Harriett G., Ph.D. *The Dance of Anger.* New York, NY: Harper & Row Publishers, 1989. Chapter 1, "The Challenge of Anger," pp. 1–16; Chapter 5, "Using Anger as a Guide," pp. 88–107.

Lerner, Harriet G., Ph.D. *Life Preservers: Staying Afloat in Love and Life.* New York, NY: HarperCollins, 1996.

Massachusetts Coalition of Battered Women Service Groups. *For Shelter and Beyond;* Second Edition. Boston, MA: The Coalition, 1992. (Available from the Coalition, 14 Beacon St., Boston, MA 02108, $10).

The Menninger Clinic. *The Menninger Letter.* Topeka, KS: The Menninger Foundation. September, 1995 (3:9); October, 1995 (3:10).

The Menninger Clinic. *Menninger Perspective,* 1996. Topeka, KS: The Menninger Foundation #4, 1995; #5.

"Mental Health: Does Therapy Help?" *Consumer Reports,* November, 1995, pp. 734–739.

National Women's Health Network. *The Network News,* March/April, 1995.
Nancy Worcester. "Health System Response to Battered Women: Our Successes are Creating New Challenges," pp. 1, 5–6.
Leslie E. Orloff. "Addressing the Needs of Battered Immigrant Women," pp. 3–4.

NOW LDEF. *A Leadership Summit: The Link Between Violence and Poverty in the Lives of Women and Their Children.* Available from Heather Ronovech, NOW LDEF, 99 Hudson St., New York 10013-2815.

Torres, José Chegui. "Let's Stop Glorifying Bullies." *Parade Magazine,* October 6, 1995, pp. 14–15.

Sources of Help

National Domestic Violence Hotline: 1–800–799–7233 (1–800–799SAFE). A 24-hour toll-free line that provides crisis assistance, counseling, and local shelter referrals throughout the 50 states, the Virgin Islands, and Puerto Rico. Funded under the Violence Against Women Act; operated by the Texas Council on Family Violence. Help is available in several languages. For the hearing impaired: Tel TDD 1–800–787–3224.

National Institute of Mental Health (NIMH) panic helpline: 1–800–647–2642.

Rape, Abuse, and Incest National Network (RAINN): 1–800–656–HOPE. A 24-hour, 7 days-a-week national hotline for victims of sexual assault. When the 800 number is called, a computer reads the area code and first three digits of the incoming call, then immediately routes the call to the nearest rape crisis center. The nearby center can then provide counseling and support for the victim. There is no charge for this service.

Adults Molested as Children (AMAC), P.O. Box 608, Pacific Grove, CA 93950.

American Coalition for Abuse Awareness: 202–462–4688. 1858 Park Rd., NW, Washington, DC 20010.

American Medical Association. "AMA Guidelines on Sexual Assault." Chicago, IL: AMA, no date.

The Citizen's Committee for Children of New York, 105 East 22 St., Dept P, New York 10010 (Information about child abuse).

Civitas Child Trauma Program, Attn.: Dr. Bruce D. Perry, Baylor College of Medicine, Dept. P, One Baylor Plaza, Houston, TX 77030 (Information about child abuse).

Clearinghouse for Child Abuse Prevention: 513–721–8392. 2314 Auburn Ave., Cincinnati, OH 45219.

Dept. of Justice: 1–800–421–6770. (Information about Violence Against Women Act (VAWA)).

National Council to Prevent Child Abuse, 332 S. Michigan Ave, Suite 1600, Chicago, IL 60604.

National Council on Child Abuse and Family Violence: 202–429–6695. 1155 Connecticut Ave., NW, Suite 300, Washington, DC 20036.

National Resource Center on Domestic Violence: 1–800–537–2238. Can provide list of domestic violence coalitions and phone numbers for each state coalition.

Physicians for a Violence-Free Society (PVS): 214–590–8887.

Women Against Sexual Harassment (WASH), 102 Plymouth Park S/C, Box 181, Irving, TX 75061. This nonprofit organization provides help to people who are experiencing sexual harassment and also conducts on-site seminars to assist companies and agencies in developing sexual harassment policies. (Internet address: http://www.pic.net/w-a-s-h)

REVIEW AND SELF-CHECK

Part I. Complete each of the following statements, using information from Unit 10.

1. The best protection a person can have against the difficulties of life is

    _____

    _____

    _____ .

2. It is important to develop skills for dealing with daily problems of living

    because _____

    _____

    _____ .

3. Six milestones in life that require changes in behavior or the formation of new patterns of behavior include:

    _____   _____

    _____   _____

    _____   _____

4. Beside each life stage above, name one significant change.

5. Three types of experience that represent a major life change include ___

    _____ , _____ , and _____ .

6. Four ways in which we can deal with threats to adjustment include:

    _____

    _____

    _____

    _____

7. Three reasons the victim of a traumatic experience may need counseling:

    _____ , _____ , and _____ .

8. Two reasons a health care provider should be aware of the effects of a traumatic experience on the victim: _____ and _____ .

9. Five examples of traumatic experiences that may occur during childhood: _____ , _____ , _____ , _____ , and _____ .

10. Two possible effects on a child whose daily life includes numerous negative experiences: _____ , and _____ .

11. Four types of child abuse: _____ , _____ , _____ , and _____ .

12. Three long-term effects of child abuse: _____ , _____ , and _____ .

13. Five terms used to refer to deviant sexual behavior:

    _____

    _____

    _____

    _____

    _____

14. Three examples of a traumatic experience that may occur during adolescence: _____ , _____ , and _____ .

15. Explain why peer pressure is a powerful influence on adolescent behavior.

16. Five types of traumatic experience that may occur during adulthood: _____ , _____ , _____ , _____ , and _____ .

17. Three traumatic effects of discrimination: _____ , _____ , and _____ .

18. Three traumatic effects of rape: _____ , _____ , and _____ .

19. Three traumatic effects of domestic violence: _____ ,

    _____ , and _____ .

20. Explain the phrase, "blaming the victim."

Part II. Define the following terms in your own words, based on information in Unit 10.

Abuse	Incest	Rape
Blended family	Paraphilia	Sex offender
Discrimination	Pedophilia	Sexism
Domestic violence	Perpetrator	Sexual deviation
Heterosexual	Perversion	Sexual variation
Homosexual	Prepubescent	STD

Part III. The following words may already be part of your vocabulary; use a dictionary to find the meaning of any that are unfamiliar to you. Write out the meaning of each word, then use the dictionary to check your definitions.

Atypical	Innate	Psychological
Custodial	Morality	Reprisal
Derogatory	Mores	Taboo
Deviation	Prevalent	Trauma
Hyperactivity	Psychiatric	Victim
Impulsivity		

ASSIGNMENT

1. Consider several of your life experiences that involved new situations. Try to recall how you felt during the early days in the new situation. Which of your familiar behaviors were inappropriate in the new situation? What changes did you make in your behavior patterns as you adapted to the new situation?

2. Consider the most uncomfortable experience you have had since entering this health occupations program. Why were you uncomfortable? What was your behavior? List changes in behavior that helped you return to a state of adjustment.

3. Make a list of rules to guide you in future situations of the following types:
   a. A radical change in your life situation.
   b. A new job in which many of the techniques used are somewhat different from those you learned as a student.
   c. A new job in the health field for which your present learnings provide a foundation, but your job responsibilities require that you learn many new techniques.

4. Obtain the name of the agency and the emergency phone number for obtaining help in your community or state for the following situations:
   a. reporting child abuse
   b. reporting a rape
   c. reporting domestic violence
   d. obtaining emergency shelter for a battered woman
   e. obtaining legal aid for a battered woman
   f. filing a complaint about sexual harassment in the workplace (after the employer's established procedures have been followed, without results)

5. Consider any life experience that was emotionally traumatic for you. Did you receive encouragement and support from friends and relatives? Did any health care personnel who cared for you show concern about the emotional effects of your experience? Do you experience fear, anger, or other strong emotions when you think of that experience? If so, consider the possibility that you could benefit from professional counseling. If the instructor schedules time for class discussions related to Unit 10, consider whether or not the class could learn from your sharing of this experience. Discuss it with the instructor first, however.

6. In reading the sections on domestic violence, did you recognize the behavior of anyone in your family? If so, what would be appropriate actions on your part?

7. Consider the following situations in terms of the trauma experienced by the victim and appropriate action by you as a friend or a health care provider:

    *   A child is brought to the emergency room by both parents, who report that the child fell down the stairs. After determining that the arm is broken, the physician asks you to take the child to the cast room and directs the parents to the waiting room. En route to the cast room, the child whispers to you, "I did *NOT* fall down the stairs." What is an appropriate action for you?

    *   Your best friend has been married almost a year. At first you and she continued your custom of having lunch and going to a movie once a week. Then, she began to cancel at the last minute; once, she didn't cancel but failed to meet you. Today, she arrives at the restaurant wearing dark glasses. She says she cannot stay for the movie, as her husband expects her home in an hour. When she adjusts her glasses, you notice bruises on her arm. What are some appropriate statements you could make to her? Or, should you just ignore what you have seen?

    *   Your co-worker tells you she has a problem and asks if you will meet her after work. She reveals that, as a child, she was sexually abused by her father. She left home as soon as she finished high school and visits her parents (in a nearby city) only on special occasions. She is divorced and has custody of her ten-year-old daughter. Now, her parents are insisting that she allow the daughter to spend one weekend a month with them. The daughter is excited about this, but has told you that Grandpa kissed her on the lips during their last visit. What factors should influence your co-worker's decision?

    *   Sylvia, a recently divorced nurse, occasionally mentions that her ex-husband would beat her about once a week. She always follows such comments with, "But I know I deserved it." What would be an appropriate response for you, the next time you hear her make that statement?

    *   Adele asks if a male colleague has ever said anything "inappropriate" to you. He has not, but you realize that he sometimes comes up behind you and runs his hand up or down your back. When you tell her this, she suggests he is checking to see if you are wearing a bra. What would be an appropriate action on your part the next time he runs his hand up or down your back?

Unit 11

Defense Mechanisms and Behavior

OBJECTIVES

Upon completion of this unit, you should be able to:

- Define defense mechanism.
- State three purposes of defense mechanisms.
- Name six common defense mechanisms.
- Define rationalization, projection, displacement, daydreaming, escape into illness, repression, and withdrawal.
- State how occasional use of a defense mechanism can contribute to good adjustment.
- Compare escape into illness and malingering.
- Compare substance dependency and defense mechanisms.
- State three guidelines for improving adjustment by modifying one's use of defense mechanisms.
- Define alcoholism, addiction, tolerance, drug dependency, and co-dependent.

KEY TERMS

Aberrant	Abstinence	Addiction
Alcoholism	Autism	Co-dependency
Dependency	Dysfunctional	Enabler
Fantasy	Fetal Alcohol Syndrome (FAS)	Habituation
Hallucinogenic	Hypnosis	Imminent
Malingering	Perception	Psychoanalysis
Psychotherapy	Self-deception	Traumatic
Withdrawal		
(drug related)		

There are certain mental devices that all of us use at times in order to feel more comfortable and make our behavior seem reasonable to ourselves and others. These devices are known as *defense mechanisms.*

REACTIONS TO THREAT

When we find ourselves in a situation that we cannot handle effectively, feelings of threat are aroused: fear, anxiety, hostility, frustration, or other negative feelings. Inability to handle the situation is a threat to one's self-esteem, in addition to the possibility of physical or psychological harm. When there is a

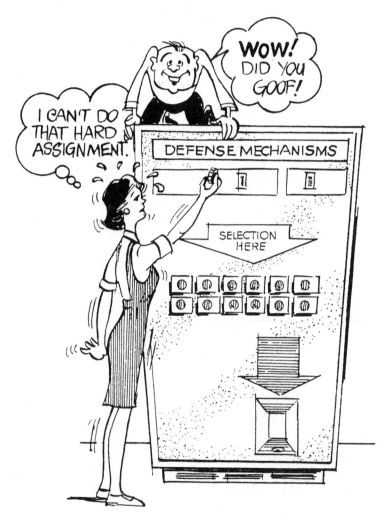

Overuse of defense mechanisms can be costly in terms of adjustment.

lack of competence for dealing with a situation, a defense mechanism may be used.

THE PURPOSE OF DEFENSE MECHANISMS

Defense mechanisms are attempts to protect against anxiety and loss of self-esteem in the face of defeat. They help us handle feelings of discomfort, make it possible to "save face," provide an *apparently* logical reason for the behavior used, and enable us to maintain self-respect in spite of the outcome. Obviously, defense mechanisms are useful—provided they do not become habitual devices for avoiding reality. Defense mechanisms can help us, or they can become crutches that substitute for more effective ways of dealing with difficult situations.

COMMON DEFENSE MECHANISMS

Rationalization

In the familiar fable of the fox and the grapes, the fox found he could not jump high enough to get some grapes. So, he announced that the grapes were sour, and therefore he did not want them. Thus, the fox avoided admitting to himself

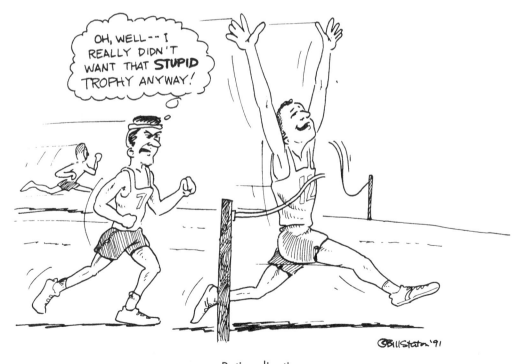

Rationalization

that he had tried but failed. This is one type of rationalization—the "sour grapes" approach to handling failure or disappointment.

Rationalization involves offering an apparently reasonable, socially acceptable explanation for behavior, when the true reason would be too painful for the individual. Thus, rationalization helps to relieve disappointment, provides a means for avoiding a situation perceived as threatening, and avoids admitting an inadequacy that would be damaging to self-esteem. Unfortunately, this device is a form of self-deception. Frequent use of rationalization is self-defeating because it displaces efforts to improve one's competence in dealing with life situations. Let us look at an example of a young girl using rationalization.

Mary has been invited to a party. She knows that the other girls know the latest dance steps. Mary does not dance. Although Mary wants to be a part of the group and have a good time, she thinks this party will place her at a disadvantage in relation to the other girls. To Mary, this is a very big problem. She believes her acceptance by members of this group will be affected when they discover she does not dance.

To Mary, missing the party is preferable to being embarrassed. Mary's mother is in poor health, but she is not so sick that Mary should stay home with her and miss the party. Yet to Mary, her mother's health provides a graceful way to avoid the party.

By rationalizing, Mary has avoided admitting to herself the degree of fear she feels at being unable to "hold her own" at the party. She has also given her hostess a socially acceptable reason for her absence. Perhaps Mary even feels somewhat proud of making a sacrifice in order to be a dutiful daughter. No conscious decision-making is involved in this situation. Mary's fears lead to seeking an escape, and her mother's poor health has provided an easy, socially acceptable way to avoid the party—and the threat it represents to Mary.

When rationalization is used habitually, it becomes an *unconscious* mechanism. Friends of the habitual rationalizer may be unaware of the fears and anxieties that are the basis for hard-to-understand behaviors. They tend to regard the habitual rationalizer as a person who always makes excuses.

Projection

Projection is a device for placing blame for one's own inadequacies on someone else or on circumstances. Projection is also used to attribute one's own unfavorable characteristics and desires to someone else; a person who is often critical of other people may be exhibiting projection. When projection is used to an extreme, the individual develops distorted perceptions of life situations and of people.

James is a health occupations student who is not making satisfactory grades. In discussing his academic standing with the counselor, he says that he cannot study at home because his mother wants him to help around the house.

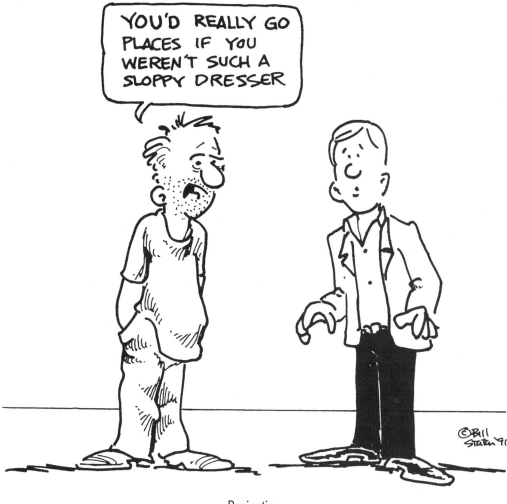

Projection

When one of the instructors corrects James on his technique in performing a procedure, he complains that the instructor does not like him. When hostility develops between James and a classmate, James explains the situation by saying that his classmate is jealous because James is dating Joanne.

Every undesirable situation in James' life is explained as the fault of something or someone other than himself. His use of projection is preventing an honest appraisal of his problems and how he himself helps to create them. Other people may be saying, "Why doesn't James wise up?" But James is more comfortable projecting blame than looking at himself. He avoids having to admit to himself that he has some shortcomings.

Lillie spends a lot of time before a mirror, working with her hair and applying make-up; because she spends so much time on her appearance, she is usually late for class and appointments. Lillie often criticizes other women for "being so vain." Lillie is unaware that she herself tends to be quite vain about her appearance. Her classmate, Suzanne, is very interested in a particular young man, even though he is dating Beth. Suzanne often attempts to get the young man's attention, especially at parties; she is quite vivacious, whereas Beth is somewhat quiet and reserved. Suzanne sometimes criticizes another woman as "always trying to steal someone's boyfriend." Both Lillie and Suzanne are projecting their own characteristics onto other people, unaware that their criticisms actually indicate disapproval of their own behavior.

Some people blunder through life using projection and other defense mechanisms instead of learning to see themselves and situations realistically. Each of use makes a mistake at times. It is no disgrace to be wrong, but it is very unfortunate to be unable to admit being wrong.

Being able to recognize how we contribute to an undesirable situation and being able to learn from our mistakes lead to growth as a person. Frequent use of projection interferes with such growth. Projection is self-deception and a distortion of reality.

Displacement

Displacement is the redirection of strong feelings about one person to someone else. Displacement occurs when there is fear or inability to direct the feeling toward the object or person who aroused the feelings. Usually, displacement involves negative feelings, but it can also occur with positive feelings.

Bob is a health care provider with hostile feelings toward his supervisor. He is well aware that the supervisor makes out the assignments and the schedule; also, the supervisor must recommend any member of the staff for a raise. It would be unwise for Bob to be openly hostile to one who has so much control over his daily work and over progress in his career. Bob recognizes this and is always pleasant to the supervisor, even doing a little "apple polishing" at times. Whenever Bob has a conference with the supervisor, the next person he sees is likely to become the object of his hostility. Sometimes Bob carries his hostility home and is irritable and short-tempered with his family or even the family pet. Bob is displacing the hostility he feels for the supervisor to others who did nothing to create his negative feelings.

Obviously, displacement creates interpersonal problems. Family and friends may be tolerant for a while, especially if they recognize that the hostility has been aroused by someone else. They may even take sides with the individual and attach unflattering names to the person who aroused the anger.

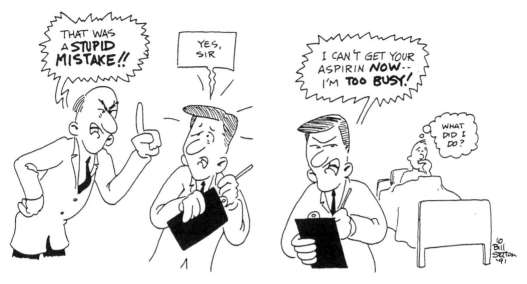

Displacement

Usually, however, the person who habitually displaces negative feelings is perceived by others as irritable and "hard to get along with."

You have learned that the energy generated by negative feelings needs to be worked off, preferably through physical activity. Displacement is an *unhealthy* method of using negative energy. It is an undesirable pattern of behavior, both because of the self-deception involved and because of unfavorable effects on relationships.

Daydreaming

Daydreaming is a device that provides escape. It is a useful mechanism if it creates dissatisfaction with things as they are, inspires the setting of goals for the future, and leads to a course of action designed to attain those goals. Daydreaming may lead to invention or inspiration for a creative activity.

If daydreaming provides an escape by substituting **fantasy** for reality, then it contributes to poor adjustment. When habitually used as an escape, daydreams can become more satisfying than life experiences. In the extreme, this escape from reality is a symptom of illness—adjustment so poor that the individual substitutes escape for dealing with life situations.

Lou, Ed, and Sue were all in high school together. None of them planned to go to college, yet all did well in their science courses and had an interest in health careers. They all tended to daydream at times, as most young people do. Lou dreamed of himself as a famous surgeon, acclaimed the world over for unusual and startling medical accomplishments. Ed and Sue also dreamed of

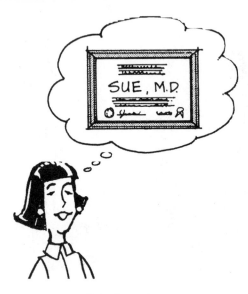

Daydreaming

themselves as physicians, but their dreams were more in line with things they had seen physicians doing. Ed's daydreams enhanced his interest in health science, and he began to save the money from his after-school job. Eventually, he entered a program for orthopedic technicians and obtained a job that enabled him to work closely with orthopedic surgeons. Sue got a job after high school and continued to daydream occasionally about herself as a physician. Soon, family responsibilities increased until she could not afford to enroll in an educational program. She continued to think of herself as a person who could have been a physician if circumstances had permitted, but she never made any real effort to achieve such a goal.

Meanwhile, Lou found his daydreams highly satisfying. He began to neglect his schoolwork. Occasionally, he imagined himself to be a famous surgeon as he performed his daily activities. Lou's first job lasted about a year: his employer said he could not keep his mind on his work. Lou's next job was quite distasteful to him; the unpleasantness of his workday made his daydreams more important than ever. Since daydreams had become Lou's main source of satisfaction in life, he was very irritable if something interrupted his daydreaming. Lou had retreated into a world of fantasy to such an extent that he could not function as a responsible adult.

Daydreaming alone is not a symptom of mental illness. However, escaping from reality through daydreams leads to increasingly poor adjustment, because it substitutes escape into fantasy for achieving satisfaction from real life experiences.

Escape into Illness

Escape into illness involves periodic illnesses that serve a definite purpose, but the individual is not aware of the purpose. Illness as an escape usually has its beginnings in childhood. Parents tend to be especially attentive when a child is sick, even if the illness is a minor one. Sometimes busy parents do not give children much more attention than is necessary for the daily routine, until a problem arises involving the child. Then the child becomes the center of attention. When the problem has been taken care of, the busy routine may be resumed, with the child again receiving only necessary attention. Thus, the child learns that illness is rewarded with parental notice and concern.

If illness during childhood is rewarded by special attention, gifts, permissiveness, sweets, or other things desired by children, then illness serves a definite purpose—the reward of being "special" and of having privileges *not usually allowed when well.* If the parents permit a child to use illness to avoid a dreaded situation and/or to gain advantages available only during an illness, then these early learnings can become an unconscious mechanism that will influence behavior throughout life. Once the child has learned that a headache, a cold, or other minor physical complaint can serve a purpose, illness may be used to get special attention or to avoid certain situations. Eventually, the purpose is no longer in the conscious mind and periodic illnesses have become "real."

Escape into illness must be distinguished from malingering. Escape is a defense mechanism, protecting the individual from threatening situations, but

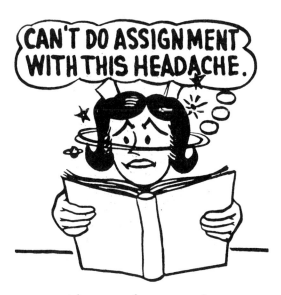

Illness can provide escape from an unpleasant situation.

operating below the level of conscious thought. **Malingering,** on the other hand, is *deliberate pretense of illness* when there is none.

Many people habitually use escape into illness as a means of avoiding some of their life problems. When the stress of accumulating problems reaches a certain point, or when an anticipated event arouses fear or anxiety, a minor illness can conveniently provide temporary escape. The symptoms experienced are real; the misery the individual feels is real. There may even be great annoyance at the inconvenience caused by this illness, yet the pattern of behavior is based on the individual's inability to face certain situations. Let us look at Joe, who is enrolled in a program for surgical technicians.

Joe is 19, a high school graduate, and somewhat the all-round American boy. He likes sports and has high ideals about team spirit and fair play. He can hold his own with his age group, whether in sports or in standing up for his beliefs.

The surgical technician program proved very interesting to Joe—until the class went into the operating room. Suddenly Joe had some feelings he did not understand. Patients on stretchers, containers of body organs, hospital staff members with masks and floppy gowns—it was a frightening and unreal world to Joe. After several days, Joe's negative feelings about the operating room were stronger than on the first day. Increasing familiarity did not relieve his intense feelings, whereas most of his classmates had become accustomed to the sights and smells of the operating room suite.

Over the weekend, Joe could think of nothing but the operating room and its effect on him. He went bowling with the gang, but he made a poor score and could not get into the jolly mood of his friends. Monday morning he could not eat breakfast. When his mother anxiously inquired about his health, he said he must have hurt his back when he was bowling. Joe, with his mother's encouragement, went back to bed and slept all day.

Joe was not pretending to be sick. His doubts and fears had mounted to the point that stress was manifested as physical symptoms. Joe really did feel terrible! His retreating into illness was an unconscious escape.

At this point, Joe's early learnings will influence the behavior pattern of the next few days. If he has learned to use illness as an escape, his back pain will become worse and he will withdraw from the surgical program because of a "bad back." If Joe is able to face life realistically, he will eventually recognize that his emotional reactions to the operating room are affecting him unfavorably. An honest and realistic appraisal of himself in relation to the job requirements of a surgical technician should be made. If Joe is not temperamentally suited to the operating room, he should feel free to withdraw from the program on that basis, without the need to project blame on his "injured back."

Sometimes a person develops insight into tendencies to use escape into illness and, through determination and effort, learns to face problems rather than trying to escape them. Many people, however, have used this device for years and are unable to develop insight into the purposes of the illnesses without professional counsel.

Repression

Repression is the forcing of an unpleasant memory into the subconscious mind. Once a memory has been forced into the subconscious mind, it cannot be recalled at will. Although deeply buried, the memory is still a powerful influence on behavior. Repression occurs most often with painful experiences of childhood, but it can also occur with an adult experience. This defense mechanism is less susceptible to conscious control than those discussed previously.

Repressed memories usually come to light only during **psychotherapy.** A therapeutic method aimed at reaching these deeply buried memories in **psychoanalysis.** Many therapeutic sessions are necessary to bring repressed memories back into the conscious level. **Hypnosis,** possibly with age regression, is sometimes used to identify and/or help a patient "relive" a **traumatic** experience that has been repressed. This is usually accomplished with only a few hypnosis sessions. These methods require the skills of a psychiatrist or psychologist with specialized training.

You, as a health care provider, should be aware of the influence of repressed memories on behavior. A traumatic experience, especially during childhood, may exert a powerful influence on adult behavior, even though the adult does not recall that experience. As a health care provider in contact with pediatric patients, try to prevent the child's experience with the health care system from being psychologically traumatic.

Withdrawal

Withdrawal as a defense mechanism involves either shutting off communication or removing oneself physically from a situation that is perceived as threatening. Withdrawal may be the strategy of choice in a situation where defeat is **imminent,** as in a disagreement when the other person becomes physically threatening. Extremes of withdrawal are characteristic of some psychiatric conditions, such as **autism** and catatonic schizophrenia. A less extreme, but quite serious, example of withdrawal is the desertion reaction of some pediatric patients if no member of the family stays with the child. Lying in the fetal position, a tendency of some chronically ill patients and many geriatric patients, is also an example of withdrawal. If your role as a health care provider will involve caring for patients who exhibit these types of withdrawal, you will study these conditions in other courses. But in every health care role and in your personal life you will see examples of withdrawal used as a coping strategy in difficult situations.

If a discussion becomes unpleasant and you refuse to participate further, you are using withdrawal. If a conference with the supervisor arouses anger and you excuse yourself from the conference, then you are withdrawing physically. If you do not do assignments and have made low grades on the tests, then drop the course the week before exams, you are withdrawing to avoid the threat to your self-esteem that a failing grade represents.

Suppose your first position as a health care provider requires that you work with someone you dislike. Every day you have one or more contacts with this person, and each encounter leaves you angry or unhappy. Except for this one person, you like your job very much. Should you resign? Should you keep the job in spite of these daily annoyances? This situation requires a decision between "fight" or "flight." You can stay on and try to cope with your reactions to this person, or you can "flee" to another job.

There are times when it is better strategy to withdraw physically from a situation than to put up with the problems it involves. There are other times when the satisfactions of a situation can balance the unpleasantness. Decisions about whether to withdraw or remain should be made on a *rational rather than emotional basis;* but, the probable long-range effects of the alternatives should enter into the decision.

Sometimes a situation can be changed or one can develop a better attitude toward it. If there is interpersonal conflict, open and honest talk may lead to improved understanding. But if a situation cannot be improved and one's feelings cannot be changed, then staying in the situation can only have unfavorable effects—the rational approach is to withdraw from that situation. If similarly unhappy experiences occur in the new setting, then a close look at oneself is indicated. Perhaps the source of the problem is self, rather than others.

SUBSTANCE DEPENDENCY

Defense mechanisms involve mental tricks—the use of the mind to deal with uncomfortable situations. Another approach to dealing with difficult experiences is the use of substances that have physical effects, thereby providing some relief from stress or diminished awareness of discomfort. Like the defence mechanisms, these substances—tobacco, alcohol, and drugs—provide an escape. With repeated use, one may develop addiction to one or more of these substances.

Nicotine Addiction

It is now known that nicotine, contained in all tobacco products, is highly addictive. During 1996, the tobacco companies have been accused of purposely adjusting the levels of nicotine in their products. Many lawsuits have been filed charging tobacco companies with creating serious health problems, including death from lung cancer and long-term disability due to emphysema. Dr. C. Norman Shealy lists six major causes of illness and death, with cigarette smoking at the top of the list.

Evidence that tobacco is a major threat to health has been increasing for several decades. As a result, many public buildings and most hospitals have been declared smoke-free environments, smoking is prohibited on airlines, and restaurants have a nonsmoking section. Many smokers refuse to give up their habit until they experience a major health problem, such as a heart attack. Others choose to give up smoking as part of a larger plan for a more healthful life-style. But for those smokers who choose to continue their habit, current societal restrictions are sources of frustration and anger.

Why do people smoke? The usual reason is that smoking provides relief from feelings of stress. For many people, the primary reason is social; this is the appeal to teenage smokers, for whom conformity to group behavior patterns is important. For an individual whose parents were smokers, the smell of a cigarette, cigar, or pipe may arouse pleasant childhood memories and feelings of comfort and security. Once a person has become addicted to nicotine, smoking is a response to subtle signals from the body that it needs a nicotine "fix."

The decision to give up tobacco may be made voluntarily or under pressure from one's physician, family, or friends. Many smokers are able to give up their habit simply by deciding to do so. When an addictive substance is no longer available to the body, physical symptoms of withdrawal occur. (This meaning of "withdrawal" is different from its meaning as a defense mechanism.) Nicotine withdrawal results in nervous agitation and intense craving for a cigarette (or whatever form of tobacco the individual uses). People who cannot tolerate withdrawal symptoms may need to use nicotine chewing gum or a skin patch. Psychotherapy also can provide assistance through hypnosis or relaxation/ guided imagery.

As a health care provider, you will encounter people who either continue to smoke or are trying to quit. These people may be patients, co-workers, family, or friends. Learn about the dangers of tobacco and the various approaches to giving up tobacco products, so you can be a source of information for anyone who seeks your help.

Alcohol Abuse/Alcoholism

Alcohol is a drug, with specific physiological effects. The use of alcohol, like tobacco, may begin as a social activity and a desire for peer approval and acceptance. It is readily available, more affordable than most drugs, and present in many homes, making it accessible to children and adolescents. The use of alcohol is so pervasive that "drinking" and "having a drink" are synonymous with "having an alcoholic drink."

Social use of alcohol can provide quick relief from stress, anxiety, guilt, insecurity, and other uncomfortable feelings. These effects may lead to occasional abuse—overindulgence to the point of becoming intoxicated. Regular use of alcohol over a period of time can result in psychological **dependency** and, eventually, physiological addiction—**alcoholism.** The distinction between occasional abuse and alcoholism is clear-cut:

1. An alcoholic's drinking is compulsive (i.e., cannot stop after a reasonable number of drinks)

2. After a period of **abstinence** (hours), the alcoholic experiences withdrawal symptoms that can only be relieved by taking a drink

Intoxication and alcoholism carry a high price tag. Intoxicated drivers are involved in over 50 percent of all highway accidents, many involving the deaths of innocent people. Automobile accidents, usually involving alcohol, are the leading cause of death among males age eighteen to twenty-five. In industry, high rates of absenteeism, errors, low productivity, and occupational accidents are attributed to alcohol. Alcohol is a factor in about one-third of all suicides. Alcohol is involved in a large percentage of crimes, especially murders, and in domestic violence, child abuse, and sex offenses. Alcoholism is now recognized by the courts as a disease (not punishable), but the individual (alcoholic or not) can be prosecuted for any crimes committed while under the influence of alcohol.

Why do people drink? Alcohol provides *escape.* Although classed as a central nervous system depressant, alcohol is considered by many people to be a stimulant, because it lowers inhibitions and releases muscular tension. Unfortunately, these relaxing effects are accompanied by diminished judgment, thinking skills, and memory—effects that make the drinker a danger to self and others. The use of alcohol to escape the feelings of despair and hopelessness that characterize clinical depression and the depressive phase of manic depressive illness is common. If such patients have also developed alcoholism, their clinical status is "dual diagnosis." Alcoholism must be treated (the individual must be "dry" for a certain period of time) before the psychiatric problem can be addressed.

Why do some people progress from social drinking to dependence on alcohol? Many factors have been implicated: physiological, metabolic, nutritional, genetic, emotional, and social. Certain personality traits seem to predominate: the individual tends to be dependent on others, harbors hostility, is somewhat egocentric, has unrealistic expectations that result in frustration and feelings of failure. Regardless of causative factors, the condition is treatable, but only when the individual can admit to needing help. This may occur only after

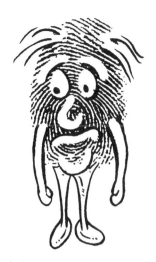 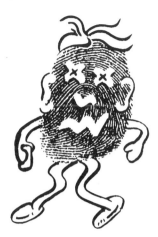

Alcohol and drugs provide escape—from the "black abyss" of depression, intolerable stress, and problems in living—but the escape is only temporary. (From Carol D. Tamparo & Wilburta Q. Lindh, *Therapeutic Communications for Allied Health Professions*. Albany, NY: Delmar Publishers Inc., 1992.)

numerous arrests, hospitalizations, and various losses (job, spouse, home) have occurred. Whereas medical treatment is required for acute phases, especially during the period when withdrawal symptoms occur, the support and encouragement of family and friends is crucial to long-term recovery of an alcoholic.

Effective treatment includes helping the individual learn to face reality and deal with life problems, instead of trying to escape them. This learning can be facilitated by counseling and participation in group therapy. Alcoholics Anonymous (AA), whose membership consists of recovering alcoholics, has proven to be effective for many people. AA emphasizes *total abstinence* from alcohol; newcomers are encouraged to avoid having a drink and to cope with one day at a time. Making it through one day is achievable for many people, but vowing to "never take a drink again" is a promise too easily broken.

The sharing of experiences at AA meetings and the encouragement and support of fellow members, all of whom "have been there and know what you're going through," enables many new members to achieve sobriety and become a recovering alcoholic. Once the alcoholic is sober and his or her body is free of alcohol, attention shifts to healing mind and emotions by following AA's "Twelve Steps to Recovery." The Twelve-Step program has been so successful during the sixty years of AA's existence that organizations devoted to other specific problems (i.e., gambling) have adapted the twelve steps to their own purpose.

Anyone may attend an open AA meeting, but closed meetings are for alcoholics only. In recognition that alcoholism is a family affair, support groups for family members have been established. Al-Anon is a self-help group for all family members; Alateen, for adolescent children of an alcoholic parent, is sponsored by Al-Anon, as is a group for adult survivors of alcoholic families. Adult Children of Alcoholics (ACOA) is a separate group, specifically for adult children of an alcoholic parent.

One tragic consequence of drinking has emerged during the last two decades: **Fetal Alcohol Syndrome (FAS).** This disorder is the result of a woman's drinking during the prenatal period. Even one or two glasses of wine per day during early pregnancy increases the probability that the baby will be born with FAS, since alcohol penetrates the placental barrier and enters the fetal bloodstream. Serious damage to the brain results, so the baby is born with an *untreatable disability.* The newborn infant is small, has characteristic cranial and facial features, and may have deformities of the limbs. Growth and development will be inhibited; mental retardation may be diagnosed when the child is old enough for testing. **Aberrant** behavioral patterns make it difficult for the child to form satisfying relationships or participate in meaningful activities. This condition is so definitely related to drinking during pregnancy that the National Institute on Alcohol Abuse and Alcoholism issued a statement in 1980 that *pregnant women should totally abstain from alcohol consumption.* In some states, establishments that serve alcohol are required to display warnings about the relationship of alcohol to birth defects.

Drug Abuse

The use of drugs is so pervasive in modern society that few people are unaffected. A *drug user* is any person who takes drugs, regardless of the purpose or type of drug, so that term applies to almost everyone at times. *Drug misuse* refers to taking doses that exceed the prescribed amount or taking medication prescribed for someone else. *Drug abuse* occurs when someone uses a drug for a nonmedical purpose. Drug abuse usually involves a class of drugs referred to as "recreational drugs," because they are often used in a social setting. That phrase is unfortunate, because it gives the false impression that these drugs are fun and harmless.

Any drug can be abused, but those most likely to be abused are drugs that relieve pain, alter one's mood, have a stimulant effect (provide a "high"), relieve anxiety, or have a **hallucinogenic** effect. Regular use of these types of drug leads to **habituation,** which is psychological dependence on the drug. If usage continues over a period of time, *tolerance* may develop, meaning that larger and larger doses are required to get the desired effect. **Addiction** exists when there is a physiological need for the drug at regular intervals. *Drug dependency* and *chemical dependency* are now the preferred terms, without concern about whether the patient's condition is habituation or addiction. *Withdrawal,* when used in relation to drug dependency, refers to the symptoms that occur

TABLE 11-1
Abused Drugs: Symptoms and Effects

DRUG	STREET NAME	SYMPTOMS	ADVERSE EFFECTS
Hallucinogens marijuana	grass, weed, maryjane, tea, pot, reefer, joint, hemp, hashish, hash, rope	sense of well-being; possible anxiety; talkative; relaxed; exhilarated; happy; altered time sense	reduced memory recall; impaired coordination and moral judgment; easily distracted, highly suggestible; long-term effect not known
LSD	25, acid, cubes, sunshine, the big D, trips, the chief, the ghost, the hawk	heightened and distorted perceptions; euphoria; altered time perception; dreamy, floating state, enlarged pupils; bizarre sensations	chromosomal damage; loss of control over normal thought processes; violence, self-destructive feelings; highly unpredictable behavior; slowed reaction time and reflexes; personality changes; paranoid symptoms
PCP	angel dust	lapse of memory; difficulty concentrating; convulsions; partial paralysis	effects highly unpredictable
Inhalants glue gasoline spray paint aerosols		similar to alcohol intoxication; sense of floating or spinning; blurred vision; confusion; staggering gait; slurred speech	brain damage; lead poisoning; damage to liver, heart, kidneys, and bone marrow; death

(From Natalie Kalman & Claire G. Waughfield, *Mental Health Concepts;* Third Edition. Albany, NY: Delmar Publishers Inc., 1993.

when a drug is withheld. These symptoms range from nervous agitation and anxiety to psychotic behavior and convulsions, depending upon the specific drug being withdrawn.

Drug use may be legal or illegal. The use of a prescription drug in accordance with the physician's directions is legal. The appropriate use of over-the-counter (OTC) drugs is legal. Misuse of a prescription drug or OTC may or may not be illegal, but is certainly unwise, unethical, and immoral. Drug abuse usually involves drugs that fall into one of the eleven categories of "controlled substances" as defined in the Controlled Substances Act of 1970. Certain controlled substances are prescribed for management of pain, anxiety, mood disorders and other medical conditions. Other controlled substances, used for nonmedical purposes, are most often obtained illegally; these are known as "street drugs."

The most commonly abused drugs are some that are socially acceptable and completely legal: caffeine, nicotine, and alcohol. Most people do not think of these three as drugs, but each has physiological effects, each is addictive, and each is subject to misuse and abuse. The coffee drinker who decides to forgo caffeine knows all-too-well the severe headache that lasts for several days—a symptom of caffeine withdrawal. The smoker who decides to quit knows well the symptoms of nicotine withdrawal. For an alcoholic, withdrawal of alcohol can have such serious consequences that it should be accomplished only under medical supervision, preferably with the patient hospitalized. And these are legally, socially acceptable drugs!

The treatment of dependency is complex and long-term. The individual must become drug-free, known as being "clean," and then must learn the coping skills required for dealing with life situations, rather than using drugs as a form of escape. For persons with a dual diagnosis, dependency must be treated and then a treatment protocol developed for the psychiatric condition. Such patients present an especially difficult situation, since the psychiatric condition often involves noncompliance with the physician's prescribed therapy. The following figure shows various approaches used in treatment of drug dependency.

The problem of drug abuse is now so pervasive that it has become a societal issue; full discussion is beyond the scope of this textbook. Yet, every health care provider should be informed about drug abuse, both from the standpoint of health care and legal/societal concerns. The Assignment section of this unit will suggest activities to help you become better informed.

Co-Dependency

Co-dependency is a situation in which the **dysfunctional** behavior of an alcoholic or drug abuser meets some need of the spouse or other close family member. The role of rescuer or protector becomes such an important part of the

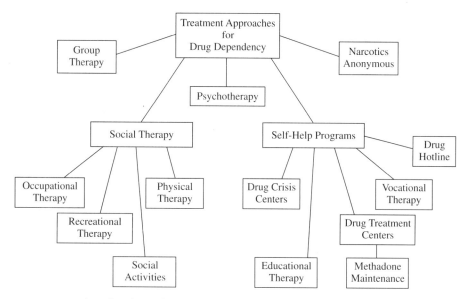

Treatment approaches for drug dependency. (From Natalie Kalman & Claire G. Waughfield, *Mental Health Concepts;* Third Edition. Albany, NY: Delmar Publishers Inc., 1993.)

co-dependent's life that the possibility of giving up that role is quite threatening. Family members may have spent years "rescuing" the addict and pleading for a change in behavior. They cling to the belief that life would be good it and when the addict takes control and gives up the addictive substance. Eventually this interaction becomes an important part of life activities; the rescuer role fulfills an important need. At that point, family members *unconsciously* encourage and support the addiction. If the addict undergoes treatment, family problems increase because family members who are co-dependent cannot cope with the new behavior of the former addict.

A co-dependent's *conscious* belief is that the family's problems will be resolved when the addiction has been treated. The reality is that a co-dependent *unconsciously* functions as an *"enabler"* by facilitating the addiction. Enabling takes many forms, such as "lending" the addict money that the enabler knows will be used for drugs, even though the addict promises to use the money for food and rent. In the case of alcoholism, the enabler may insist on going to parties where alcohol will be served or continue to keep liquor in the home for personal use, knowing that its presence is a temptation for the alcoholic. In the mental health field, co-dependency is itself considered an addiction that requires intensive psychotherapy.

Obviously, where co-dependency exists, treatment of the addict must include treatment of the co-dependent person also. Ideally, the entire family will be involved in therapy, so that any dysfunctional family dynamics may be corrected. The addict must learn to cope with life problems effectively, without escaping into a drug-induced euphoria or relying on the co-dependent for solving his or her problems. The co-dependent must learn to encourage the addict to be self-reliant and be willing to give up the role of rescuer, protector, and care-giver. Effective treatment of an addict, then, must involve family members. Otherwise, the "cured" addict will return to a dysfunctional family situation that does not support the addict being drug-free.

Tough Love

The parenting technique known as "Tough Love" was developed by Phyllis and David York as an approach to coping with out-of-control teenagers, especially those who are abusing alcohol and/or drugs. The title is derived from the notion that parents are manifesting love for their child when they get tough:

> *They set limits on what behaviors will be tolerated in the home,*
> *They require that the limits be respected,*
> *If the child fails to respect those limits, they arrange for the child to live elsewhere; and*
> *The alternative living arrangement is one in which the child is more likely to accept limitations and begin to make behavioral changes.*

The Yorks are family counselors who work with clients and their families and also train other counselors. They are considered to be experts in the field of drug and alcohol rehabilitation counseling. During the 1970's, the Yorks were trying to deal with some of the same problems as their clients—their own children were out of control.

They tried numerous approaches: counseling for the children and for themselves and various enrichment activities for the children. They tried being more permissive, tougher, and more understanding, but nothing seemed to work. When a daughter was arrested for armed robbery, they searched for a new approach to parenting in hopes of restoring harmony within their family. The result was a combination of philosophy and specific actions that came to be known as "Tough Love."

Tough Love involves expressing love and concern for the child's well-being while being very specific about what behaviors will be tolerated in the home. If an adolescent has a drug problem, the parents state, "We will not tolerate drugs or a drug user in our home." If the child chooses not to respect this limitation, then the parents make arrangements for the child to live elsewhere. This is usually the home of a relative or friend who understands Tough Love, is willing to accept the adolescent in their home, and agrees to require that the parents' limits be observed. The parents assume responsibility for any costs involved, including rehabilitation counseling and other health care expenses.

The specific limits that are set depend upon the behavioral problems the child has exhibited; examples of appropriate limits include:

"We will not tolerate verbal abuse." ("that type of language")
"We will not allow drugs in our home." ("alcohol")
"We will not allow a criminal in our home."
"We will not allow promiscuous sex in our home."

Every parent has a right—a responsibility, in fact—to establish limits on what behaviors will be tolerated in the home. Arrangements for alternative living arrangements should include setting goals—the behavioral changes that must be achieved before the child can return home. These goals should be made clear to the child:

"You will remain drug-free."
"You will not consume alcoholic beverages."
"You will stay in school."
"You will get a job."
"You will not socialize with people who . . . (do not behave in accordance with the limits
  established for the child).
"You will participate in a program for . . . (substance abusers)"
"You will attend the counseling sessions set up for you."

As adults other than the parents assume parenting responsibilities, the child must accept the limits that have been established. This is easier when the child is away from whatever dysfunctional dynamics exist in the home situation. As the child adapts to the alternative "home," new patterns of interacting with adults can develop—accepting limits no longer gets confused with rebelling against parental authority. Adults other than the parents now model the desired behaviors; the child may accept these role models and find it easier to respect the limits that have been established. Tough Love requires weeks, months or even several years to bring about the desired behavior changes.

The Yorks started a support group for parents of their clients and wrote a manual for other parents to form self-help groups. There are now Tough Love groups all over the United States and Canada and several foreign countries. Parents who cannot cope with the behavior of an adolescent child can contact a Tough Love group and learn about this approach. It is not easy—for parents or child. Anyone who is considering Tough Love should become well-informed, talk with others who have used the method, and join a Tough Love support group. Friends or relatives who are to participate should be carefully chosen, based on their probable effectiveness in establishing a good relationship with the child and their willingness to learn the Tough Love method. It is especially important that everyone involved understand that "throwing him or her out of the house" is not Tough Love, nor is it a manifestation of love. Throwing the child out of the home is unloving, total rejection of a child, and avoidance of parental responsibility.

DEFENSE MECHANISMS AND ADJUSTMENT

All of us need to use adjustment mechanisms of many types, including defense mechanisms. At one time or another we all have unhappy experiences, problem situations to face, and obstacles to overcome. We all experience disappointment and failure at intervals. We all need to feel good about ourselves, but our self-esteem is always at risk—vulnerable to negative experiences. When circumstances threaten self-esteem, we tend to become defensive.

A situation that you perceive as threatening may not bother your best friend. Conversely, you may be puzzled about your friend's defensive reaction to a situation you consider to be ordinary. Some of us become defensive whenever we are criticized. Some of us become apprehensive when we are expected to show achievement. Some of us become uncomfortable in the presence of an authority figure. Some of us distrust others, always expecting a put-down or criticism. Threat, then, is quite personal. It is based on our own specific areas of sensitivity, the psychological scars that are the result of hurtful experiences in our past.

The Patient

As a health care provider, keep in mind that illness and hospitalization represent a threat to most people. Therefore, you are likely to see many examples of defense mechanisms as you work with patients. If you work with psychiatric patients, you will need to learn about other mechanisms and about behavior deviations that psychiatric patients manifest. In the meantime, observe behavior and learn to recognize defense mechanisms.

When you become aware that someone is using a defense mechanism, realize that the person feels threatened by a situation. It is *not your role to point out the defense mechanism.* Your role is to *reduce the degree of threat the individual feels.* Through reassurance, acceptance, and sincere interest in the patient's well-being, you can usually reduce a patient's need for defensive behavior.

The Health Care Provider

How can you use knowledge about defense mechanisms to improve your own adjustment? First, keep in mind that defense mechanisms can be useful in relieving discomfort or negative feelings. Suppose a friend drops in just as you are about to leave home for a movie. At first, you feel quite irritated, but then you tell yourself, "I didn't really want to see that movie anyway." Having thus rationalized, you disposed of the angry feelings toward your friend and are free to enjoy the unexpected visit.

The key to healthful use of a defense mechanism is awareness. If you are aware of using a defense mechanism and of your reason for using it, then you are probably using it healthfully.

Suppose, on the other hand, your supervisor criticizes your performance frequently, but each time you place the blame on someone else or on circumstances. For example, the supervisor comments that you should have explained a procedure to your patient before carrying it out, but your reaction is, "I didn't have time." For every criticism you have an excuse. Then your use of projection is an obstacle to improving your performance as a health worker. Self-deception and distorted **perception** of situations are incompatible with learning and improved performance.

In striving to improve your own adjustment, be aware of the frequency and purposes of the defense mechanisms you tend to use. As you learn to recognize your use of each defense mechanism, you will be able to identify the types of situations that are threatening to you. Then you can seek ways of effectively dealing with such situations. If you have a habit of projecting blame, you may have to force yourself to admit a shortcoming now and then. Eventually, you will find it easier to admit being wrong or having made an error. By discarding the defense mechanism, you open the way to learn from experience.

As you become more aware of your tendencies to use defense mechanisms, you will begin to recognize those you have previously been using unconsciously. This awareness will not come overnight, nor will it come without some effort on your part to study your behavior patterns.

With increased understanding of yourself and your use of defense mechanisms, you will be ready to eliminate **self-deception,** learn to face reality, and use appropriate behavior in a variety of situations. Through practice in dealing with problems rather than "fleeing" from them, you will improve your skill in solving problems—even those that involve some unpleasantness. At that point, you will have less need for defense mechanisms.

References and Suggested Readings

Beattie, Melody. *Codependents' Guide to the Twelve Steps.* New York, NY: Prentice Hall Press, 1990.

Kalman, Natalie & Waughfield, Claire G. *Mental Health Concepts;* Third Edition. Albany, NY: Delmar Publishers Inc., 1993. Chapter 10, "Alcoholism," pp. 232–251; Chapter 11, "Drug Dependency," pp. 252–274.

The Menninger Clinic. *The Menninger Letter.* Topeka, KS: The Menninger Foundation, January, 1996 (4:1). "Dual diagnosis complicates treatment, caregiving," pp. 6–7.

Shealy, C. Norman, M.D., Ph.D. & Myss, Caroline M., Ph.D. *The Creation of Health: The Emotional, Psychological, and Spiritual Responses that Promote Health and Healing.* Walpole, NH: Stillpoint, 1988.

Yoder, Barbara. *The Recovery Resource Book.* New York, NY: Simon & Schuster, 1990. Contains a directory of self-help clearinghouses, state agencies, and state departments of rehabilitation.

York, Phyllis, York, David, and Wachtel, David. *Tough Love.* New York, NY: Bantam Books, 1982.

York, Phyllis, York, David, and Wachtel, David. *Tough Love Solutions.* Garden City, NY: Doubleday, 1984.

Sources of Additional Information

AA General Service Office, Box 459, Grand Central Station, New York, NY 10163.

Al-Anon Family Grand Headquarters, Inc.: 1–800–356–9996. 1600 Corporate Landing Parkway, Virginia Beach, VA 23454-5617.

The US helpline for abusers and their families: 1–800–COCAINE

Narcotics Anonymous: 1–800–282–2686, Ext. 998. World Service Office, P.O. Box 9999, Van Nuys, CA 91409.

REVIEW AND SELF-CHECK

Complete the following statements, using information from Unit 11.

1. Defense mechanisms are _____ .

2. Three purposes of defense mechanisms are

   _____ ,

   _____ ,

   _____ .

3. Rationalization is a defense mechanism that involves _____ .

4. Projection is a defense mechanism that involves _____ .

5. Displacement is a defense mechanism that involves _____ .

6. The basic purpose of daydreaming is _____ .

7. Daydreaming is useful if it _____
    and _____ .

8. Excessive use of daydreaming has the danger of _____ .

9. Escape into illness is a defense mechanism that involves _____ .

10. The primary difference between escape into illness and malingering is
    that _____ .

11. Repression is a defense mechanism that involves _____ .

12. Withdrawal is a defense mechanism that involves either _____
    _____ or _____ .

13. The occasional use of a defense mechanism aids adjustment by _____
    _____ .

14. Three guidelines for using defense mechanisms constructively are

    _____

    _____

    _____ .

15. Substance dependency is similar to defense mechanisms in that it _____
    _____ .

16. Substance dependency differs from defense mechanisms in that it _____
    _____ .

17. The term "co-dependent" refers to someone who is addicted to _____
    _____ .

18. Alcoholism is characterized by (1) _____
    and (2) _____ .

19. Alcohol appeals to many people because its effects provide _____ .

20. Dual diagnosis means _____ .

21. Fetal alcohol syndrome (FAS) is caused by _____ .

22. A drug user is someone who _____ .

23. Drug misuse refers to _____ or _____ .

24. Drug abuse occurs when _____ .

25. Habituation means _____ .

26. The term "recreational drug" is misleading because _____

    _____ .

27. Addiction means _____ .

28. Withdrawal (drug-related) refers to _____ .

29. Tolerance (in regard to drugs) refers to _____ .

30. Habituation and addiction are both included in the two terms

    _____ and _____ .

31. Three commonly abused, but socially acceptable and legal, drugs are

    _____ , _____ , and _____ .

32. Treatment of drug dependency requires that the individual become

    drug-free and then _____ .

ASSIGNMENT

1. Explain the difference between daydreaming as used by Lou, Ed, and Sue.

2. Explain the difference between malingering and escape into illness.

3. Use the following as a checklist to set objectives for modifying your use of defense mechanisms. The first item is explained to show you how to think through an item before applying it to yourself.
   a. I tend to use rationalization when I must choose between duty and pleasure. *Explanation:* This is true of me to a large extent. When I want to watch television, I convince myself that I have studied enough and understand the material. The next day, I wish I had studied. Therefore, I shall check this item as an example of a habit I need to modify.   ____
   Or,
   This is not particularly true of me. I like to do my work and fulfill my responsibilities. Then I can enjoy my free time without worrying about what I should be doing. I will not check this item.

b. I think of myself as a very capable person, yet I become anxious when a test is scheduled (or substitute another type of threatening situation). If I do not do well, I tend to rationalize. I do not like to admit that I did not do something well. _____

c. I do not like to be criticized, even when I know the criticism is true. _____

d. I am easily hurt by other people's remarks. It seems to me that people are too ready to be critical or to say unkind things. _____

e. I have a lot of trouble with teachers (parents, supervisors, etc.) because of things other people did. I also have a lot of bad luck. _____

f. Other people often make me angry (or unhappy) but I usually do not let them know it. I wait until I am home and then "let off steam." _____

g. Sometimes my daydreams are more pleasant than what is going on around me. Then I have trouble keeping my mind on my work. _____

h. It seems as though my colds always come when we have a big test scheduled (substitute some other type of threat if it is more applicable to you). _____

i. I don't believe in getting upset. When the going gets rough, I leave. _____

j. Some people irritate me, so I don't talk to them unless I have to. _____

4. Select one item you checked in activity #3 (or substitute a specific defense mechanism that you tend to use). State how you will modify your use of this mechanism.

5. Select a defense mechanism you have used in the past week.
   a. Explain the defense mechanism in your own words.
   b. Describe the situation in which you used this mechanism.
   c. Explain why that situation elicited defensive behavior.
   d. Consider the situation from your own viewpoint and, as best you can, from the viewpoint of other people who were present.
   e. List two or more ways you could have dealt with the situation without using a defense mechanism.

6. Participate in a class discussion on the topic: "Watching television serves as an escape for many people."

7. Your Uncle Bob was an alcoholic. The family often expressed sympathy for "poor Mary Lou," who put up with his drinking for many years. When Uncle Bob died unexpectedly, the family believed Mary Lou could now enjoy life, free of the problems Uncle Bob had created. Several

months later the family was amazed to learn that Mary Lou had married Joe, who was known to be an alcoholic. Explain Mary Lou's behavior.

8. You work at Community Hospital. A family friend, Joe (who married your Aunt Mary Lou in #7), often seeks your company at family gatherings. Today he says to you, "I really want to stop drinking. I've tried several times, but sooner or later I fall off the wagon. Can you help me?" Describe three things that must happen in order for Uncle Joe to become a recovering alcoholic.

9. What will be your first step in helping Uncle Joe?

10. What role could you play over the next year as Uncle Joe works on controlling his drinking? List specific actions you could take and indicate who you could involve.

11. List five dangers of alcohol abuse.

12. Consult your local telephone directory and obtain phone numbers for each of the following:
Alcoholics Anonymous
Alcohol abuse 24-hour helpline
Drug abuse 24-hour helpline

NOTE: Some toll-free (800) numbers provide information, some provide a local phone number for obtaining assistance, and some are private organizations seeking clients. Optional activity: Call each toll-free number and determine which ones offer guidance for locating community services and which ones are for-profit agencies. If they ask about your health insurance, they are probably a for-profit agency.

13. Obtain the location and phone number of your local community agency for alcohol and drug abuse.

14. Participate in a class discussion on one or more of the following topics:
Why health care providers should be free of addictions
Effective ways to stop smoking (give up coffee, alcohol, drugs)
Indications that an adolescent is using drugs
Indications that a co-worker is using drugs (illegal)
Examples of the destructive effects of alcohol
Examples of the destructive effects of prescription drug abuse
Examples of the destructive effects of drug abuse (illegal)

$\mathcal{U}nit$ 12

Inner Conflict

OBJECTIVES

Upon completion of this unit, you should be able to:

- Define inner conflict.
- List five influences on inner conflict.
- List and explain three types of inner conflict.
- State one requirement for dealing with inner conflict.
- List seven steps for resolving inner conflict.

KEY TERMS

Alternative	Analgesic	Collaborating
Debilitating	Digital	Incompatible
Indecision	Manipulative	Narcotic
Proficient	Prognosis	Prosthesis
Vacillate		

You have learned that habitual use of defense mechanisms can cause poor adjustment. Another common cause of poor adjustment is inner conflict.

THE MEANING OF INNER CONFLICT

Perhaps you are accustomed to thinking of conflict as a fight or argument. Such conflicts involve two or more people and are *interpersonal* conflicts. This unit is concerned with inner conflict—that which exists *within one person.* Other people may contribute to a person's inner conflict and others may be affected by the behavior resulting from inner conflict, but it is the individual with the conflict who is most affected.

Inner conflict creates inner discomfort. It is difficult to understand. It may arouse strong emotions. Until the conflict has been resolved, the individual may experience a variety of emotions, especially negative ones. Inner conflict, then, may cause much unhappiness unless one learns to recognize it, use a rational approach to identifying the needs that are in conflict, and then use good judgment in resolving the conflict.

Inner conflict exists when an individual has two **incompatible** needs or goals, or when the individual must choose between two or more **alternative** means for meeting a need or achieving a goal. The conflict arises because of the incompatibility of these needs, goals, or means, but other behavior influences may also be involved. One's value system, standards of behavior, beliefs, interests, personality traits, character traits, and self-concept may all contribute to inner conflict.

The person who has an inner conflict is usually aware of the need to choose between two goals or two courses of action. However, the individual may be unaware of the basic needs, values, interests, beliefs, and other factors that contribute to the conflict.

Conflict Between Needs

Adolescents are often faced with a conflict between the need for acceptance by the peer group and the need for maintaining their beliefs about "right" and "wrong" behavior. Suppose someone in Bill's crowd proposes a risky adventure involving behavior Bill believes to be wrong. Bill must choose between participating in the adventure or refusing to participate. His need to belong, feel accepted, and be approved by members of his peer group is in conflict with his need for maintaining his standard of behavior, beliefs, and self-concept—"I am a person who does not do things that are wrong." Going along with the adventure requires lowering his standards of behavior, which is a threat to his beliefs, values, and self-concept. Opposing the proposed adventure involves risking his status with the group, which is a threat to his need to belong. Through no fault of his own, Bill is in a situation that requires a decision between two alternative actions, both of which threaten something he values.

Conflict Between Means

Conflict also exists when a goal can be reached in two or more ways. Mrs. P. has a chronic condition that causes her much discomfort. She usually relies on **analgesic** drugs, but more and more often she must have a **narcotic** to obtain full relief from pain. Her physician now warns her that continued use of drugs will have undesirable effects. He recommends surgery to correct her problem.

Mrs. P.'s goal of restored health requires choosing between habitual use of drugs and surgery. To be free of pain, she must use one means or the other. When Mrs. P. was a child, her oldest brother died during an operation. Since

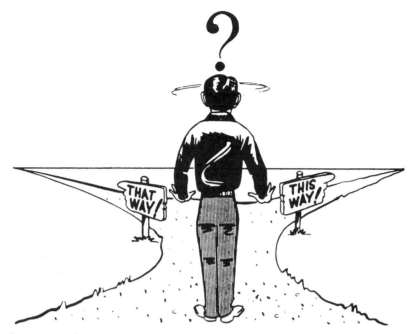

Inner conflict exists when one must choose between alternative means for meeting a need.

then, she has heard numerous stories about unsatisfactory surgical results, each one adding to her fear of surgery. Now, the thought of going to the operating room terrifies her, yet she desperately wants to be free of pain. To Mrs. P., with her deep-seated fear of the operating room, this conflict between two remedies for her health problem may be far more distressing than the physical discomfort associated with surgery.

TYPES OF INNER CONFLICT

Regardless of whether a conflict is between needs, goals, or the means for achieving them, the individual must choose between alternatives. These alternatives may be positive (desirable) or negative (undesirable). Even in a choice between two positives, unhappiness may result from giving up one alternative. The degree of difficulty in making a decision is often influenced by whether the alternatives are both positive, both negative, or positive accompanied by a negative outcome.

Approach-Approach Conflict—Two Desirable Goals

Approach-approach conflict involves two needs or goals that are incompatible. Al is working in the local hospital as a nursing assistant. He enjoys his work and is especially good with elderly patients. His supervisor calls him into the office and states that he has been recommended to the director of the practical nursing program. The supervisor points out the advantages of being a licensed nurse and indicates belief in Al's potential for succeeding in the program. Al is proud that the supervisor has so much faith in him. He is suddenly fired up with ambition to improve himself through educational preparation for a career.

When Al tells his girlfriend about his exciting opportunity, she says, "But how can we get married if you are not going to have any income for a year?" Al is eager to get married and has been carefully saving for the costs of setting up a home. Any delay in these plans will be just as disappointing to him as to his girlfriend.

Al has two goals, each of which he would like to reach as soon as possible. He is eager to get married, but he is also aware of the advantages of educational preparation for his job. He cannot get married immediately and, at the same time, enroll in the practical nursing course. Al has a conflict between two strong but incompatible needs—they cannot be met at the same time.

Approach-Avoidance Conflict—Desirable Goal With a Negative Effect

Phil is enrolled in a dental laboratory technology course. He is having difficulty developing some of the **manipulative** skills necessary for constructing dental **prostheses.** His teacher discusses the problem with him, emphasizing that he must spend more time on laboratory practice to develop the necessary **digital** skills. The only time Phil has for this extra practice is the period the basketball team practices. Phil is top scorer for the team.

Phil wants to pass his lab course, but to do so he has to miss basketball practice. To achieve his goal of becoming **proficient** as a dental laboratory technician, Phil has to accept the negative aspects of giving up his prized position on the team, of feeling he has been disloyal to the team, and of relinquishing an activity that gives him much satisfaction. Regardless of which choice he makes, Phil will lose something that he values.

Approach-avoidance conflict is a special type of conflict involving a desirable goal with undesirable effects. The individual **vacillates** between trying to reach a certain goal and abandoning the goal. The decision to abandon a goal usually occurs as the individual approaches achievement of the goal or when the time for a desired event approaches.

Betsy is a dental assistant who is engaged to Larry. Betsy gets along well with her parents. She especially likes her room, which she decorated and furnished during her first year as a "career woman." When she comes home from her job, mother has dinner ready. Betsy's only home responsibility is cleaning her own room. She is able to save a large portion of her paycheck. Getting married and moving into an apartment requires that Betsy give up these benefits of living with her parents. On the other hand, she loves her fiancé, wants her own home, and wants to have a family.

Betsy has set the wedding date several times. Repeatedly, when ordering the wedding announcements could not be delayed any longer, she has broken the engagement. Larry is persistent and has accepted each delay with good humor. But each time the date approaches for achieving her goal (getting married, having her own home, starting a family), Betsy develops intense negative feelings (anxiety? panic?) that she relieves by breaking off the engagement. Thus, she avoids achieving the goal that would involve giving up the advantages of living with her parents.

Avoidance-Avoidance Conflict—Two Negative Alternatives

Avoidance-avoidance conflict exists when an individual must choose between two alternatives, both of which will have a negative outcome. Carolyn is a student in a medical assistant program. Last week her best friend in the class broke an expensive piece of equipment and returned it to its storage case without reporting the breakage. Carolyn was present at the time, and her friend insisted that Carolyn promise not to tell anyone. Today, Carolyn learns that another student in the class has been blamed for the broken equipment and told to pay for it.

Carolyn has strong feelings about loyalty to friends. She also has strong feelings about keeping promises, honesty and truthfulness, and fair play. Carolyn knows who actually broke the equipment, but the guilty person refuses to report herself. Carolyn can break her promise to this friend and report the incident, or she can keep silent and permit an innocent person to take the blame. Carolyn's values are involved, yet either course of action will violate personal traits on which she places a high value. Carolyn's self-concept is also involved: she does not want to be a person who breaks promises, nor does she want to be a person who permits an injustice when she could prevent it. She has to choose between loyalty to her friend and her sense of fairness. She has to choose between telling the truth, which includes breaking a promise, and keeping silent, which involves **collaborating** with her friend in a dishonest situation. To maintain her self-concept, Carolyn needs to uphold these personal traits she values. Therefore, either alternative involves a threat to her self-concept. Regardless of which alternative she chooses, there will be negative effects.

How Carolyn handles this situation will probably be determined by her values. She must place a higher value on one set of traits than on the other in order to select an alternative. If she reports the breakage, then honesty and fair play assume a higher place in her value system than loyalty to friends and keeping promises.

Carolyn's behavior patterns will affect how she works through this conflict. She may put off a decision and, by her inaction, allow the wrong person to be blamed. She may project blame by saying to herself that it is her friend's responsibility to tell the truth. She may rationalize by telling herself it is not really her business. Which choice she makes and how she justifies that choice to herself will result from many years of forming behavior patterns to deal with unpleasant situations.

HOW TO DEAL WITH INNER CONFLICT

Exploring Emotional Aspects

Inner conflict may be handled effectively *only by making a decision between alternatives.* Obviously, the choice will be better if the individual recognizes that a conflict exists and identifies the competing needs or goals. Insofar as possible, the feelings and values related to the conflict should also be examined.

Suppose Ruth has cancelled her plans for marriage several times because her mother has a health crisis each time Ruth sets a wedding date. Strong emotional factors are involved: Ruth's love for her fiancé, her love for her mother, her fiancé's feelings about the delayed wedding, negative feelings toward her mother for being an obstacle, guilt feelings about having negative feelings toward her mother, feelings of loyalty, sense of duty to her parent, resentment and indignation at being deprived of living her own life, and many other feelings. Ruth, in order to use a rational approach to resolve this situation, needs to explore these feelings honestly to avoid letting any one emotion or value dominate her decision.

Thinking through a Conflict Situation

The following steps provide a rational approach to resolving a conflict:

- Recognize that there is a conflict.

- Identify the two incompatible needs (or goals).

- Examine the situation in terms of interests, values, immediate needs, long-term needs, and other relevant factors.

- Decide how each need could be met (or each goal achieved).

- Think through the probable effects of each possible action: what will be gained, what will be lost, and whether or not the action would be in accord with your beliefs, value system, interests, goals, and needs.

- After thorough consideration of the probable effects of each possible choice, make a decision.

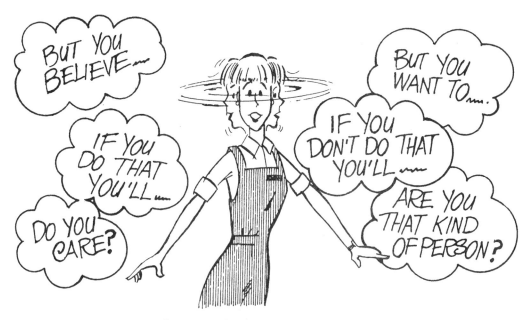

Inner conflict can only be resolved by making a choice.

- *Fully accept your decision.* One alternative has been selected; the other has been discarded. Do not flounder in doubt about whether the right choice was made. Set out to prove that you made a good decision. Do not develop feelings of guilt or failure about the alternative that was discarded. Remember: *A choice had to be made.*

Identifying Opportunity Cost

In business a concept known as "opportunity cost" may be used to assist in making decisions. This concept, when applied to inner conflict, can help the individual focus on presumed facts; by so doing, vague fears about alternative actions can be translated into information—the basis for a *rational*, rather than an *emotional*, decision. **Opportunity cost** refers to what one must give up (an opportunity) when choosing one course of action over another.

In resolving inner conflict, opportunity cost consists of what will be given up if action #1 is pursued, and what will be given up if action #2 is pursued. Opportunity cost may be the basis for anxiety about choosing either action. The cost of a specific decision, then, includes not only the obvious consequences of that decision, but also the opportunity cost involved in not following the other course of action.

Anita is working the night shift at Community Hospital; she needs to leave home by 10:15 to be on time for report. It is her birthday, but her husband still is not home at 9:00. She and her husband have only one car, and he knows she is scheduled to work tonight. She puts on her uniform so she will not have to dress after he does arrive. As she worries about why he is not home yet, she hears the car pull into the driveway. Her husband enters laughing, accompanied by Donna (his co-worker), Donna's husband, and a couple she does not know. They are carrying refreshments and exclaiming, "Happy birthday!" It is now 9:45.

Anita obtains glasses and ice for everyone, then explains that she must leave for work. She is greeted by a chorus of, "Oh, no! It's your birthday. We came to party." When Anita explains that she cannot stay and party, that she is needed at the hospital, her guests suggest, "Just call in sick. They'll never know you are having a birthday party." Leaving aside the matter of her husband's behavior, let us look at Anita's inner conflict. Should she stay home and enjoy these guests who want to give her a birthday party? Or should she go to work?

The *reward* of choosing to call in sick and stay home would be that Anita has a birthday party, enjoys socializing with friends, and becomes acquainted with the new couple. The *cost* of staying home would be that Anita uses a sick day she might need later. The *opportunity cost* of this choice could be a sense of guilt for lying to the supervisor and leaving her co-workers short-handed. Anita is conscientious; her self-esteem would be affected negatively if she fails in her duty. Possibly, her supervisor would learn that she is not sick, but stayed home to party.

The *reward* for choosing to go on duty as scheduled would be that Anita retains her self-respect, her self-esteem is not threatened; she does not harbor guilt about her behavior; she does not worry about the supervisor finding out that she lied about being sick; she does not feel guilty about leaving her co-workers to do double duty, and she does not risk hearing later that a patient did not receive some needed attention during the night. Also, Anita still has that sick day in reserve in case she needs it. The *cost* of not staying home to party was missing her own birthday party and the annoyance of her husband and the guests about her leaving. The *opportunity cost* was not having a chance to become acquainted with the new couple.

Note that identifying the rewards, costs, and opportunity costs of each alternative paves the way for a *rational,* rather than *emotional,* decision. So, adding the concept of opportunity cost to your problem-solving method can facilitate the resolution of a inner conflict.

INNER CONFLICT AND ADJUSTMENT

Common Reactions to Inner Conflict

The above approach illustrates the familiar saying, "You can't have your cake and eat it too." Even minor conflicts cause a certain amount of inner discomfort until they are resolved. If you put off doing an assignment in favor of more

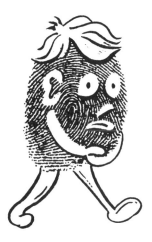

"I don't know what to do."

Many people react to an inner conflict with indecision. (From Carol D. Tamparo & Wilburta Q. Lindh, *Therapeutic Communication for Allied Health Professions.* Albany, NY: Delmar Publishers Inc., 1992.)

pleasant activities, you eventually reach the point of having to resolve the conflict. You must either decide to do the assignment instead of some preferred activity, or decide not to do the assignment and accept the consequences. You are probably a little uncomfortable as long as you continue to put off the decision.

Many people react to conflict by **indecision,** either procrastinating as long as possible or making one choice and then changing to another. Only a firm decision truly resolves a conflict. Sometimes the decision is necessarily accompanied by an unfavorable effect, either on oneself or on others. *The ideal result in handling conflict is to gain the desired goal with the least possible undesirable effect.*

Inner conflict contributes to poor adjustment in a number of ways. Some people are not able to recognize a conflict. They become upset over failure to gain some goal that actually is incompatible with other goals they are pursuing. Other people may be aware that a choice needs to be made but find it too difficult to face. Ruth, for example, knows she must choose between her mother and her fiancé: this is not an easy situation to resolve. She can choose to be the dutiful daugher and give up her plans for marriage, or she can choose to marry and hope her mother will accept this decision without permanent damage to their relationship. Ruth may continue to postpone her marriage repeatedly. Negative feelings may develop following either choice: guilt if she leaves her ailing mother or bitterness and resentment if she abandons plans for marriage.

INNER CONFLICT AND THE HEALTH CARE PROVIDER

As a health care provider, you can make good use of your understanding of conflict and its effects on behavior and emotional states. Health care providers frequently have inner conflict. The responsibilities of being a health care provider are great. Health care providers often possess confidential information. People tend to put health care providers into conflict situations by asking about patients or seeking health advice. The necessity for providing many health services on a 24-hour basis requires that some health care providers have a schedule different from that of their families. Staffing problems give rise to occasional changes in time off, sometimes on short notice. Urgent situations require working overtime, being "on call," or returning to work unexpectedly after putting in a full day's work.

The health care provider who is dedicated to serving others and has a strong sense of duty is likely to experience conflict between loyalty to the job and loyalty to the family. There may be occasions when there is a conflict between responsibilities and "rights" as a person.

Medical ethics and the policies of your place of employment can help you with some of these conflicts. For example, when a close friend asks about a patient, your *ethical responsibility* to hold in confidence what you learn about patients in the course of your job helps you resolve the conflict between responsibility and desire to have your friend's approval. At times, you may have to justify your *sense of duty* when job requirements interfere with plans involving family or friends. Thinking about such possible conflicts in advance can help you resolve them if they actually occur.

CONFLICT AND THE PATIENT

Many patients have inner conflict related to their illness. Mr. B. has orders for strict bedrest, yet he feels capable of returning to work. He has a conflict between his need for self-interest (perhaps self-preservation) and his need to fulfill his job responsibilities. Ms. J., who is having diagnostic studies, may have a conflict between the need for relief from distressing symptoms and the fear of learning something unfavorable as a result of the studies.

Family members, too, have inner conflict when decisions must be made. It is difficult to agree to painful procedures on someone you love; yet refusing permission for the procedure may contribute to continued illness or the loved one's death. The decision on whether or not to consent to surgery involves many emotions, including the possibility of guilt feelings if the outcome is unfavorable. An emotionally wrenching conflict for family members is a decision to discontinue life-support. Even if the patient's status fits the conditions specified in an Advance Directive, an inner conflict exists for each person involved in the decision. Some physicians try to protect families from decisions that may lead to guilt feelings. However, it is desirable that the family be involved in decisions about painful or **debilitating** treatments and the use of life-support systems for persons whose illness involves a hopeless **prognosis.**

USING KNOWLEDGE OF CONFLICT

As a health care provider, be aware that some of the distress you see in patients and their families is due to inner conflict. With such understanding, you are better able to accept behavior that appears unreasonable and accept emotional reactions that seem out of proportion to the seriousness of the illness. Be aware, too, that sometimes the physician has given the family or patient information that you do not have, such as an unfavorable prognosis.

Applying knowledge about inner conflict to your personal life can help you resolve conflict situations rationally to achieve the best possible outcome for you and your family. Applying your knowledge of inner conflict to relations with patients can help you be more understanding and more accepting of your patients and their families.

References and Suggested Readings

Branden, Nathaniel. *Taking Responsibility: Self-Reliance and the Accountable Life.* Edgartown, MA: S & S Trade, 1996.
Simon, Sidney B. *In Search of Values.* New York, NY: Warner Books, 1993.
Weeks, Dudley. *The Eight Essential Steps to Conflict Resolution.* New York, NY: J. P. Tarcher, 1994.

REVIEW AND SELF-CHECK

Complete each statement below, using information from Unit 12.

1. Inner conflict can be defined as a condition that exists when an individual _____ or _____ .

2. Some behavior influences that may be involved in an inner conflict are

   _____ , _____ .

   _____ and _____ .

3. Three types of inner conflict are _____ ,

   _____ and _____ .

4. Inner conflict can be handled only by _____ .

5. Steps for resolving an inner conflict are:

   1. _____

2. _____

3. _____

4. _____

5. _____

6. _____

7. _____

6. The ideal result in dealing with conflict is to _____ .

ASSIGNMENT

1. Refer to the previously described conflicts experienced by Al, Phil, Carolyn, or Ruth. Select one example and complete the following chart:
   a. What *values* does the individual probably have that should be considered in resolving the conflict? What strong *needs* does the individual probably have that should be considered in resolving the conflict? What *beliefs* does this individual seem to have? What are the two conflicting needs (or goals or means)? Indicate which example you are analyzing: Al ___ , Phil ___ , Carolyn ___ , Ruth ___

VALUES
NEEDS
BELIEFS
THE CONFLICTING NEEDS (GOALS, MEANS OF ACHIEVING A GOAL): 1. 2.

b. List two or more alternative actions that might resolve the conflict. Then anticipate the possible effects of each.

ACTIONS	EFFECTS	
	DESIRABLE	UNDESIRABLE

2. Consider one conflict you have had during the past month.
   a. Analyze this conflict in terms of the following:
      - your basic needs
      - goals that were incompatible
      - emotions you were experiencing
      - values involved
      - beliefs involved
   b. Describe how you handled the conflict.
   c. Describe the effects of your handling of this conflict.
   d. State two possible alternatives for resolving the conflict.
   e. In the light of your knowledge about inner conflict, how do you *now* think you should have handled this particular conflict? Justify your answer in terms of basic needs, value system, emotional effects, and short-term or long-term goals.

3. Refer to Carolyn's conflict situation and put yourself in Carolyn's place. You decide to talk to your co-worker about the broken equipment and your own feelings, including regret that you agreed to the promise your friend wanted from you. Describe the conditions under which you will initiate this conversation—certainly not during lunch! Next, write out what you will say:
   - Your opening statement
   - Key points you want to make
   - How you will respond if the co-worker insists you should keep your promise not to report her

- Statements you could make to encourage the co-worker to take responsibility for the broken equipment

NOTE: Your instructor may choose to schedule this situation for role-play during classtime.

4. Identify the opportunity cost involved in each of the following situations:
    a. Al decides to enter the Practical Nursing Education Program.
    b. Phil chooses to spend extra time in the lab.
    c. Betsy chooses to marry and move into an apartment.
    d. Carolyn chooses to report the co-worker.
    e. Ruth's sense of duty to her mother controls her decision, and she cancels her wedding plans.

5. You are on night duty; one of your patients, Mr. R, has an Advance Directive and a DNR order on his chart. Suddenly his wife rushes out of the room saying, "My husband has stopped breathing!" You automatically reach for the phone to call a Code. Then you remember the DNR; should you make the call?

6. Write out the meanings of the following, based on explanations in Unit 12; use a dictionary as necessary to clarify meanings.

Alternative	Incompatible	Proficient
Analgesic	Indecision	Prognosis
Collaborate	Manipulative (skill)	Prosthesis (dental)
Debilitating	Narcotic	Vacillate
Digital (skill)	Opportunity cost	

$\mathcal{U}nit$ 13

Frustration and Behavior

OBJECTIVES

Upon completion of this unit, you should be able to:

- Define frustration.
- Name four sources of frustration.
- List four environmental factors that could be sources of frustration.
- List five factors that could influence a person to obstruct another's goalseeking efforts.
- Explain prejudice as an obstacle for members of certain groups.
- Describe emotional reactions to frustration.
- Describe a general approach to dealing with frustration.
- List five guidelines for preventing unnecessary frustration in one's life.
- Use a systematic approach to study a specific situation in which frustration is occurring and make a rational decision about how to deal with it.

KEY TERMS

Aspirations	Attitude	Capabilities
Evoke	Frustration	Obstacle
Orientation	Rigor	Subtle

You are now aware that everyone experiences threats to adjustment at intervals and reacts to such threats according to learned patterns of behavior. A type of threat that tends to arouse negative emotions and **evoke** aggressive or defensive behavior is **frustration.** The effects of frustration on the individual and the tendency of the resulting behavior to be misunderstood by others can seriously interfere with interpersonal relations and adjustment.

MEANING OF FRUSTRATION

Frustration exists when progress toward a desired goal is blocked. Frustration is a threat to one's feelings of adequacy and can be an **obstacle** to reaching a goal. It is a common experience for all of us. How we react to frustration determines to a large extent whether or not we reach the desired goal.

Degrees of Frustration

Frustration may evoke irritation or a major emotional reaction. Minor frustrations occur almost daily. The car won't start when we are in a hurry; a pencil point breaks just as we begin a test; we miss the bus; someone keeps us waiting; a button pops off when we do not have time to sew it back on. Such experiences arouse feelings that range from annoyance to intense anger—these feelings are due to frustration.

Major frustrations usually involve larger aspects of living. A person whose job is not satisfying, has many job-related problems or has been passed by repeatedly for promotion—has frustrations in the workplace. A mother who wants a career but feels "trapped" by home responsibilities experiences frustration involving almost her total life situation.

Minor frustrations cause annoyance for a relatively short period of time, though a frustration encountered in the morning often sets the pattern of the day. On such days we are likely to comment, "I should have stayed in bed today." Major frustrations, however, may affect the individual's total personality—behavior patterns, values, beliefs, moods, attitudes, and general outlook on life. Major frustrations of long duration are incompatible with good adjustment.

Cumulative Effects of Frustration

Minor frustrations have great significance if they lead to a buildup of negative feelings, with sudden release over a seemingly minor incident. A series of frustrations during the day may be the underlying cause of Dad's explosion when Johnny asks for five dollars. Or, Dad may show his annoyance on Friday after giving Johnny one dollar every morning. Unknown to Johnny, his requests for money are frustrating Dad's effort to make his money hold out until payday. Knowing that Johnny has to have lunch money does not help Dad with his own frustration.

People differ in their tolerance for frustration. Some react emotionally whenever their goals are blocked, and others show the effects of frustration only when it is major. Most people react to minor or moderate frustration with some type of activity that resolves the problem; but when frustration is overwhelming, performance deteriorates.

SOURCES OF FRUSTRATION

Blocking of progress toward a goal can arise from many sources: personal characteristics, the environment, other people, or prejudice.

Self as a Source of Frustration

Frustration involves both needs and goals. Each of us is influenced by many different factors in setting our goals. Whether or not these goals are in accord with our own **capabilities** and the opportunities available to us has a bearing on the amount of frustration likely to occur.

As high school seniors, Jack and Paul shared an interest in the health field. Both boys discussed their futures with the guidance counselor, taking into consideration many types of information, including high school record, achievement and aptitude test scores, vocational interest surveys, personal interests, family finances, and other factors.

Paul's record indicated that he could probably be successful in college. Family finances were strained, and Paul did not like to think of four or more years of school. He liked the idea of becoming a laboratory assistant, so he enrolled in the nearby technical institute. After completing his course with honors, Paul accepted a position in the local hospital. Soon he asked the laboratory supervisor to teach him some of the complex procedures, but he was told that only the registered medical technologists were allowed to do these tests. Paul felt resentful and became increasingly hostile toward his co-workers. He felt he was quite capable of doing more than he was allowed to do. Paul had settled for objectives too low for his potential. As a result, he was frustrated in his job because he was not allowed to function like the more highly trained technologists. Yet, because of the expense and long-term preparation required to become a medical technologist, Paul did not set his goal in accordance with his demonstrated abilities.

On the other hand, Jack applied to a college, even though he had difficulty with high school subjects. The school counselor had encouraged Jack to plan vocational goals rather than academic ones. Jack's mother always said she wanted her son to be a doctor, so Jack had grown up with the idea of attending medical school. He refused to recognize evidence that he probably would not be able to handle the **rigor** of college courses. After failing three out of four courses at the university, Jack came home confused and upset about his failure. He had set his objectives too high, in spite of guidance that could have helped him plan more realistically.

Frustration, then, can result from trying to reach what is unreachable or from achieving unchallenging goals. It is not always easy to determine what is a realistic goal. A career goal should be carefully selected on the basis of all information available about the individual and occupations in which the person is interested. Career goals are extremely important to achievement, development of one's potential, job satisfaction, and ultimately, to adjustment, and happiness.

Goals are also involved in short-term aspects of living. To some youngsters, failure to make the Little League team is a shattering experience. Athletic ability is, to a great extent, based on physical characteristics and motor skills. If one's goal is to make the football team in spite of small physical build and limited stamina, then frustration is sure to occur. If one enjoys singing, the short-term goal of being accepted into the school chorus is probably realistic. On the other hand, the goal of becoming an opera star is realistic only for those few who have rare talent, resources to develop the talent, and the determination and perseverance to strive many years for that goal.

Goals are more realistic when related to what we enjoy and learn readily. Satisfaction is greater if goals continue to offer challenge. In measuring goal progress, it is better to compare yourself today with yourself in the past, rather than with other people. Thus, progress can be noted and a sense of achievement experienced. **Aspiring** to be "the best" in anything is more likely to lead to frustration than aspiring to "continue to improve."

Environment as a Source of Frustration

Environment—either physical or social—can be a source of frustration because of a lack of opportunities or resources and obstructions. The environment is less subject to control than one's goals and *aspirations.* Rain on the day of a picnic or lack of snow for skiing are frustrations one must learn to accept. The opportunities an environment offers should be considered in making long-range plans. If one elects to follow a career for which there is no locally available opportunity, frustration will occur unless resources can be made available or a move to another community can be arranged.

Sometimes the customs and practices of a community are the source of frustration. The health care provider who wants to improve health habits in a community must give careful consideration to the established beliefs, values, and customs of that community. Cultural aspects of the social environment may block efforts to change established practices.

Other People as a Source of Frustration

Many obstacles can be overcome through persistence, problem-solving techniques, or an approach that removes the obstacle or allows one to get around it. When the obstacle is a person, however, overcoming the obstacle is likely to be difficult.

Paul's laboratory supervisor was an obstacle to his learning advanced techniques, even though the supervisor was basing the decision on hospital policy, role differentiation, and Paul's lack of educational foundation for the judgments required by advanced procedures. For Ruth, whose mother did not want her daughter to leave her, the mother was an obstacle to marriage. Suppose Jack had been refused admission to college. Then, the admissions committee would constitute an obstacle to his attending college. If a man firmly believes "a woman's place is in the home," then his belief is an obstacle to his wife's having a career.

Many people who represent obstacles, and thereby contribute to someone's frustration, do so as a job responsibility. This is especially true of school admissions committees, personnel directors, teachers, supervisors, or anyone whose evaluation or judgment determines whether or not a person will have some specific opportunity.

In other cases, people are obstacles because of their beliefs, prejudices, attitudes, superior ability, dependency, and many other factors. When achieving a goal requires changing an **attitude** or belief of the person who is an obstacle, then the frustration is not likely to be overcome easily; people do not readily change their values and beliefs. In competition, the abilities of other persons determine whether or not an individual makes the team, wins a gold medal, or gets a promotion. When the obstacle is a competitor's superior ability then personal effort to surpass such ability is necessary to reach the goal. Members of minority groups are all too familiar with the obstacle represented by prejudice.

Illness as a Source of Frustration

Illness may cause either minor or major frustration, depending upon the duration of illness and the patient's life situation. A minor illness that lasts a few days may simply be an inconvenience, or possibly a welcome relief from the daily routine—a chance to stay home and take it easy. But even a minor illness can create intense frustration if it interferes with some important event.

If the illness is serious, or life-threatening, the patient experiences numerous frustrations. There may be a feeling of losing control of one's life. Suddenly someone else (i.e., doctors) are telling the patient what he or she must do. Often these mandates include major life changes: stop smoking, change jobs to minimize stress (or physical exertion or exposure to chemicals), stop playing tennis, eat fresh vegetables, do not eat red meat, stop drinking alcoholic beverages, stop drinking sodas, exercise at least 20 minutes every day, stay in bed a minimum of ten hours a day, have at least two rest periods, stay out of the sun between 11 a.m. and 3 p.m., agree to a course of chemotherapy (or radiation), go to such-and-such medical center for special tests or treatment. Whatever the mandate includes, it will have some impact on the patient's life-style. The significance of each thing that must be given up determines the degree of frustration. The specific treatment may also be a source of frustration, especially if there are side effects.

Frustration is experienced as anger. When you, as a health care provider, realize that a patient's behavior seems to be an expression of anger, consider what impact the illness is having on the patient's life. Show interest in the patient's life situation with an expression of caring and concern, such as, "I suppose this illness is really changing your life." If the patient is willing to talk about the effects, it will help to diffuse the anger. As you carry out your responsibilities for health care, be aware that the recipient of your services is a person who may be angry and/or sad about the losses involved as his or her life is being disrupted by illness.

Prejudice as a Source of Frustration

The Congress of the United States has attempted to remove prejudice as an obstacle to educational and job opportunities. Unfortunately, the passage of a law does not change deeply rooted beliefs or the behavior patterns of a lifetime. Yet, this legislation has increased awareness of the extent to which prejudice creates obstacles for women, minority groups, youth, elderly, handicapped, and those with low income. Such prejudices of employers and school officials continue to create obstacles for many people, but in more **subtle** ways than in the past. At this time, a person who has been discriminated against because of one of the conditions covered by equal rights legislation may petition the courts to remove the obstacle. Some professional groups and consumer advocate organizations provide legal assistance to people whose rights to equal opportunity have been violated.

Perhaps with increasing opportunities for various groups to work and learn together, there will be greater readiness to accept each person as an individual and judge each on the basis of personal attributes, rather than the group (age, religion, nationality, race, sex) affiliation. This ideal can serve as a guide for us as we strive to better ourselves and our environment.

EFFECTS OF FRUSTRATION

Each of us reacts to frustration according to patterns we have learned throughout life. These reactions, therefore, vary from one person to another, but they usually involve either hostile behavior or withdrawal. Frustration arouses negative emotions: fear, anger, disappointment, anxiety, resentment, or a combination of these. Both behavior and emotional reactions to frustration are

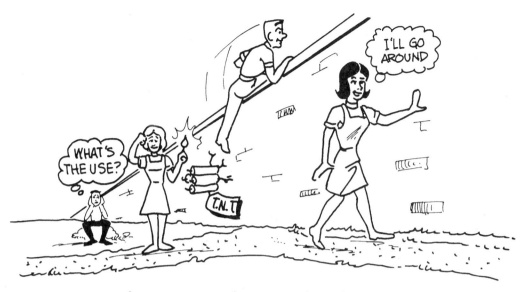

Each person reacts to frustration in his or her own way.

influenced by the importance attached to the goal as well as the individual's adjustment. A person who is insecure and inclined to perceive frustration as a threat is likely to feel a mixture of fear and anger. A person who is self-confident is likely to feel some degree of anger, with little fear. The person who is easily discouraged is likely to give up when there is an obstacle to success. Quitting, remember, is a form of withdrawal. The person who is stimulated to try harder in the face of difficulty is likely to react to an obstacle by increased effort or a change in strategy. Why should there be such extreme differences in reactions to frustration? The answer lies in those early learnings that influence the formation of behavior patterns.

FRUSTRATION AND BEHAVIOR PATTERNS

Early Learnings

Experience with frustration may begin almost with birth. The infant who is fed according to a rigid schedule, rather than when hungry, experiences frustration as well as the physical discomfort of hunger. Each developmental task (such as turning over, sitting, and standing) requires many efforts before success is realized. Early efforts to perform such activities are frustrating, but the infant persists until bodily control has been mastered. Many infants show distress when these early efforts result in failure.

Toddlers know what they want long before they can state their wants verbally. When a toddler is unable to make wants known, the reaction may involve falling to the floor, kicking, or crying. The child's frustration is due to inability to communicate verbally—a lack of competence for the task attempted. The parent who does not understand frustration may punish the child. Then the child feels anger as the result of frustration and fear as the result of punishment. Such experiences affect the child's learnings about frustration and also about the "right" to express feelings. The parent, without realizing it, is teaching the child that it is "wrong" to express negative feelings. This can be the beginning of ineffective patterns for dealing with frustration. It can also be the beginning of a pattern you have already learned as undesirable—suppression of emotions.

Childhood

During childhood, many frustrations result from the child's lack of competence for tasks being attempted, parental restraints, and rules at school, in clubs, and other organizations. Adults should make a conscious effort to help children understand the necessity for placing limits on behavior, especially where there are groups of children. Yet, even when the need for rules is understood, the child is frustrated when these limits interfere with a desired activity. If the frustration is great, the child may feel resentment toward the source of the rule— a parent, teacher, club sponsor, or whatever authority figure seems to be preventing some desired activity. If punishment is also involved, fear and distrust of authority figures may develop. Rebelliousness or hostility toward authority, beginning with such childhood experiences, may later interfere in relationships with authority figures such as supervisors in the job setting.

Adulthood

Adults experience frustration in many forms and in every aspect of living. For the majority of people, probably the most common frustration is lack of enough money to have the material possessions desired. The major adaptations required by marriage, parenthood, and a job all involve numerous frustrations. Even after one has learned to function within the various roles of adulthood, frustrations periodically occur in each role.

COPING WITH FRUSTRATION

You will experience frustration at intervals throughout life. This is a good time to evaluate your behavior patterns and decide whether you need to find new ways of dealing with frustration. By learning to handle frustration effectively, you can spare yourself much unhappiness and increase the proportion of satisfying experiences in your living.

There are numerous ways of dealing with frustration. The most desirable method of handling one particular frustration may be quite inappropriate for handling another. The general approach requires three steps:

1. Expect a certain amount of frustration in living and avoid overreacting emotionally or using defense mechanisms to avoid dealing with the problem.

2. Recognize frustration when it occurs.

3. When experiencing frustration, evaluate the total situation and use the systematic procedure described below to select an approach for dealing with the obstacle.

Effective Ways of Dealing with Frustration

There is no guaranteed way to overcome any and all obstacles. Recognize that the negative feelings of the moment are due to frustration, then use a rational approach to solve the problem at hand. The following questions can help in planning to overcome the obstacle:

- Exactly what goal am I trying to reach?

- What is preventing my reaching that goal? (Identify the obstacle.)

- How can I overcome or get around this obstacle? List *all* possible ways to deal with the obstacle.

- How is each possible solution likely to affect my achieving the goal?

- How is each possible solution likely to affect the way I feel about myself?

- How is each possible solution likely to affect other people?

- Is this *my* goal? Or, did someone else set this goal for me?

- Which solution is most likely to help me reach my goal?

- Is the goal important enough to me to justify the expenditures (time, effort, energy, money) required for reaching the goal?

- What other benefits (such as new competencies, widened experience, and future opportunities) am I likely to gain from continued efforts to achieve the goal?

- Shall I persist in striving for this goal? Or, shall I substitute another goal?

- Make a decision.
    a. If you decide to continue to strive for that goal, select a means for dealing with the obstacle and follow through with it.

  b. If it does not remove the obstacle, try another approach.

  c. If you decide not to continue to strive for that goal, modify the goal or substitute a different goal.

Preventing Frustration

It is also desirable to use a preventive approach to frustration. As illustrated by Jack and Paul, unrealistic goals can be the source of much frustration. If one sets unreachable goals, major frustration is inevitable. If one sets goals that offer too little challenge, especially if reaching that goal limits future goals, then frustration is inevitable. Goals should be realistic and yet sufficiently challenging to provide satisfaction when they are achieved.

  Long-term goals, such as preparing for a career, usually include numerous short-term goals. There may be many frustrating experiences before the long-term goal is reached. If the short-term goals provide stepping stones to be reached one by one, then frustration is offset by achievement of these intermediate goals.

  The philosopher Socrates once advised his students, "Know thyself." This is good advice to apply in setting one's goals. Striving to know yourself can also help you recognize sources of frustration within yourself. Does your behavior arouse negative feelings in others, which they then express by opposing you? Is your reaction to defeat so satisfying to others that they enjoy winning in a competition with you? In numerous ways, we create obstacles for ourselves. With a change in our own behavior, frustrations may be fewer.

  Lack of a particular skill for achieving a goal is an obvious obstacle. Sometimes it can be corrected by personal effort, but in some cases assistance from others is necessary. Undertaking a new activity is almost invariably frustrating during a period of **orientation.** Your courses that were frustrating at first become satisfying, rather than frustrating, as you acquire basic knowledge and develop skills. If you fail to acquire the necessary basic knowledge, then course assignments become more and more frustrating.

  The most important principle in preventing unnecessary frustration is to direct your living so that you succeed in achieving some of your goals. It is also desirable to know your environment and the people in it. You can change some things in the environment through your own efforts; others are beyond your ability to change. You can "win over" some of the people who obstruct you; however, a certain proportion will oppose you. When it is appropriate to make changes, and it is within your ability to do so, then make those changes in order to reach your goal. If you cannot change the situation, do not "burn out your bearings" trying to change what cannot be changed.

  As indicated above, many people create a certain amount of frustration for themselves, resulting from what they attempt to do. Frustration is involved in the very process of achieving. Some frustration is involved in dealing with the everyday problems of living. Frustration cannot be avoided, but we can learn not to create *unnecessary* frustration for ourselves. In that sense, we have some control over the amount of frustration we experience. Ultimately, however, our skill in coping with frustration influences the degree of satisfaction and happiness we experience in life.

References and Suggested Readings

Backer, Barbara A., Hannon, Natalie R., And Gregg, Joan Young. *To Listen, To Comfort, To Care.* Albany, NY: Delmar Publishers Inc., 1994.

Glass, Lillian. *Toxic People: Ten Ways of Dealing with People Who Make Your Life Miserable.* New York, NY: Simon & Schuster, 1995.

Kaufman, Barry Neil. *Happiness is a Choice.* New York, NY: Fawcett, 1991.

Potter-Efron, Ron and Potter-Efron, Pat. *Letting Go of Anger.* Oakland, CA: New Harbinger, 1995.

Taubman, Stan. *Ending the Struggle Against Yourself: A Workbook for Developing Self-Confidence and Self-Acceptance.* New York, NY: Putnam, 1994.

REVIEW AND SELF-CHECK

Complete each statement below, using information from Unit 13.

1. Frustration may be defined as a state that exists when _____ .

2. The feelings aroused by frustration range from _____

   to _____ .

3. Four sources of frustration are_____ , _____ ,

   _____ , and _____ .

4. Some personal factors that influence achievement of one's goals are

   _____ , _____ ,

   and _____ .

5. Some environmental factors that can be obstacles, thereby creating frustration, are _____ , _____ ,

   _____ , and _____ .

6. When people are obstacles to another person's goal achievement, it is usually because of their _____ , _____ , _____ , or _____ .

7. Groups most likely to experience prejudice as an obstacle include _____ , _____ , _____ , _____ , and _____ .

8. Emotions that may be aroused by frustration include _____ , _____ , _____ , _____ , and _____ .

9. Behavior and emotional reactions to frustration are influenced by _____ and _____ .

10. A general approach to dealing with frustration includes three steps:

   1. _____

   2. _____

   3. _____

11. Four guidelines for preventing some of life's frustrations are:

   1. _____

   2. _____

   3. _____

   4. _____

ASSIGNMENT

1. Your goal for a particular course is a "B." The examination is two weeks away. In the meantime, you have three laboratory reports and a term paper due. Develop a plan that will increase the probability of your feeling prepared for the exam and also completing the other assignments. Explain how your plan would minimize the frustration likely to occur.

2. Suppose you receive a "D" in that course, which means that you must make an "A" in the next course in order to graduate. Explain how each of the following might affect attaining that "A":

    a. Projecting negative feelings about your grade onto the subject matter of the course.

    b. Conflict between your need to study and your need for approval from friends who expect you to participate in the usual social activities.

    c. Hostile feelings toward the teacher.

    d. Use of a problem-solving approach to completing course requirements.

3. Look up each of the following words in a dictionary. Then write the meaning in your own words.

aspiration	dependency	nonverbal
attitude	evaluation	prejudice
competitor	evoke	verbal
manifestation	rigor	

4. You have a two-year-old male patient who is to be hospitalized for about a month. During the first days in the hospital, the child tries to talk to those caring for him, but no one can understand him. He frequently throws himself down in bed and kicks violently; sometimes he bangs his head on the crib.

    a. Explain the child's behavior.

    b. How should you as a health care provider react to this behavior?

    c. How could those in frequent contact with this child best help him?

    d. Describe this child's primary need.

    e. List some possible long-term effects on the child if health care providers

        (1) label the child "spoiled" and avoid the child whenever possible, or

        (2) make a sincere effort to understand what the child is trying to say.

5. You have accepted a well-paid position in a large health agency. Job descriptions have been written for each position. The job description for your position lists the procedures you will be permitted to do, omitting several that you learned in your health occupations course. You resent not being allowed to perform these procedures.

    a. What are some possible approaches to dealing with this situation? Describe each approach fully in terms of your goals, possible actions, possible effects of each action, and the solution you believe most likely to help you reach your goal.

    b. Contrast the probable outcome of each of the following actions:

        (1) Ignoring the job description and doing the procedures whenever you have a chance.

    (2) Accepting these restrictions without objection and functioning in a more limited role than that for which you are educationally prepared.

    (3) Functioning in a limited role but voicing your feelings about the restrictions at every opportunity.

    (4) Developing hostile feelings toward administrative personnel of the agency who, you believe, are responsible for restricting your role.

    (5) Quitting your job in protest over the restrictions.

6. Harriett is a graduate of a two-year Medical Office Assisting program. She began work at a large clinic immediately after graduation. This clinic has family practice physicians plus eight different specialists, its own laboratory and a physical therapy unit. As part of her orientation, Harriett worked for one week in each department and is now assigned to Patient Admissions and Intake. Her responsibilities include an interview and initial history, scheduling appointments with specific services, and setting up the new patient's chart. Most of the scheduling is done by telephone.

    There are frequent mix-ups in patients' appointments and other problems related to inter-departmental communications. Harriett is efficient and well-organized, but noticed during her rotation that some departments did not function efficiently. Some of the clerical personnel were careless about messages and viewed the paper work as a nuisance. Harriett believes that some relatively simple changes in procedure would improve communications and increase efficiency. She schedules an appointment with her supervisor and offers three suggestions; the supervisor nods and says she will "take care of it." A month passes with no changes in procedures. During her break today, a co-worker comments, "I hear you don't like the way we do things." Harriett is increasingly unhappy with her job, as the same problems occur time and again.

    Participate in a class discussion dealing with the following questions:

What is Harriett experiencing?
What are some possible ways of dealing with her feelings?
Why did the supervisor not implement the changes Harriett suggested?
  (Brainstorm to list all possible reasons.)
What actions might Harriett take to prevent these problems?
If conditions do not change and Harriett feels more and more unhappy about the problems, what are her options?

Striving to Become an Effective Health Care Provider

The technological advances of the health field tempt the health care provider to become absorbed in complex equipment and the details of technique. To the patient, however, the *social climate* that health care providers create has great importance. Each contact with a member of the health team affects the patient's peace of mind, emotional state, and outlook. *Scientific breakthroughs and sophisticated procedures cannot replace the human element in patient care.*

Section IV is designed to help you learn ways to promote a favorable outlook for the patient. Make it your aim to relate to each patient as a human being and develop your own personal technique for identifying patient needs. As you consciously learn to select the behavior that will promote favorable reactions in others, you will also be learning to enrich your personal living. Thus, you can grow not only as a health care provider, but also as a thoughtful, self-directing person, gaining increased satisfaction in living and at the same time enriching the lives of others.

Unit 14

Illness and Patient Behavior

OBJECTIVES

Upon completion of this unit, you should be able to:

- List six physical effects of illness.
- Name five possible emotional reactions to illness.
- List five behavior indications of a patient's emotional reaction to illness.
- List seven influences on a patient's reaction to illness.
- State six guidelines for providing effective care for a hospitalized child.

KEY TERMS

Counteract	Lethargy	Mind set
Incapacitated	Verbalize	Separation anxiety
Desertion reaction	Disguised	

Illness is always a threat to one's sense of security. Even a minor illness or injury is a threat to physical and emotional well-being. The pattern of life is disrupted. There is discomfort and inconvenience. The threat arouses feelings—perhaps fear, anger, or grief. These feelings are often manifested through the patient's behavior, but are not **verbalized.**

In other courses you are learning about specific illnesses: symptoms, diagnostic procedures, therapeutic techniques. Such knowledge is essential to safe and efficient performance as you provide patient care. Your *effectiveness* as a health care provider, however, is dependent upon your skill in applying knowledge about human behavior to relationships with patients. An effective health care provider/patient relationship promotes the patient's well-being. For one patient, reassurance in large amounts is needed to **counteract** fear and anxiety. For another patient, you may need to build confidence in the health team in order to gain the patient's cooperation in following the therapeutic plan.

Trying to provide a therapeutic atmosphere that is favorable for each patient is a never-ending challenge. Human variability is so great that no one method will serve for all patients. By applying your knowledge about human behavior and the effects of illness, you can become sensitive to patient behaviors and their possible significance in terms of mental and emotional needs.

PHYSICAL EFFECTS OF ILLNESS

Patients not only experience the signs and symptoms of a specific illness, but also various physical effects related to emotional reactions, change in daily routine, drugs, and numerous other factors. Examples of such general physical effects are fever, pain, nausea, lack of appetite, urinary problems, and difficulty with elimination. The overall effect may range from extreme **lethargy** to extreme restlessness. These general effects may be just as distressing to the patient as the symptoms of a specific illness. *The patient's complaints about general or vague effects should be noted.* These general symptoms may indicate either physical or emotional needs. Since interpretation may be beyond the scope of your role, report such complaints to your team leader or supervisor.

EMOTIONAL EFFECTS OF ILLNESS

Most people react to illness with some degree of negative emotion. These emotional reactions vary in type and intensity. Some patients are mildly annoyed at being sick; others are quite angry. Some patients are apprehensive; others are almost in a state of panic. Some feel somewhat sorry for themselves; while others react with pronounced self-pity. Some people feel bitter about their misfortune; bitterness is a combination of anger and self-pity.

Some patients readily verbalize their feelings. The patient who says, "Why me?" is probably expressing anger. The patient who says, "It seems as though everything happens to me!" is probably expressing self-pity. Obviously, the words alone do not carry the full message. Be alert for additional evidence about the patient's emotional reaction to illness: facial expression, tone of voice, body posture, choice of words, and emphasis given to certain words.

Negative feelings may also be expressed through *disguised* behavior. The patient who is very talkative may be covering up fear. The patient who is eager to please may be covering up fear, hostility, or other negative feelings. Such patients are just as much in need of understanding and interest from health care providers as those who verbalize their feelings. Do not make the mistake of thinking that the patient who is pleasant does not have fears and anxieties; for these patients, too, illness is a threat. *Each patient reacts to threat in a very individual way.*

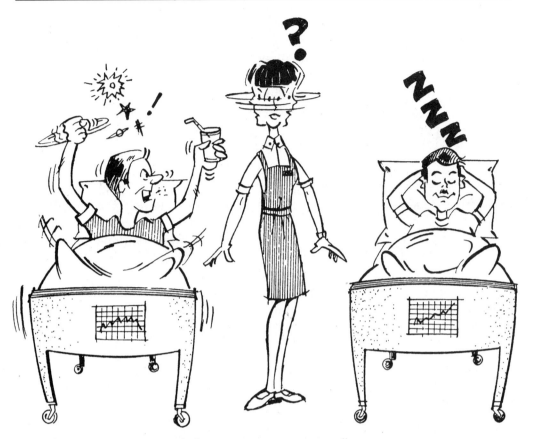

People have various reactions to illness.

GENERAL EFFECTS OF SERIOUS ILLNESS

During serious illness there is some depression of mental and emotional functioning. The individual's energy resources are being utilized to cope with the physical stress of illness. There is likely to be decreased awareness of surroundings and lessened concern about life problems. One exception to this is the patient with coronary occlusion. These patients often are alert, very much aware that life is hanging in the balance and, therefore, extremely fearful. A calm, interested, and caring manner on the part of health care providers is essential to provide these patients with emotional support, reassurance, and, hopefully, some relief from fear.

Sometimes a patient who has been very cooperative during the serious stage of illness shows a marked change in behavior as convalescence begins. Energy resources are no longer fully required for coping with physical demands. The patient is now more aware of discomfort. There is energy for emotional reactions and for conscious attention to symptoms and life problems. You may find it difficult to cope with this change in behavior, because you probably believe the patient should now exhibit a positive emotional state. Accept a patient's behavior as indicative of needs and problems, rather than condemning behavior because it is different from what you think it should be.

INFLUENCES ON PATIENTS' REACTIONS TO ILLNESS

As a health care provider, you will see situations involving pain, discomfort, disability, and even death. The atmosphere of the health agency is your work environment. The equipment you use daily has meaning to you in terms of its purpose. The clinical sights, smells, and sounds that are so familiar to you may be quite frightening to other people. The strangeness of the health agency, equipment, protective apparel, and procedures contribute greatly to the emotional reactions of some patients. Most patients will benefit from your taking time to explain a procedure and to answer questions, no matter how routine that procedure has become for you. By dealing with the strangeness of a situation and by helping the patient understand, you can have a positive influence on patient behavior. Be aware that numerous other influences may affect the behavior of a specific patient.

Childhood

Age influences patient reactions to illness, especially if the patient is at either extreme of the life span. The young child reacts to illness as a child, with all the characteristics of the stage of development, in addition to the child's fear of strange places, the discomfort of illness, and expectations developed from past experiences with health care providers.

Hospitalization may result in a "desertion reaction" or "separation anxiety," unless some member of the family stays with the child. **Desertion reaction** is a form of withdrawal in which the child retreats to a corner of the crib or curls up into the fetal position. The child is unresponsive when caregivers try to communicate. **Separation anxiety** is a type of panic reaction when the child realizes the parent is going to leave him or her in a strange place. A young child cannot understand the need for hospitalization; nor does a small child understand that he or she is not being abandoned and the family will return later. Because of these two common reactions of small children, most hospitals now allow, or even encourage, a member of the family to stay with a small child.

How to work effectively with sick children of various ages is a full course of study. By observing some general rules, however, you will improve your effectiveness with young patients. Accept each child according to their current stage of development. Allow the young patient to express feelings—do not suggest that a three-year-old "be brave" and not cry when something hurts. Do not expect cooperation from those who are too young to understand. Be aware that the child does not understand what is happening. Accept that the child is afraid. Remember that children often sense the feelings of adults. If you have negative feelings, the child is likely to sense your true feelings. Some child behavior is actually a reaction to the feelings of an adult.

As a health care provider, it is your task to win the child's confidence. *When a treatment or diagnostic procedure must be done, indicate that you accept the child's feelings and are sorry that he or she is having pain.* Be aware that any traumatic experience will influence the child's behavior throughout this illness, create negative feelings toward health care providers in general, and influence behavior in future illnesses.

Senescence

Most elderly people have great fear of becoming bedridden or otherwise losing their independence. For the senescent patient, any illness is especially threatening. This may be the illness that will render the patient helpless. An elderly patient may have greater anxiety than you think is justified by the particular illness. Such patients need your sincere interest and concern as they cope with the threat their illness represents.

Life Role

One's life role assumes great importance during illness. The mother with small children has anxiety about their care while she is **incapacitated.** Possibly, there is also anxiety about her ability to fulfill her responsibilities as a wife and mother. Her reaction to illness may be quite different from that of a woman with the same illness whose family is less dependent on her.

Occupational role also influences the degree of threat. Illness can seriously threaten job security; even if one's job is secure, there may be loss of income. Sick leave, salary continuation plans, whether or not one works on commission, whether or not insurance will help with the costs of illness—all influence the amount of anxiety the patient feels. If there is permanent disability, a change of occupation may be necessary. For most of your patients, you will not know the details of their life situation; hence, you cannot know what their worries are. You can, however, be sensitive to manifestations of anxiety, and you can listen when a patient indicates a need to talk.

Adjustment

The usual adjustment of a patient has much influence on reactions to illness. The patient who has a sense of security and usually copes with life problems

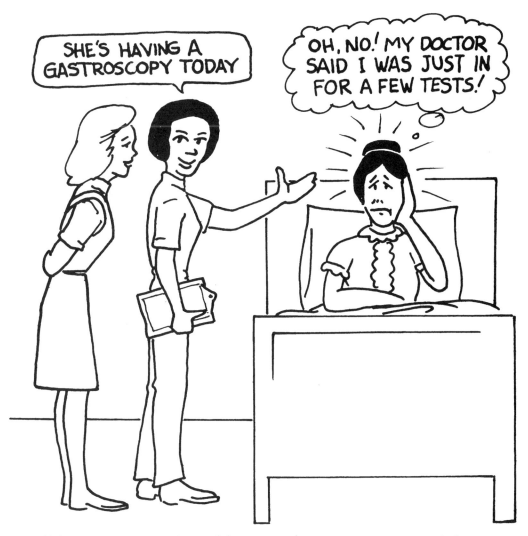

Help your patient to understand the situation by using appropriate vocabulary.

effectively is very likely to cope with illness effectively also, even though adjustment will not be as good as usual. *Even for the well-adjusted person, illness is accompanied by inconvenience and discomfort which alters the degree of adjustment.*

Those same personality traits and patterns of behavior that influence adjustment also influence how one reacts to illness. A person who is inclined to use defense mechanisms will continue this pattern during illness. The person who is inclined to find escape from unpleasantness will try to avoid facing the reality of illness. Sometimes the defense mechanisms fail the individual during illness; then, the patient may be unable to cope with the situation. When the usual patterns of coping fail, the individual may become fearful and may even panic. Patients who seem overly anxious may not know how to cope with illness.

Dependency

Some people are quite independent, in the sense of being self-reliant. Others are inclined to lean on someone else whenever possible. This trait is known as dependency. People who are extremely dependent may react to illness in a way that reflects this characteristic. It is expected that the sick be dependent on others; therefore, illness justifies dependency. During illness, *a dependent person* escapes the self-reliance normally expected of adults. Therefore, *unconsciously* wishing to prolong an illness, they find it difficult to admit they are improving. New complaints may be offered as evidence that they are still sick.

It is easy to be critical of such patients. Yet, if you had that patient's life problems, background, and patterns of behavior, then you would probably be using the same behavior pattern the patient is using. Instead of being critical, the health team should plan ways for such a patient to resume self-care progressively during convalescence.

Cultural Background

Another influence on patient reactions to illness is cultural background. The patient who is from a foreign country and has a poor command of English needs careful explanations to promote an understanding of instructions and to relieve fear. Sometimes it is desirable to have an interpreter present to be sure the patient understands. The patient whose religious beliefs influence diet and other practices needs assurance that the practices will be respected. The patient from a minority group may expect prejudice from caregivers. Efforts to show that they are accepted may even arouse suspicion. There is no room for prejudice in providing health care, however. Your philosophy of individual worth should guide you in providing quality care for each patient, regardless of cultural background.

Past Experience

Experience creates in each of us a "mind set" toward certain types of experience. **Mind set** influences how we perceive a situation. How we perceive the situation influences how we react. The patient who has had unfavorable experiences with sickness, health care providers, or health agencies is likely to perceive greater threat than a person who has not had such unfavorable experiences. The patient who has a mind set that health care providers are cold and impersonal may perceive coldness even in a friendly care provider. If the patient expects inefficient care, then examples of inefficiency will be found.

Evidence of defensiveness, distrust, hostility, or fear toward health care providers may indicate traumatic past experiences.

You cannot undo past damage quickly. Mind set is a fixed expectation that is not easily modified; it creates readiness to behave according to the *expectation,* rather than according to the specific situation. When you encounter a patient who seems to have had unfavorable experiences with health care providers, do not expect to establish rapport immediately. However, your efforts may be more effective than you realize and pave the way for new and more favorable attitudes in the future.

THE CHALLENGE FOR HEALTH CARE PROVIDERS

As a health care provider, you will sometimes be extremely busy performing all the procedures required to complete your assignment. Both time pressure and work load can be quite stressful. At such times you may tend to focus on task completion, rather than identifying patients' needs, being aware of patients' emotional reactions to their illnesses, and understanding that certain behaviors are reactions to illness. Actually, *giving your attention to human relations as you perform various procedures* will help you manage your own stress. You will be able to enjoy interacting with each patient and be less aware of job pressures.

Relating to the Patient

Practicing effective human relations is not time-consuming; it is a matter of *where you focus your attention.* Familiar procedures do not require a lot of concentration, so you can focus on relating to the patient while you carry out a procedure. If you do need to concentrate on the task, you can simply state to the patient, "I really need to focus on what I'm doing; we'll talk some more when I have finished."

Relating to your patients effectively requires certain attitudes: genuine concern for others, the belief that other people are important, and willingness to see a situation from the patient's point of view. Actually, these three attitudes are essential to feel empathy for another person. The care-giver who truly feels empathy for a patient is likely to be perceived by the patient as warm and caring.

Certain personal traits also contribute to effective relationships, especially sincerity, truthfulness, and honesty. In addition, behavior patterns affect relationships. Attentiveness, giving one's full attention to the patient, is absolutely necessary to convey caring and concern. Two health care providers who carry on a conversation with each other while performing a procedure on a patient are sending the message: "We are not really interested in you as a human

TABLE 14–1
Statements That Show Caring

ACTIVITY	EXAMPLES OF STATEMENTS TO PAIR WITH ACTIVITY
Bring something for the patient	"I brought you a book to read. It's one I thought you'd like."
Covering the patient with a blanket	"It feels chilly in here. Perhaps this blanket will help."
Assisting the patient to dress	"I really like that robe. It brings out your color," or "I noticed you're having a little trouble getting your robe on. Perhaps I can help."
Feeding the patient or serving a tray to the patient	"It's time to eat. I hope you're hungry because it really looks good."
Giving the patient a drink of water	"Here's some nice fresh water for you," or "I bet some nice cool water would taste good right now."
Offering the patient a chair	"You look tired. Why don't you sit down?"
Offering the patient assistance	"Here, let me help you. Perhaps together we can arrange these flowers."
Leaving a room	"Is there anything more I can do for you before I go?" or "I'm leaving now, but I'll be back in twenty minutes."
Moving the patient up in bed	"You look so uncomfortable. Let me move you up in bed."
Making the patient's bed	"There is nothing like a nice fresh bed, is there?" or "Now you have a nice fresh bed."
Regulating the temperature of the environment	"It seems very warm in here. Perhaps if I turn the air conditioner up, it will help."
Rubbing the patient's back	"A back rub always feels so good, doesn't it?"
Turning the patient in bed	"Changing position really makes a difference, doesn't it?"
Straightening a pillow	"Let me straighten your pillow for you," or "That ought to feel better now."

(From Natalie Kalman & Claire G. Waughfield, *Mental Health Concepts;* Third Edition. Delmar Publishers Inc., 1993.)

being. We are just here to do this task." Making eye contact at frequent intervals also conveys attentiveness. Have you ever tried to have a conversation with someone who looked over your shoulder or kept glancing around the room while you were talking? If so, you probably felt that the other person was not really interested in you or what you had to say. Probably the most important of all caring behaviors involves just "being there" when someone

TABLE 14-2
Reasons for Ineffective Communication

- The sender does not send the message he or she think he or she is sending.
- The receiver may not hear the message the sender intends.
- Verbal and nonverbal messages conflict.
- The message is disguised by the sender.
- Many English words have multiple meanings.
- The message is abstract and therefore confusing.
- The receiver is prepared to hear another message.

(From Natalie Kalman & Claire G. Waughfield, *Mental Health Concepts;* Third Edition. Delmar Publishers Inc., 1993.)

needs comfort and emotional support. Being there may or may not include conversation. It may involve simply taking the patient's hand in yours for a moment, or simply asking, "Do you need anything?"

Attitudes, personal traits, and behavior patterns all influence your effectiveness in relating to others. Effective communication, the subject of Units 17 and 18, is another essential component of effective human relations. The paragraphs below present key aspects of effective communication within the context of effective patient care.

Communicating with the Patient

Your purpose in communicating with a patient affects your communication style. Interviewing a patient to obtain information, instructing the patient in self-care, explaining a procedure or the patient's care plan, or conveying empathy are examples of different purposes that would require somewhat different approaches. Regardless of purpose, however, it is important to convey caring and concern for the patient. Communication includes both verbal and nonverbal messages, so you should become aware of your own communication style, especially your use of body language as you communicate verbally.

Spoken communication should make use of appropriate vocabulary for the patient's age, educational level, linguistic skills—the patient's ability to understand the message you wish to send. Enunciate clearly and speak loudly enough for the patient to hear. Look directly at the patient while speaking; one who has hearing problems may use lip-reading to supplement hearing. Make eye contact at frequent intervals. Be sensitive to the patient's desire to respond or ask questions.

When the patient does speak, *listen!* Look at the patient, not at the chart in your hand. Allow plenty of time for the patient to finish speaking; do not interrupt and do not use this time for cleaning the bedside table or filling the water pitcher. Follow up on statements that seem to signal unspoken concerns of the patient:

- "I'm not sure I understand what you mean by that."

- "Are you saying that . . . ?"

- "I sense that you are feeling . . . "

In responding to the patient, convey respect for what the patient has said, but tactfully correct any errors or apparent misunderstandings. If the patient has a complaint, listen respectfully without becoming defensive. If you can resolve the complaint, do so; otherwise, assure the patient that you will inform the appropriate person of the complaint. Then check back with the patient after a reasonable period of time to see if the problem has been corrected. It is especially desirable to avoid the types of statement that tend to shut-off communication, as shown in Table 14–3.

In talking with patients whose diagnosis is serious or life-threatening, avoid statements that offer false hope. It is very easy to say, "Now don't you worry. I'm sure everything will be all right." This type of statement may make you feel better, but it conveys to the patient that you do not want to hear his or her concerns and fears. This type of situation calls for effective listening, in which your comments encourage the patient to continue to talk. In Units 17 and 18, you will have the opportunity to practice communication skills, both nonverbal and verbal.

So, the ongoing challenge throughout your career as a health care provider will be to practice effective human relations, including clear communication, as an essential part of your overall performance.

References and Suggested Readings

Anderson, Carolyn. *Patient Teaching & Communicating in An Information Age.* Albany, NY: Delmar Publishers Inc., 1990. Chapter 2: "Purposes of Nurse-Patient Communication," pp. 35–36; "Trust in Nurse-Patient Relationships," pp. 36–38; "Empathic Components in Nurse-Patient Relationships," pp. 38–40; "Listening Behaviors to Promote Effective Communication," pp. 40–45; "Building a Helping Relationship," pp. 45–47.

Kalman, Natalie & Waughfield, Claire G. *Mental Health Concepts;* Third Edition. Albany, NY: Delmar Publishers Inc., 1993. Chapter 7: "Attitudes that Affect Communication," pp. 141–149; "Purpose of Communication," pp. 137–138; "Ineffective Communication," pp. 136–137; "Blocks to Communication," pp. 140–141.

TABLE 14–3
Communication Blocks

TECHNIQUE	EXPLANATION	EXAMPLE
Belittling	statement which tends to make light of the patient's beliefs or fears	Patient: "I won't leave here alive." Nurse: "That's ridiculous. You shouldn't even think that way."
Disagreeing	response indicating that the nurse believes the patient to be incorrect; generally relates to the cognitive rather than the affective message	Patient: "Why am I here? Nothing is being done for me and I'm not getting any better." Nurse: "You are getting better."
Defending	statement used to repel a verbal attack	Patient: "I had my light on for fifteen minutes." Nurse: "I am doing the best I can. You are not the only patient I have."
Stereotyped statement	common statement made without sincerity	Patient: "I am really worried about the children. I came to the hospital so quickly and I didn't get to see them. They just won't understand. I wish I could have talked to them" Nurse: "I know exactly what you are going through."
Changing the subject	different subject introduced to prevent talking about a topic that causes anxiety	Patient: "They are doing a biopsy tomorrow. I hope it isn't cancer." Nurse: "Are these your children? That's such a nice looking family."
Reassuring cliché	reassuring statement that is not sincere	Patient: "What will I do if it is malignant?" Nurse: "Don't you worry. Everything will be all right."
Giving advice	statement telling the patient what the nurse thinks the patient should do	Patient: "I broke my arm when I fell off a skateboard." Nurse: "At your age, I would suggest you give up skateboards."
Agreeing	statement showing that the nurse believes the patient's cognitive message is correct; may not be the patient's real concern	Patient: "I am afraid the doctor won't discharge me tomorrow." Nurse: "I am sure you are correct. I doubt he will let you go home so soon."

(From Natalie Kalman & Claire G. Waughfield, *Mental Health Concepts;* Third Edition. Delmar Publishers Inc., 1993.)

REVIEW AND SELF-CHECK

Complete each statement below, using information from Unit 14.

1. In addition to the signs and symptoms of a specific illness, a patient may experience other physical effects, such as _____ ,

   _____ , _____

   _____ , _____ , and _____ .

2. Emotional reactions to illness vary in type and intensity. Examples of the range of such feelings include

   From _____ to _____ ;

   From _____ to _____ ;

   From _____ to _____ .

3. Some behaviors that may reveal a patient's emotional reaction to illness are _____ , _____

   _____ , _____ , and _____ .

4. Some of the factors that influence a patient's reaction to illness are:

   _____

   _____

   _____

   _____

5. Desertion reaction refers to the tendency of small children to _____

   _____ .

6. Separation anxiety refers to a small child's reaction to _____ .

7. Some general rules for improving a health care provider's effectiveness with young patients are:

   _____

   _____

   _____

   _____

ASSIGNMENT

1. Consider some past illness you have experienced. Describe your reactions to this illness in terms of the following:
   a. perception of threat
   b. emotional effects
   c. physical discomfort
   d. your behavior when you were uncomfortable
   e. inconvenience of the illness
   f. effects on your daily habits
   g. effects on your state of adjustment
   h. patterns of behavior you used to cope with the illness
   i. influence of one or more personality traits on how you reacted to illness
   j. expectations or mind set that affected your relationship with those caring for you

   NOTE: Reactions to illness occur even if the illness is a minor one. If you have never had any illness that could provide a basis for this assignment, interview a friend or member of your family who has had a recent illness.

2. You have been having annoying symptoms for several months. Then a new symptom appears—one that you know is a warning sign of cancer. When you consult your physician, he recommends hospitalization for diagnostic studies. Picture yourself on admission to the hospital. Using "a" through "j" in assignment one, think through the reactions you might have under these circumstances.

3. As a health care provider, you probably would react somewhat differently from a lay person when you have a potentially serious illness. How is being a health care provider an advantage? How is being a health care provider a disadvantage?

4. It has been said that doctors and nurses make "poor" patients. Why?

5. Your neighbor comes to you to talk about her recent experiences with diagnostic studies. She states, "The doctor says there is nothing physically wrong. He says I should stop being so nervous. I don't know what he means." How could you help this neighbor understand what the doctor means, without exceeding your role as a health care provider?

6. A member of your family has a disorder that can only be treated by extensive life-style changes. List specific suggestions for helping this relative make the necessary changes.

7. A friend informs you that her husband has a malignancy and describes some changes in his behavior. How could you help her to understand her husband's behavior?

8. You are assigned to a patient whose treatment includes bedrest. As you prepare to give a bedbath, you put on gloves. The patient says angrily, "Am I so dirty that you can't touch me with your bare hands?" How will you respond?

$\mathcal{U}\textit{nit}$ 15

Coping with Patient Behavior

OBJECTIVES

Upon completion of this unit, you should be able to:

- State the primary requirement for improving one's interpersonal relations.
- List and explain eight guidelines for improving health care provider/patient relations.
- List nine behavior patterns commonly manifested by patients.
- Recognize manifestations of emotional reactions to illness.
- Convey acceptance, concern, and willingness to listen.
- List five communication techniques that can be used to make appropriate responses to patients.
- React appropriately to nine common behavior reactions to illness.

KEY TERMS

Aggression	Antagonize	Covert
Disoriented	Egocentric	Individualistic
Inebriated	Psychotic	Overt
Passive aggression	Valid	Regression
Reverting		

Behavior is highly **individualistic.** Each person has typical patterns of behavior for various types of situations. Each person has specific patterns for reacting to stress, including the stress of illness. Do not expect to know exactly why each person behaves in a certain way. You can, however, be aware of *possible* reasons for behavior and thus be more accepting of whatever behavior the patient does exhibit. Through such understanding, you can avoid a judgmental attitude toward your patients, thus eliminating one big obstacle to effective relationships.

It is the purpose of this unit to provide some guidelines for forming effective relationships. Recognize, though, that learning to form effective relationships does not come from reading a book or even from completing a course of study. Such learning begins with knowledge and understanding of human behavior, *but skill in interpersonal relations comes through a conscious effort to apply your knowledge and understanding to every relationship with another person—at work, at home, and in all activities involving other people.*

With experience, you can develop sensitivity to the feelings behind specific types of behavior. Once you begin to develop this sensitivity, you can strive to adapt your own behavior to each patient, in an effort to provide the kind of relationship that promotes the patient's well-being. The following guidelines describe ways to improve your relationships with patients.

GENERAL GUIDELINES

Accepting the Patient

Each patient needs to feel approval and acceptance by providers of health care. Many patients are quite sensitive to any evidence of irritation, impatience, indifference, or hostility on the part of a health care provider. Accepting each and every patient may require effort, because each of us has some prejudice or lack of understanding toward those who are different from ourselves. Through increased experience with a wide variety of people, you can grow in understanding of others—provided you avoid a critical or judgmental attitude. This is the key to learning to accept others—*recognize that other people are like you in many ways, even though different in other ways.*

Accepting someone includes accepting that person's behavior—even if it is not pleasant. There may be good reason for a patient's irritability or criticism. It is not realistic to expect everyone to be pleasant all of the time; such an expectation is especially unrealistic in regard to people who are sick.

Occasionally, a patient's behavior *is* unacceptable. Then, without showing anger or fear, the health care provider can use an "I" statement to indicate that such behavior is unacceptable. If the behavior is repeated after limits have been set, the supervisor should be consulted. Obviously, with patients who are **inebriated, disoriented, psychotic,** or otherwise irresponsible, it is more difficult to obtain cooperation in observing limits.

Showing Interest and Concern

While you are caring for a patient, give that patient your full attention. Address the patient by name, listen, respond appropriately, and show willingness to act on any requests. In many situations, hospital routine requires that things be done at a certain time; usually, an explanation will gain the patient's

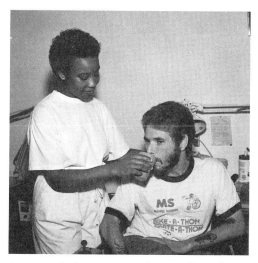 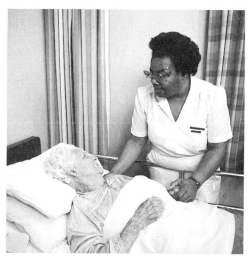

You can help patients adjust to their illness by showing acceptance, caring, and concern.

cooperation. In other situations, health care providers unnecessarily force patients into a routine. If a patient customarily bathes at bedtime, why insist upon a morning bath while in the hospital? Some patients deeply resent unnecessary interruptions or changes in their daily routine. Before insisting that such patients conform to the usual hospital routine, be sure that such insistence is *really necessary.*

Listening and Observing

The patient who has fears and anxieties can benefit from talking out these feelings. Most patients, however, do not readily "open up." Be sensitive to subtle indications that something is bothering the patient. Linger in the patient's unit to chat casually and respond to any hint of anxiety by showing interest in how the patient feels. Be available as an interested listener. A patient's readiness to express feelings to you is, in a sense, a test of the effectiveness of your relationship with that patient. Usually acceptance, demonstrated interest, and concern pave the way for a patient to express fears, anxieties, and uncertainties.

Recognizing Significant Behavior

Nonverbal behavior often provides a clue to the patient's feelings. Nervous movements, restlessness, unwillingness to participate in conversation, and many other behavior indicators of inner feelings signal that a patient needs extra attention.

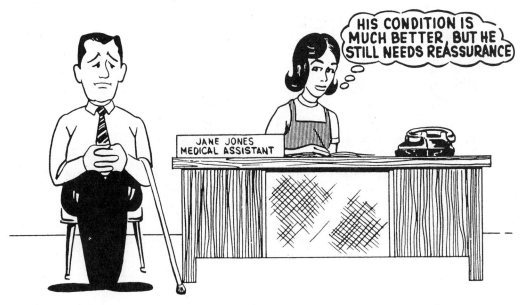

Observation of behavior can help you recognize a patient's needs.

The patient who states, "My doctor says I should have surgery," is probably signaling a need to talk about it. You can shut off conversation, or you can encourage it by your response. Saying, "I know that. I took your preoperative orders from the doctor," may be interpreted by the patient to mean, "This health care provider doesn't care how scared I am." On the other hand, if you respond, "How do you feel about having surgery?" or "The thought of having surgery is disturbing," the patient is more likely to verbalize feelings about the impending surgery.

When you encourage patients to express feelings, you are providing a valuable service. A patient may gain far more from verbalizing anxieties than from taking a tranquilizer.

Using Appropriate Responses

When patients make "loaded statements," it is usually effective to repeat what the patient has said, using essentially the same words but with a questioning inflection. This type of response, known as *echoing*, is a safe response; it does not give information, and it does not show your reaction to what the patient said. It merely says to the patient that you heard; the rising inflection in your voice implies, "Please continue. I am listening." Some patients will not understand the meaning of the rising inflection and simply be annoyed by your use of echoing.

It is good to have a range of communication techniques so you can use the most appropriate one for a particular situation. Some other useful techniques are: reflecting, clarifying, validating, questioning, and confronting. *Reflecting* is similar to echoing, but requires that you restate what the patient said, indicating that you have heard the message and are aware of the patient's feelings. Your response may begin with a phrase such as, "it sounds like . . . " or "it seems like you . . ."; this type of response is also called *mirroring*. When you use reflecting, you are essentially providing a mirror for the patient to view what he or she just said. The patient then has an opportunity to confirm, deny, or modify the meaning of the comment.

Clarifying is a technique used to test your interpretation of what has been said. After stating something like, "Let me see if I understand what you mean," you state the message, as you understand it, in your own words. The speaker can then confirm or deny that you understand the intended meaning. This may require several repetitions before the speaker will agree that you understand the message.

Validating is a technique used to check the meaning of certain nonverbal behaviors of the speaker. Often, the spoken message conveys one meaning, but certain nonverbal clues indicate a different meaning or indicate that the speaker's emotional state is different from what the verbal message implies. The technique for validating involves such statements as, "I sense that . . . " followed by a description of a feeling state, or "I notice that . . . " followed by an observation of some behavior, posture, or facial expression. This technique invites the patient to express feelings, doubts, anxieties, worries, annoyances, and frustrations.

Questioning is often required in the performance of patient care, usually to obtain specific information. Questioning can also be used as a therapeutic tool and as a means of avoiding a misunderstanding. Questioning should be done with a caring attitude. It is better to ask only one question, allow time for the patient to answer, then converse briefly before asking another question. It is especially important that you *listen* while the patient responds and allow the patient to finish before you speak again.

Confronting is a technique that challenges the patient's statement. It must be done in a calm and friendly manner, not in the adversary manner associated with the word "confrontation." Confronting can be used to clarify a message discrepancy (verbal/nonverbal), challenge a belief, or examine an attitude that may block effective therapy. A summary of these five communication techniques is shown in Table 15–1.

TABLE 15–1
Techniques of Helpful Communication

TECHNIQUE	EXPLANATION	EXAMPLE
Validation	a statement which attempts to verify the nurse's perception of the patient's message in both content and feeling areas	"You really look distressed. Something must be wrong."
Clarification	a statement used to clear up possible misunderstandings or to seek information necessary for understanding	"If I understand you correctly, you are upset because your daughter has just told you she is getting married."
Reflection	stating the nurse's perception of the patient's message in both content and feeling areas	"You are afraid you won't be needed after your daughter marries."
Broad questions	questions used to encourage the patient to talk	"Would you like to tell me about it?"
Confrontation	attack on the patient's belief in an attempt to get the patient to rethink his or her ideas	"What proof do you have that your daughter is making a mistake?"

(From Natalie Kalman & Claire G. Waughfield, *Mental Health Concepts;* Third Edition. Delmar Publishers Inc., 1993.)

Maintaining Confidentiality

Ethics require that you hold in confidence some information revealed by patients. An exception is information *relevant to the patient's well-being.* For this reason, it is unwise to commit yourself to promises. If a patient offers to tell you something that requires a promise "not to tell," do not be flattered that the patient wants to share a secret. Even more important, do not make such a promise. Simply state, "Whatever I learn about a patient is kept in confidence, unless the patient's well-being requires that I share the information with the health care team." Then, indicate that you are listening if the patient wishes to talk.

Suppose you made such a promise to Mr. Zel, a very personable young man who has been admitted to the hospital with a possible bleeding ulcer. After extracting a promise of secrecy from you, he confides that his brother is bringing clothes tonight, and they are going to slip out of the hospital and "hit the bars." What should you do, once you know that his "secret" involves a plan that would be harmful to Mr. Zel? Should you break your word and report his plan to your supervisor? Should you keep your word and not tell his secret? Suppose he really does slip out of the hospital? Suppose you report his plan;

when your supervisor confronts him, he denies everything. The next time you enter the room, he says, "Well, your word isn't worth a wooden nickel. How does it feel, being a traitor?" Avoiding any promise of secrecy can prevent getting caught in such a trap.

Being Sensitive to Feelings

Unpleasant behavior is usually due to a negative emotional state, ignorance, or an unfavorable attitude. Few people are "mean" in the sense of gaining satisfaction from being unpleasant.

When patients behave in undesirable ways, it is almost always the result of inner feelings. These feelings affect the patient's well-being. *Whenever you encourage a patient to adopt a positive, realistic outlook, you contribute to that patient's well-being.* Negative feelings indicate a need. Try to identify the need and respond appropriately.

Striving to Identify Patient Needs

Any behavior that may indicate a negative emotional state should signal to the health team that the patient needs additional attention. All too often, such behavior results in the patient being labeled "difficult," and the patient is avoided as much as possible. The health care provider who labels a patient with an unflattering term (i.e., "impossible") demonstrates ignorance of needs and lack of caring about that patient.

For experienced health care providers who have mastered the routine procedures and techniques, the real challenge of patient care lies in identifying needs of patients and establishing a therapeutic caregiver/patient relationship. The patient's behavior provides the clues for identifying a need. Once identified, a need may require medical intervention, but many patient needs can be met through nursing interventions.

Mrs. K. was in a room at the end of the hall, many steps away from the nurses' station. She turned on her call light every few minutes. Sometimes, the person who answered her call could not return to the desk before Mrs. K. had her light on again. The staff was irritated about the extra mileage being walked to take care of trivial requests. Sunday morning, Roberta had a few minutes before giving out medications, so she went—unsummoned—to Mrs. K.'s room. She found little things to do for Mrs. K., rearranged her flowers, and showed interest and concern. It was about an hour before Mrs. K. turned on her call light again. As other members of the nursing team spent more time with her, Mrs. K. volunteered the information that a neighbor, who had recently been discharged from the hospital, told her, "It is impossible to get any attention in the hospital." Mrs. K. feared she would not be able to get a nurse if she needed one. When the staff demonstrated interest and showed that they were available, Mrs. K.'s fear was relieved and she no longer made excessive demands.

Being Willing to Serve Patients

Linda was a student in the dietary aide program. She noticed that one patient always asked for several things to be done each time she carried a tray in. Linda was increasingly irritated since it was not her responsibility to "wait on" the patient. She decided to get in and out of the room before the patient could ask her to do something. She was still asked to do things, in spite of her great haste. When she mentioned this to the head nurse, she was told, "Never appear to be in a hurry. Never talk about how busy the staff is. This makes some patients think they must ask for things while someone is in the room, for fear help will not be available later."

Linda then tried walking into the patient's room in a leisurely way, putting the tray in position and then asking, "Is there anything I can do for you?" The surprised patient answered, "No, I can't think of anything."

Linda's haste in getting out of the room had contributed to the patient's anxiety and distress. Linda found that she could complete her assignment just as quickly by appearing calm and unrushed as by dashing in and out of patients' units.

COMMON BEHAVIOR PATTERNS OF PATIENTS

Egocentrism

Most people become **egocentric** during illness. This means that the patient becomes self-centered—the primary concern is with self. Much of the demanding behavior that health care providers (and families) resent in patients is actually a manifestation of the egocentric reaction to illness. In the extreme, this type of behavior can test your acceptance of the patient, yet egocentrism is just as much a reaction to illness as physical symptoms. If you accept egocentrism as a reaction to illness, you will find it easier to tolerate a patient's self-centered behavior.

Regression

Regression, another common reaction to illness, involves **reverting** to behaviors that are appropriate to an earlier level of development. The most extreme form of regression is lying in the fetal position and not responding to one's surroundings. This is often seen in elderly patients who have been bedfast for a long period of time.

In the home, a young child may regress when a new baby arrives. For example, a toddler who has mastered drinking from a cup may ask for a bottle.

Many examples of regression can be seen with patients of all ages. Dependence on others for personal care, when one is capable of self-care, is an example of regression. Understanding regression as a common reaction to illness can help you avoid impatience and a judgmental attitude toward a patient who exhibits regressive behavior.

Unfriendly Behavior

Place yourself in the following situation. Today you are assigned to Mr. A., who is totally indifferent to all your efforts to be pleasant. You feel annoyed and wonder why you are wasting good cheer on this cold, unfriendly person.

Then you tell yourself that there may be reasons for Mr. A.'s behavior. Your thoughts run through some of the possible reasons. "Maybe Mr. A. fears his illness, but he does not want me to know he is frightened. Perhaps he does not admit to himself that he is frightened. He may have had unfavorable experiences with health care providers and is transferring hostility from his previous experiences to me. Perhaps his unfriendliness is a form of **passive aggression.** On the other hand, he may perceive health care providers as cold, indifferent, unsympathetic, or incapable of understanding how he feels."

If you are really trying to understand Mr. A.'s behavior, your thoughts might be: "My behavior may have annoyed Mr. A. Was I too cheerful when he felt there was nothing to be cheerful about? Maybe he just wants to be left alone! I should accept him and acknowledge his right to behave according to his present feelings. I will not perceive his lack of responsiveness as a personal affront."

There is no one way to cope with an unfriendly patient. Every person reacts as an individual and may or may not be aware of the reaction or its effects on other people. Do not allow unfriendliness to affect your own mood. Accept it for what it is, namely, a manifestation of how the patient feels at the moment. Maintain your own pleasant manner. Continue to show interest and concern. Visit the patient's room at intervals, but not so frequently that you are an annoyance. Sometimes your efforts will pay off without your knowing. The patient will be aware of your interest and this, in itself, will contribute to a sense of well-being. Sometimes your persistence pays off—your sincerity and interest lead to trust and the patient begins to respond to you.

Aggressive Behavior

Aggression, a form of behavior that usually indicates hostility, may be physical or verbal. Physical aggression is most likely to occur if the patient is a child, is emotionally or mentally disturbed, is inebriated or in an irresponsible state. A simple aggressive act such as pushing your hand away may indicate fear, anger, or other negative emotional reactions to you or to what you are planning to do. It may be an effort at self-defense. If the aggression is more serious—an actual attack on you, for example—you must handle the situation as best you can to avoid being hurt and then summon help from a professional worker. *Since there are legal and ethical implications in handling aggression, avoid any action that could result in your being accused of assault on the patient.* Therefore, protect yourself from injury, but secure the assistance of your supervisor as quickly as possible.

A child is likely to use physical aggression defensively, due to the expectation of pain. The child's age, condition, and other factors determine the best way to handle aggressive behavior. If you are in doubt about how to work with a particular child, discuss the problem with the pediatric supervisor and obtain specific instructions. Your general approach, however, must include an accepting attitude. Never say to a child, "You are bad." Instead, tell the child you cannot accept kicking, biting, or whatever form the aggression is taking. Set limits to the behaviors you will accept. Even if the child does not respect these limits (i.e., no more kicking), he or she will understand why you are using restraints during a procedure. When you have finished working with the child, demonstrate acceptance with friendly behavior. Keep in mind that the child who fights you is manifesting an intense emotional state.

With adults, aggressive behavior is usually in the form of verbal attack or resistance. Verbal aggression may involve criticism, loud talking, profanity, or arguing. If the patient is critical, listen to the complaint and how it is described. If there is a valid complaint, corrective steps should be taken immediately. If the complaint does not seem to be **valid,** consider the complaint to be an expression of feelings. Arguing may be a disguised request for an explanation: the patient is challenging you to justify some aspect of the therapeutic plan, some policy of the health agency, or some procedure.

Passive aggression, on the other hand, is likely to consist of overt or covert noncooperation. In **overt** noncooperation, the patient balks—refuses to take medicine, accept a treatment, undergo a diagnostic procedure, or carry out some self-help routine. **Covert** noncooperation involves deceit. The patient wants the health team to think he or she is cooperating, but actually is not. Patients who ask that their medication be left on the bedside table ("I'll take it later") may intend to flush it down the commode. If you discover that a patient has been covertly noncooperative, you will probably feel anger. It is hard to accept that someone has deceived you. But consider for a moment: why would a patient not cooperate with the therapeutic plan?

Perhaps the patient fears drug reactions and believes that quietly disposing of the drug is easier than trying to explain to health care providers "who do not understand how I feel about drugs." Perhaps the patient's religion discourages the use of drugs. Perhaps the patient knows (or thinks) that this is a terminal illness and does not want to prolong life, if the cost is pain and helplessness or

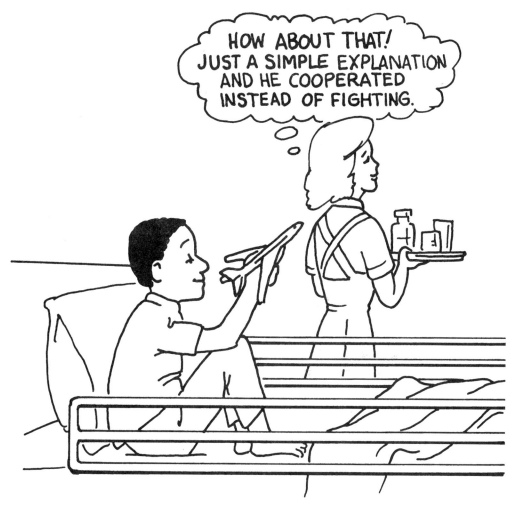

A patient who understands a procedure is more likely to cooperate.

depleting the family's financial resources. Whatever the reason for this noncooperation, you may be sure it makes sense to the patient. It is your responsibility to (1) refer this problem to the professional staff, (2) remain nonjudgmental toward this patient, (3) accept that you may never understand the reasons for the patient's behavior, and (4) remember that this noncooperation serves a purpose for the patient.

The Hostile Patient

Dealing with verbal or passive aggression is largely a problem of dealing with hostility. Team planning is more likely to be effective than isolated efforts by one or two members of the team. In general, each health care provider should give undivided attention to the hostile patient; listen without defensiveness or argument; indicate respect for the patient's feelings; show concern; and encourage expression of thoughts and feelings. Sometimes, it is effective to reflect what the patient has just said: "You think the food is terrible." At other times it may be more appropriate to question, using the patient's ideas but adding your own interpretation followed by "Is that what you mean?" It may be more appropriate to test your guess about the feelings behind the patient's comments: "Are you unhappy about this?" Or, "You seem to be quite angry about this." Use a pleasant tone and phrases that help the patient feel free to express feelings. Your responses should convey acceptance, caring, and willingness to listen. Sometimes such an approach has unexpectedly good results. The patient, after airing feelings, may say something such as, "I guess that's a pretty small thing to be fussing about."

The worst thing you can do with a hostile patient is to return hostility. This, simply confirms the patient's belief that you do not care or understand—your hostility has justified the patient's hostility. To avoid hostile behavior toward the patient, you *must* avoid hostile feelings. Accept the patient's hostility as indicative of a need, perhaps a need to develop trust in the health care team. If you recognize that you are developing negative feelings toward a patient, avoid defensiveness, criticism, arguing, short answers, or otherwise showing your negative feelings. If the patient detects your negative feelings, someone else should be assigned to care for that patient.

The Crying Patient

Crying can result from any degree of anger, fear, or grief. Some people cry whenever they experience sentimental feelings. Crying is an emotional release and should not be stifled. Women tend to cry more readily than men. This is a result of cultural influence: little boys are taught that it is unmanly to cry. Do not make the mistake of thinking that men do not have emotional reactions just because they do not cry readily. Any male patient may be experiencing just as much fear, anger, or grief as the woman crying in the next room.

When you find a patient crying, avoid such comments as, "Let's stop crying now," or "You are much better, so there is nothing to cry about." These remarks may make you feel better, but they indicate to the patient that you are not trying to understand the patient's feelings.

Sometimes it is appropriate to ask the reason for the crying. At other times, it is better just to show acceptance, encourage freedom to express feelings through crying, and wait for the patient to volunteer information. It is not difficult to find out if the patient is crying because of pain and discomfort, fear, or sadness. If the crying seems to be due to personal problems, avoid prying questions, which could be an invasion of the patient's privacy.

With the crying patient, always indicate that you approve of crying as a means of relieving feelings. Sometimes holding the patient's hand or placing your hand over the patient's hand provides reassurance and conveys your interest and concern. Offer to stay, but if the patient shows a preference for being left alone, then say you are available if anything is needed, and leave. But, return after 15 to 20 minutes and use appropriate behavior to respond to the patient's status at that time.

Each situation with a crying patient must be handled according to your best judgment and knowledge about the patient. The preceding suggestions may guide your behavior. Exactly what to say and do is dependent on the patient's situation.

1. Do not offer false hope.

2. Do not make promises you cannot keep.

3. Do not minimize the patient's cause for crying.

4. Do not express disapproval of crying.

Crying is sometimes exhibited by patients suffering from mental/emotional disturbances. These patients need your reassurance, caring, and concern, in addition to specific approaches that are part of the therapeutic plan. If your course includes care of the psychiatric patient, you will learn additional techniques for dealing with crying.

The Uncooperative Patient

When an adult patient is uncooperative, there is usually a reason. Most adults recognize that cooperation with the health team is in their interest. Some possible reasons for noncooperation are lack of understanding, misinformation, suspicion or distrust, and preference for one's own way of doing things. Negative feelings can also cause noncooperation; for example, resistance may be due to underlying hostility.

To understand a patient's failure to cooperate, inquire in an interested but uncritical manner about the reason for the patient's behavior. You may find that an explanation is needed, the patient needs to be taught a health principle, a false belief needs to be corrected, a misunderstanding needs to be cleared up, or feelings of fear or distrust need to be relieved.

Suppose your patient refuses a medication. Perhaps the patient believes the physician intends to discontinue that medication. The patient may have grown up with the belief that taking pills is a sign of weakness. Perhaps the patient

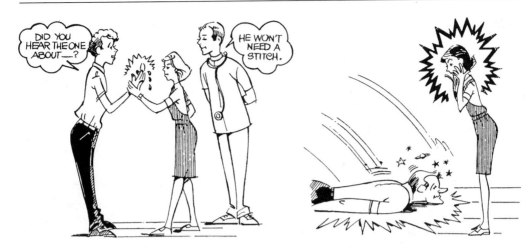

Some behaviors are a cover for fear.

has heard about health care providers giving patients the wrong medication. (Let's admit it! Medication errors do occur and are inexcusable.) The patient may be convinced that the "little red pill" is causing nausea or some other discomfort. (And, it may be!) Maybe the patient resents the health team's expectations that the patient adapt personal habits to their routines. The patient who is accustomed to going to bed at midnight may resent being told to take a pill and go to bed at 10 o'clock.

Patients cannot be forced to cooperate. Cooperation must be gained by eliminating the cause of noncooperation. If you are unable to learn why the patient is not cooperating, discuss the situation with your supervisor. Sometimes the problem must be referred to the patient's physician. If cooperation is essential to recovery, then it must be secured in some way. If the patient is objecting to a procedure that is not essential to recovery or well-being, then the physician may discontinue it rather than **antagonize** the patient.

The Overly Cheerful Patient

Convalescent patients usually are optimistic and happily anticipating full recovery from illness. Such cheerfulness is genuine and can be accepted at face value.

Any patient who is awaiting surgery or the results of diagnostic studies, however, probably has some anxiety. Some of these patients appear quite cheerful, in spite of great anxiety. Do not allow apparent cheerfulness to make you indifferent to needs of such patients. Some may handle their anxiety quite effectively without help. Others may need to talk about their feelings. Your observation skills and awareness of subtle signs of stress can help you know which patient is handling feelings effectively and which one is covering up with outward cheerfulness that is inconsistent with inner feelings. By being available and encouraging patients with anxiety to bring their fears into the open and talk about them, you can contribute to their well-being. Secret fears loom very large. When brought out into the open and discussed, they often become less frightening.

The Overly Friendly Patient

Occasionally, you may have a patient who is overly friendly. Such behavior may consist of personal questions or physical contact. The person who begins to ask personal questions may be innocently trying to make conversation or may be attempting to establish an overly familiar relationship. It is better to avoid discussing your personal life and your own experiences with patients. Instead, direct the conversation to the patient or to impersonal topics.

Unnecessary physical contact may indicate a need for reassurance or it may be an attempt at familiarity. If you are sure the behavior is an attempt to be familiar, calmly state that you prefer that the patient discontinue the behavior. Whenever behavior exceeds desirable limits, make the limits clear. Do not, however, be so expectant of familiarity that you misinterpret a patient's plea for reassurance. To many patients, touch provides a source of strength and comfort.

Situations involving familiarity should be discussed with your supervisor. *Be sure to report facts—what actually happened.* Do not color your report with what you would have liked the situation to be, with judgmental statements, or with opinions. The supervisor can best assess the situation if you give an

---

TABLE 15–2
Coping With Problem Behaviors of Patients

BEHAVIOR PATTERN	COPING STRATEGIES
Egocentrism	Accept egocentrism as a common reaction to illness; practice tolerance and patience.
Regression	Recognize regression as a common reaction to illness; encourage the patient to perform tasks he or she is capable of doing; avoid a judgmental attitude.
Unfriendly behavior	Do not perceive unfriendly behavior as a personal affront; maintain a calm and friendly approach; occasionally ask if there is anything you can do for the patient.
Aggressive behavior/ Child	Recognize that the child is probably frightened, may expect you to perform a painful procedure, be angry, or have had bad experiences with health care providers in the past. Maintain a friendly and caring attitude; explain procedures; express regrets

	if the procedure is painful; set limits on what behaviors you will tolerate (i.e., no kicking, no biting); obtain assistance or use restraints in accordance with policies of your agency.
Aggressive behavior/ Adult	If the patient is physically aggressive, protect yourself but avoid any behavior that could be construed as assault on the patient; call for assistance if needed; consult the supervisor.
Verbal assault	Firmly but pleasantly state that you do not wish to be spoken to in such a manner. Consult the supervisor if the behavior continues.
Criticism	Consider whether or not the criticism is valid. If so, take steps to correct the problem. Offer an apology if one is due. If the criticism is unreasonable or does not have a basis in fact, confrontation may result in the patient reconsidering the criticism.
Arguing	Does the patient need an explanation? Is the arguing really based on unexpressed fear or anger? Use various communication techniques, but avoid the attitude that you have to "win" an argument.
Hostility	Listen without defensiveness or argument; show respect for the patient's feelings; show acceptance, concern, caring; use various communication techniques to encourage expression of feelings. Avoid hostile feelings toward the patient.
Crying	Express concern; show acceptance of patient's feelings; consider whether the crying may be due to pain or discomfort; ask if the patient would like to talk; indicate approval of crying as an expression of feelings; offer to stay or, if the patient prefers, leave; if you leave the patient, return in 15–20 minutes to express concern and caring.
Uncooperative	Use various communication techniques to determine the reason for noncooperation. (Remember: a patient's right to refuse a medication or procedure is protected by federal law). Ask if the patient has any questions; offer to explain. Consider: Does this patient resent not being included in decisions about his/her care?
Overly cheerful	Is the patient using cheerfulness to cover up fear about impending surgery or the outcome of diagnostic tests? Use various communication techniques to encourage expression of feelings.
Overly friendly	Is the patient merely showing interest with questions about your personal life? Does the patient's touch indicate a need for reassurance? Or is the patient being "too familiar"? If needed, calmly state limits on what is acceptable behavior between a patient and care-giver. Show caring and concern, provide reassurance. Discuss the behavior with your supervisor.

accurate account of what the patient said or did and what you said or did. The supervisor's professional judgment can provide guidelines for members of the health team who are caring for the patient.

References and Suggested Readings

Anderson, Carolyn. *Patient Teaching and Communicating in an Information Age.* Albany, NY: Delmar Publishers Inc., 1990. Chapter 2, "Positive Nurse-Patient Relationships through Communication," pp. 28–47; Chapter 3, "Promoting Effective Communication," pp. 49–73.

Burley-Allen, Madelyn. *Listening: The Forgotten Skill.* New York, NY: John Wiley & Sons, 1995. Chapter 3, "Barriers between Listener and Speaker," pp. 46–80.

Kalman, Natalie & Waughfield, Claire G. *Mental Health Concepts;* Third Edition. Albany, NY: Delmar Publishers Inc., 1993. Chapter 7, "Effective Communication," pp. 135–160.

Tampara, Carol D. & Lindh, Wilburta Q. *Therapeutic Communications for Allied Health Professionals.* Albany, NY: Delmar Publishers Inc., 1992. Module III—Unit 2, "The Therapeutic Response in Age Groups," pp. 135–146; Module III—Unit 3, "The Therapeutic Response to Frightened, Angry, and Aggressive Clients," pp. 150–155; Module III—Unit 4, "The Therapeutic Response to Stressed and Anxious Clients," pp. 159–173.

REVIEW AND SELF-CHECK

Complete each statement below, using information from Unit 15.

1. The primary requirement for improving one's interpersonal skills is to

   _____   _____

   _____ .

2. Eight guidelines for improving relations with patients are:

   _____

   _____

   _____

   _____

   _____

_____

_____

_____

3. Nine behavior patterns commonly manifested by patients are:

    _____   _____

    _____   _____

    _____   _____

    _____   _____

    _____

4. If a patient's behavior is unacceptable to a health care provider, the
    appropriate action is to _____ .

5. If a patient persists with unacceptable behavior, the health care provider
    should _____ .

6. Some ways a health care provider can show caring and concern include:

    _____   _____

    _____   _____

7. When a patient makes a "loaded" statement to a health care provider, it
    is usually effective to _____ .

8. List five communication techniques that can be used to make an appro-
    priate response:

    _____

    _____

    _____

    _____

    _____

9. Examples of regression that might be seen in an adult patient are:
    _____ and _____ .

10. The types of patient most likely to behave aggressively are: _____ ,
    _____ , _____ , and _____ .

11. Four statements to avoid saying to a crying patient are:

_____

_____

_____

_____

12. Some possible reasons for a patient's noncooperation are:

_____

_____

_____

_____

13. The best way to gain a patient's cooperation is to _____ .

14. In reporting a situation involving familiarity, the health care provider should be careful to _____ and _____ .

ASSIGNMENT

1. List four examples of *nonverbal* behavior that may indicate that the patient is worried or upset.

2. List four examples of verbal behavior that may indicate hostility.

3. List four examples of "loaded" statements that appear to be "small talk" but could indicate underlying anxiety.

4. For each statement in assignment three, list two or more "safe" responses that a health care provider could make to the patient's statement.

5. In a whining tone, Mrs. Z. often asks a member of the health team to do things she could do for herself. List four other behaviors that would be a manifestation of regression.

6. Mrs. H. is crying. She tells you her husband is not paying any attention to her while she is sick. You have noticed that he visits each day for about

30 minutes. Mrs. H. told you when she entered the hospital that her husband would be trying to work and manage their home while she is hospitalized. There are two school-age children. Is Mrs. H. being unreasonable? Be prepared to justify your answer.

7. Mr. R. is scheduled for a lobectomy because of lung cancer. He tells you he has smoked two packs of cigarettes a day for twenty years. He is very cheerful, joking with all members of the health team. You have been caring for him for several days and notice that he paces back and forth in his room when he is alone. Discuss this patient in terms of his probable emotional state, his needs as a patient, and the health team's responsibilities to him.

8. Write a brief description of a situation in which a patient exhibited a pattern of behavior discussed in this unit. Indicate the response or behavior you think would be most appropriate for a health care provider.

Unit 16

Human Relations and the Health Care Provider

OBJECTIVES

Upon completion of this unit, you should be able to:

- List three guidelines for improving one's interpersonal skills.
- List seven ways a health care provider can help patients adjust to illness.
- Explain the health care provider's role in identifying a patient's needs.
- List three ways a health care provider can provide emotional support for a patient.
- State five guidelines for becoming an effective member of the health care team.
- List three beliefs that contribute to a favorable work attitude.
- State three ways in which a health care provider can maintain up-to-date knowledge and skills.

KEY TERMS

Adverse	Amateurish	Compensation*
Counterpart	Dynamic	Flawless
Horizontal communication	Vertical communication	

You are now more aware of human behavior than you were at the beginning of this course. You should be using your knowledge about human behavior to better understand yourself and others. You should be consciously evaluating the outcomes of your life experiences in an effort to understand how your behavior influences such outcomes. You should be eliminating ineffective behaviors and developing behavior patterns that produce favorable results. If

*As used in this unit; different from its use in Unit 5.

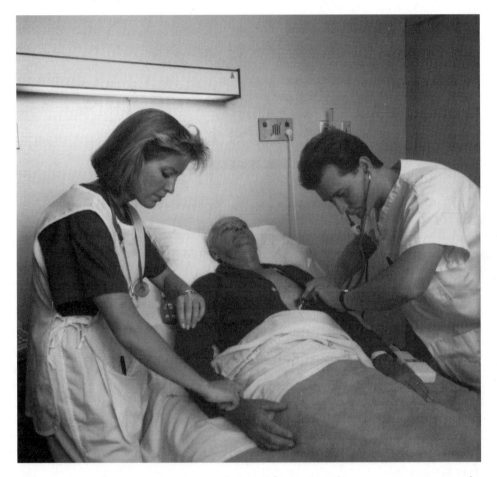

When a co-worker is assisting you with care of a patient, keep your attention on the patient and the procedure. Do not have a personal conversation with the co-worker, while ignoring the patient as a person.

you are making such efforts, then you have gained from this study of human behavior.

Skill in interpersonal relations does not develop overnight, nor does it suddenly appear as a result of wishful thinking. It develops through continuous striving to evaluate one's own behavior, understand the behavior of others, and using various ways of coping with problems and life situations to find those patterns of behavior that achieve the desired results. Slow and steady progress in developing human relation skills is your goal, rather than sudden and complete achievement. The approaches described can help you apply your present knowledge to various areas of living.

HELPING PATIENTS ADJUST TO ILLNESS

Recognizing the Effects of Illness on the Patient

Your patients come to the health agency with the effects of illness added to their usual problems. There are some—perhaps many—stressors in their life situations; illness is an additional stressor. To some people, the health agency is a strange place. For some, it is so threatening that the patient enters only as a desperate effort to get help. In a stressful situation such as the hospital, the patient uses patterns of behavior that have proven useful in past threatening situations. Then, the patient meets you.

You are at home in this environment. The instruments and equipment are useful and meaningful items that make up a large part of your daily routine. You may or may not like your work. You may or may not like your co-workers. You may feel good, or you may feel terrible today. You may have problems at home. You have your own frustrations and conflicts.

Rising Above Your Own Problems

Do you have the right to inflict your personal problems on this troubled patient? Your role is to provide health care. To do so effectively, you must handle your own problems of living well enough to give your full attention to your patients. When you report for work each day, the problems of your personal life must be set aside until you have completed that day's work. *You cannot deal with job problems and home problems at the same time.* Try to form a habit of putting personal matters aside while you are on the job. Then, give your full attention to your patients.

Identifying a Patient's Needs

You have learned about some influences on patient behavior. Use this knowledge to understand and accept each patient as a person. You do not serve Mrs. Jones' needs when you tell your co-workers "she just acts like that because she has a conflict." You may or may not be right about the cause of her behavior. Your role is to be aware of *possible* meanings of behavior in terms of patient needs. Recognizing some of the possible influences on behavior is the key to identifying patient needs, not the source of conversational topics.

If you think a patient's behavior indicates unmet needs, discuss the patient's behavior with your supervisor. Sometimes, the health team needs to study a patient situation in an effort to identify needs. Striving to understand the behavior of your patients should be approached *in a thoroughly ethical and responsible way.* An **amateurish** attempt to provide a full explanation of a patient's behavior could result in serious misunderstandings.

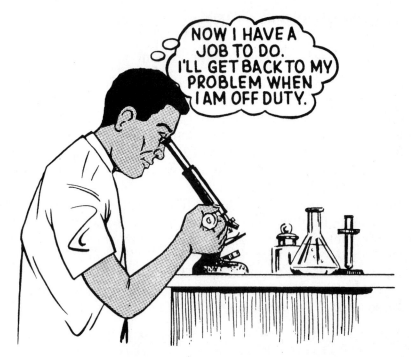

Do not carry your personal problems to work with you.

Introducing Patients to the Health Agency

Each new patient should have health agency procedures explained so the patient knows what to expect. Explain a procedure before doing it. Answer the patient's questions or refer the question to the appropriate person. Through careful orientation of a patient to the health agency, its policies and procedures, and the plan of care, misunderstandings can be minimized. These measures can relieve a patient's fear of the unknown. The interested, sincere, and pleasant manner of the health care provider can build the patient's confidence in members of the health team.

Adapting Your Behavior

Accept each patient as a worthy person. Remember that the patient's behavior is an effort to deal with the present situation. If it becomes apparent that you are having an **adverse** effect on the patient, change your behavior. Some patients enjoy a cheerful, talkative health care provider; others find cheerfulness annoying. As you become more sensitive to the feelings of others, you will be able to adapt your behavior to each patient. If you insist on being the same with all patients, you will be accepted by some but not others.

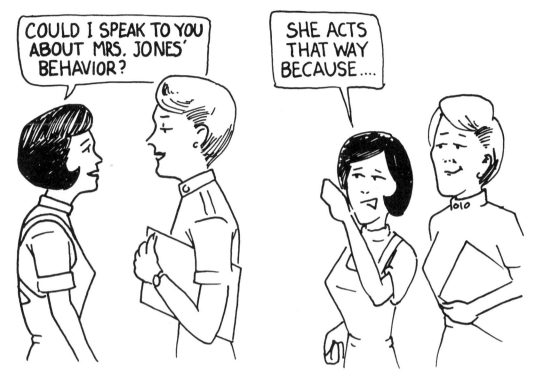

There are ethical and unethical ways to use knowledge of human behavior.

Providing Emotional Support

Some patients need emotional support; others draw on their own resources. With increasing sensitivity, you will be able to detect a patient's need for emotional support. Give extra time and attention to such patients, be available to listen, and accept their feelings and behavior. *True emotional support comes more from your availability and acceptance of the patient than anything you actually say.*

Using Good Judgment

With increasing experience, you will learn which observations should be reported to the appropriate person and which provide clues regarding your appropriate behavior. It is better to report an observation the supervisor considers unimportant than to fail to report something significant. Good judgment in this respect comes from applying learnings from all your courses and from having experience with many different patients.

BECOMING A MEMBER OF THE HEALTH TEAM

As a health care provider, your interpersonal skills will be a major factor in determining how effective you are.

Understanding Your Role

The primary requirement for getting along with your co-workers is to know your role and stay within it. Your preparatory course is helping you understand your role as a health care provider. When you accept a position with a specific health agency, you should clearly understand your role within that agency. Most health agencies and hospitals have job descriptions for each position.

If you accept a position in a solo practice office, or even in a small clinic, you may find that roles and responsibilities have not been specified in writing. If there is no job description, discuss your role with the person who employs you and with your intermediate supervisor. Take notes, and write out a list of your responsibilities as you understand them. Then, ask your supervisor to sign it. Several revisions may be required. Your goal is to have a *written* list of responsibilities. Role confusion can be the cause of misunderstandings, so a written list is your best protection.

It is possible that policies of the employing agency will not permit you to perform some procedures you learned during your course. Many new health care providers are appearing in the health field; responsibilities have not been clearly defined for some of them. In agencies that use several levels of care providers, the division of responsibilities is often based on the availability of prepared workers at each level. If there is an adequate supply of professional workers, those at the technical level are not given as much responsibility as when there is a shortage of professional personnel.

Your exact role in the agency, then, is influenced by the functions of that agency within the community, by the policies and practices of that agency, and by the availability of personnel. If you accept employment with a clear understanding of your role, do not complain later about that role. If an agency offers you a position that does not allow you to use your educational preparation fully, consider whether or not you should accept that position. Being overqualified for a position usually leads either to frustration and job dissatisfaction or to violating existing policies and job descriptions by performing beyond the prescribed role. Both are undesirable situations. It is usually preferable to obtain employment where your role will be consistent with your educational preparation.

Do not assume responsibilities for which you have not had educational preparation. If the employing agency expands your role, then educational

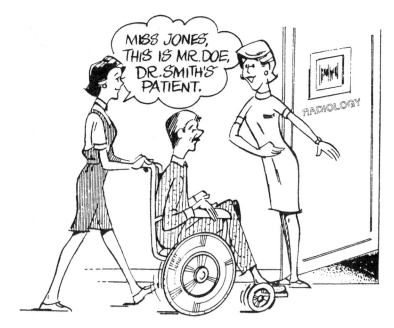

Report to the proper person.

preparation for your expanded duties must be provided; do not assume your expanded duties until after your additional training.

Maintaining Good Relationships

Satisfactory job relationships include working cooperatively with members of other services in the agency. *All* services have responsibilities for serving patients. Respect the role of each service. Recognize that staff members of a service are responsible to the supervisor of that service. Do not give orders to people from another service. Give information if it is needed, but not orders. If there is a problem, your supervisor should discuss it with the supervisor of the other service. This may appear to be a roundabout way to solve a problem, but observing lines of authority prevents confusion and interdepartmental conflict.

Understanding Organizational Structure

Communication channels in an organization are referred to as vertical or horizontal. When the supervisor communicates with you, that is **vertical communication.** If someone works under your direction, then your communication with that person is vertical. Your supervisor's communications with the top administrative level are vertical.

When your supervisor communicates with the supervisor in another department, that is **horizontal communication.** Usually horizontal communication does not occur below the supervisory level. This does not mean that you cannot talk to people from other departments. It means that problems, policy changes, and other matters affecting two or more departments are handled through horizontal communication at the supervisory level or above. Therefore, if you are aware of a problem involving your **counterpart** from another department, do not approach that person directly. Instead, inform your supervisor who can then use either vertical or horizontal channels of communication to correct the problem.

Interdepartmental conflict can result if appropriate lines of communication are not observed. As a member of the health team, you occupy a position on the vertical organization of your own department and a horizontal position in relation to health care providers of your same level in other departments. *Your communication lines for assignments, problems, reports, and complaints are limited to vertical relationships.*

Be aware of the organizational position of your specific job. Be clear about who is in a vertical relationship to you and who has a horizontal relationship. It is possible, even probable as a new health care provider, to learn from experienced workers whose relationship to you is horizontal. But, you receive your orders from the person who has a vertical relationship to you—your supervisor or team leader—and you report to that person.

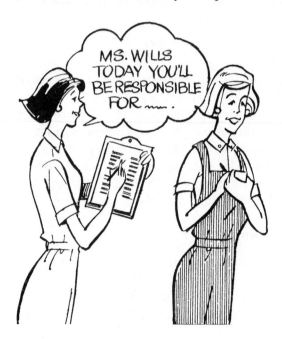

The health care team functions best when each member understands the channels of authority and lines of communication.

The principles of effective human relations and effective communication that you have studied in Section IV also apply to your interactions with co-workers, friends, and relatives. As you strive to improve your human relations skills, practice interacting and communicating effectively with everyone, not just patients. Over time, your communication skills will improve and you should find it easier to form satisfying relationships with others.

Job Satisfaction, Standards, and Self-Respect

It is each health care provider's responsibility to know the extent and limitations of a role, how to carry out the responsibilities of that role, and maintain high performance standards. You will see health care providers who use **flawless** technique in all that they do. You may see others who take every shortcut they can. If you set high standards for yourself and live up to them throughout your career, you will be able to take pride in your work.

If you set high standards for your performance, you may be told occasionally that you are being too particular. Some people not only make minimal effort themselves, they also try to get others to do as they do. It requires determination to hold high standards. In the health field, high standards protect patients from errors or the results of poor technique. Through practice, high standards of performance become part of one's value system. By upholding high standards at all times, a person can become incapable of violating good technique. On the other hand, if one uses sloppy technique most of the time, any attempt to use good technique seems to require much effort. Actually, good technique requires no more effort than sloppy technique, and it enables one to take pride in a job well done. Such pride contributes to self-respect and job satisfaction. There is no substitute for the satisfaction that comes from doing a job well.

Attitudes

Attitudes consist of a mixture of feelings, beliefs, and behaviors. Many attitudes are learned early in life by imitating adults. Some attitudes are formed unconsciously on the basis of experience. A boy who was often severely punished by his redhead first grade teacher may go through life with a bad attitude toward redheaded people, but he may not associate his attitude with those early painful experiences.

Your attitudes affect your adjustment as a health care provider. If you have a strong prejudice, you may find it difficult to work with some of your co-workers or care for some patients. Each of us has an attitude toward work. It may be a favorable attitude, such as "one can find much satisfaction in work." It may be unfavorable, such as "work is what you have to do to get some money."

If you have the attitude that work is worthwhile, that it is satisfying to serve others, that it is desirable to do every task to the best of your ability, then your attitudes will help you find much satisfaction from day to day. Dissatisfaction among workers is often the result of poor attitudes toward work and/or persons in authority.

Compensation

Salary is sometimes a cause of dissatisfaction in a job. Salaries of health care providers are not as high as those in some types of industry. The choice to work in a health occupation should have been made on the basis of complete information, including knowledge that health agencies usually do not pay salaries comparable to those offered by profit-making organizations. Much progress has been made in recent years, however, and today's health care providers are receiving better salaries than ever before.

Compensation other than money can be found in serving others, especially the sick. Only you can decide whether or not the degree of job satisfaction you experience is sufficient to make up for a smaller salary than you might be able to make in some other type of work. Job satisfaction is a highly personal matter. If you know someone who is making a high salary but hates the job, then you are already aware of the importance of job satisfaction to one's happiness. Salary alone is not enough to provide job satisfaction.

THE CHALLENGE

One exciting aspect of the health field is that it is **dynamic.** Research produces new knowledge every day. No one knows for sure what the treatment for certain diseases will be in the future.

If you wish to be an alert and informed member of the health team, you will need to read your professional journals, be active in your professional association, attend staff development programs, and become active in community health programs. It is highly satisfying to be well informed, but remaining well informed in the health field requires continuous effort. If you sit back and admire your diploma for twenty years, you will not remain up-to-date in your field.

Look around you at the health workers you see every day. Some are interested in their work and are up-to-date on information and techniques. Others come to work each day, but do not make an effort to continue learning. Which type of worker do you want to be in fifteen years? Your attitudes toward work and your efforts to be informed will determine which type of health care provider you become.

PRACTICING EFFECTIVE PATIENT RELATIONS

Becoming an effective health care provider includes knowing your job, performing well all tasks within the scope of your responsibilities, understanding and applying the concepts and facts relevant to each task, and observing safety precautions (including asepsis as appropriate). Most of the courses you are now studying prepare you to fulfill these requirements. But to be *truly effective*, you must also focus on developing human relations skills—a never-ending challenge. In this Section, you have studied several topics that will help you be sensitive to the needs of a patient and understand common behaviors of patients.

- Physical and emotional effects of illness

- General effects of serious illness

- Influences on a patient's reaction to illness (age, life role, usual state of adjustment, dependency, cultural background, past experience)

- Common behavior patterns

- Strategies for coping with certain problem behaviors

You have also studied several topics that are relevant to you as a health care provider—*the beliefs and attitudes that you personally bring to the role.* These are an important aspect of your personal effectiveness.

- Acceptance of each patient as a worthwhile human being (including tolerance for those who are different from you)

- Interest in and concern for each patient

- Willingness to listen

- Accuracy in observing

- Ability to recognize significant behaviors

- Respect for confidentiality

- Being sensitive to a patient's feelings and providing emotional support as needed

- Willingness to try to identify needs and serve each patient in accordance with those needs

- Ability to put your personal problems aside while caring for patients

- Willingness to adapt your behavior as needed to interact effectively with a variety of patients exhibiting many different behavior patterns

These topics deal with how you relate to your patients. Another major aspect of good human relations is how you communicate, verbally and nonverbally. In Unit 14, you learned how to convey caring, some reasons for ineffective communication, and responses that tend to block further communication. In Unit 15, you learned several specific communication techniques: echoing and reflecting, clarifying, validating, questioning, and confronting. Becoming a skillful communicator requires conscious effort and practice.

In Section V, you will have the opportunity to practice improving your communication skills. In Unit 17, you will practice interpreting nonverbal behavior and in Unit 18 you will learn additional aspects of effective verbal communication. In each of these units, you will have the opportunity to participate in role play situations as a means of polishing your communication skills and increasing your sensitivity to the *real messages* sent to you by another person.

References and Suggested Reading

Anderson, Carolyn. *Patient Teaching and Communicating in an Information Age.* Albany, NY: Delmar Publishers Inc., 1990. Chapter 9, "Nurses' Communication within the Health Care Organization," pp. 185–204; Chapter 10, "Nurses' Communication with the Health Care Team," pp. 208–215.

Kalman, Natalie & Waughfield, Claire G. *Mental Health Concepts;* Third Edition. Albany, NY: Delmar Publishers Inc., 1993. Chapter 7, "Effective Communication," pp. 135–163.

REVIEW AND SELF-CHECK

Complete each statement below, using information from Unit 16.

1. Developing interpersonal skills requires continuous striving to

   _____

   _____

   _____ .

2. Recognizing some of the possible influences on a patient's behavior is the key to _____ .

3. The study of a patient's situation to identify needs may require _____
   _____ .

4. One way to minimize misunderstandings between a patient and health
   care provider is to _____ .

5. A health care provider who believes that a particular patient needs emotional support should _____
   _____
   _____ .

6. Some ways a health care provider can help patients adjust to illness
   include _____
   _____
   _____
   _____
   _____ .

7. Five guidelines for becoming an effective member of the health team are:
   _____
   _____
   _____
   _____
   _____

8. Some beliefs that contribute to a favorable attitude toward work are:
   _____
   _____
   _____

9. Some ways a health care provider may continue to learn are:
   _____
   _____
   _____

ASSIGNMENT

1. List five benefits of improving your interpersonal skills.

2. List five ways you can minimize a new patient's fears.

3. Describe how you may relieve a patient's anxiety associated with strange places and uncomfortable procedures.

4. List three examples of inappropriate behavior by health care providers. Explain why each is inappropriate for the situation in which it occurred. Suggest a more appropriate behavior.

5. Describe a situation in which a health care provider used knowledge about human behavior to identify a patient's unmet need.

6. Explain vertical lines of communication (and authority) in relation to your role on the health team within the health agency affiliated with your educational program.

7. Identify your counterpart (horizontal relationship) on another service within the affiliated health agency.

8. Explain why you should discuss patient problems with your supervisor rather than with co-workers.

9. List ten guidelines for continued growth as a health care provider after you have become employed in a health agency.

10. One of your co-workers has been employed at your health care agency for fifteen years when you arrive as a new employee. In spite of having seniority, this person has a horizontal relationship to you and others with your job title. Two or three times a week, this co-worker tells you to do some task or take over the care of a specific patient. Since she speaks with an authoritative tone, you tend to comply with her instructions. Yesterday, your supervisor said, "You are not assigned to Mrs. X. Why are you taking care of her?" When you explain, the supervisor says, "You get your assignments from me."

Today, this co-worker says, "You take care of Mr. Z for the remainder of this shift." How will you respond?

NOTE: Your instructor may choose to allow class time for role playing this situation or a full class discussion.

11. Develop a chart to show how your job title relates to other job titles in the agency where you are getting your clinical experience.
     a. Using the format below, insert job titles to show vertical relationships:

The person to whom your supervisor reports

_____

Your supervisor

_____

Your job title

_____

Any persons who report to you

_____

_____

_____

_____

_____

_____

b. List job titles that are in your department but have a horizontal (equal) relationship to your job title.

Section V

Practicing Effective Communication

You have learned a number of things about human behavior: ways people are alike and different; the basic needs of people and how they attempt to meet these needs; how people try to protect themselves against real or imagined threats to security, happiness, peace of mind, or general well-being; and ways people react to physical illness and the problems that accompany it.

Applying knowledge about human behavior to relationships with others is easily talked about, but difficult to practice. There must be a beginning, however, and that beginning can lead to a high level of skill for those who continuously strive for improvement. This section will provide opportunities for practicing three skills that are basic to understanding human behavior: observing the behavior of others, observing your own behavior, and adapting your behavior according to how you "read" another person's behavior.

Unit 17

Observing Nonverbal Behavior

OBJECTIVES

Upon completion of this unit, you should be able to:

- Explain the meaning of "skill in interpersonal relations."
- Explain "selective observing."
- List five examples of nonverbal behavior that may convey a message.
- State five steps for improving one's use of nonverbal communication.
- Observe nonverbal behavior.
- Interpret the message of nonverbal behavior.
- Recognize one's own patterns of nonverbal behavior.
- Relate one's nonverbal patterns to reactions to various situations.
- Use nonverbal communication purposefully to improve interpersonal relations.

KEY TERMS

Consistency	Impending	Jeopardy
Misinterpretation	Quality control	Random
Selective observing	Stance	Tentative

You have heard much about "good human relations" since you began your preparation for a career in the health field. Have you thought about the *real meaning* of that expression? Does it mean that knowing about influences on human behavior makes it easy to develop good human relations? Perhaps you already recognize that such is not the case, because good human relations requires far more than just knowing *about* human behavior. Actually, good human relations involves a conscious effort to *select your behavior* for a given situation, rather than allowing habit or emotions to determine what you say and do.

Skill in interpersonal relations may be thought of as *controlled* interaction with others. It means control over what happens by *consciously deciding* what to say or do to bring about the response you desire from another person. Of course, it is seldom possible to control what happens completely, but you can have an influence. When your behavior arouses positive feelings in others, then it is likely that the behavior of the other person toward you will be favorable. On the other hand, your behavior can arouse negative feelings in others: anxiety, anger, a sense of threat, self-pity, feelings of being "put down," or just plain irritation. When your behavior arouses such negative feelings, then the behavior of the other person toward you may be unpleasant: noncooperation, complaints, withdrawal, or disagreement with whatever you say.

To learn how to select appropriate behavior, you must first learn to use any available evidence to determine the other person's feelings. Some of the evidence lies in *what* is said and *how* it is said. Some consists of the other person's behavior. Much of the evidence, especially in a stressful situation, lies in nonverbal communication. And so, your learning to influence the outcome of a given situation must start by learning to observe nonverbal behavior—a form of communication that is often more meaningful than spoken communication.

OBSERVING AND INTERPRETING NONVERBAL BEHAVIOR

Most of us think we are observant and that our observations are reasonably accurate. **Selective observing** means that we notice some details of a situation, while completely missing many other details. Left to chance, observations are likely to be made according to one's interests or curiosity. To become skillful in observing nonverbal behavior, you must bring nonverbal signals within the range of your selective observing.

Most people communicate feelings through nonverbal behavior, often unconsciously. But regardless of whether or not the nonverbal behavior is conscious, it signals that the person is responding to something—perhaps to you as a person, something you said or did, your tone of voice, the expression on your face, and the other person's interpretation of what it means. It is also possible that the behavior indicates the individual's response to the total situation: the stress of a job interview, anger at being ill, fear of **impending** surgery, or the expectation of an unfavorable diagnosis. Nonverbal communication, then, provides a clue to a person's inner feelings. In some cases, it is also a signal that more specific behavior, such as an angry outburst, is about to occur.

The message of nonverbal behavior is lost unless you note it and interpret the meaning correctly. To improve your use of nonverbal communication, consciously practice observing the nonverbal behavior of others. Next, practice interpreting that behavior and check your interpretation against further evidence. Whenever you are interacting with another person, note any changes in facial expression, slight movements of facial muscles, position of the lips, direction of gaze, position of the eyelids, body movements, **stance,** general posture, and the hands—position and movements.

After noting the nonverbal clues, try to interpret that behavior. Does a twitching facial muscle indicate stress? Or repressed anger? If stress, why does the individual feel stressed in this situation? Do the restless movements of the hands indicate nervousness? If so, why does the person feel nervous in this situation? What is the person's emotional state? What expectations does the person have? Are you sending nonverbal messages to which that individual is responding nonverbally? By associating the nonverbal behavior of a specific person with additional evidence as it becomes available, you can learn to "read" that person with a reasonable degree of accuracy.

Interpretation of nonverbal behavior carries the risk of **misinterpretation.** This is a serious risk, for *misinterpretation can lead to more misunderstanding than simply ignoring the nonverbal communication.* The risk of misinterpretation can be decreased by following five steps:

1. Note the nonverbal behavior.

2. Make a **tentative** interpretation.

3. Continue to observe for more evidence, especially evidence that is easily interpreted—a display of anger, statements of disapproval, objections, or complaints.

4. Revise your interpretation if there is evidence that the first interpretation was not accurate.

5. Watch for **consistency,** i.e., occurrence of a specific nonverbal behavior every time that individual is in a particular situation, such as making a decision, doing something new, speaking before a group, or coping with conflict.

Once you have detected the pattern and determined that certain nonverbal behaviors consistently indicate a specific feeling state of that person, you have learned "to read" that person's nonverbal behavior.

With friends and co-workers, you may become quite accurate at reading their feelings without any words being exchanged. Accuracy in interpretation is achieved only over a period of time and through frequent opportunities to observe an individual in a variety of situations. Even then you may find it difficult to interpret some nonverbal behavior. You may practice trying to read one of your co-workers over a long period of time, and finally say, "Look, I have noticed that you often pick up a pencil and roll it between your fingers. At first I thought you do this when you feel irritated; then it seemed that you do this when you are bored; but just now you did it after laughing at Joe's story. Tell me, just why do you pick up a pencil and twirl it?" Your friend may give you an answer that indicates one of your interpretations was correct, may indicate a lack of awareness of the behavior, or may admit not knowing the reason for it. Your friend may say that all of your attempts at explaining the behavior are wrong: "I formed that habit when I quit smoking. Now, every time I see someone light up, I pick up a pencil and twirl it. I suppose it serves the purpose my smoking used to serve." Note that in this case you still do not have an interpretation of the *feeling state* when this behavior occurs. So, continue to watch your friend's use of this particular behavior in different situations.

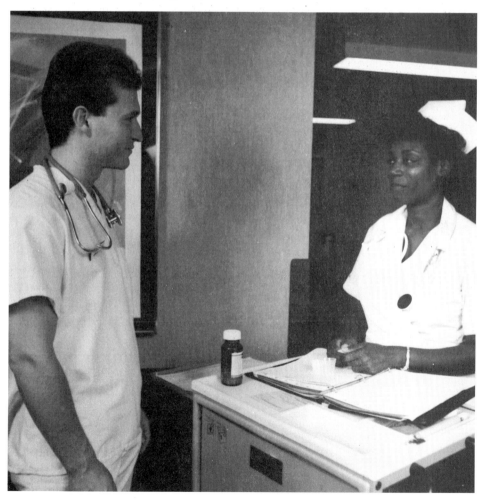

Careful observation of nonverbal behavior can help you determine if someone understands what you have just explained.

With people you see less frequently, you will not be able to learn the meaning of their nonverbal clues as readily. And, with people you see only occasionally or for brief periods of time, you must make your best judgment of the probable meaning of nonverbal behavior and try to confirm that interpretation as the relationship proceeds.

In relating to patients and their families, look for nonverbal behavior that may mean a buildup of feelings, especially fear, anxiety, confusion, and anger. When you detect such signals, it is likely that the patient would benefit from extra attention in the form of sincere interest, concern, consideration, and emotional support while adapting to strange surroundings and illness.

The special attention you provide may encourage the patient to talk. You might invite questions with, "Is there something you would like me to explain? I will try to answer any questions you have." You may be able to answer some questions, but find it necessary to refer others to appropriate persons—the patient's physician, the supervisor, or another department of the health facility. You will be safe in giving information about routines and the facility itself. Questions about the patient's condition should be handled by others, usually the physician. Your role is to provide emotional support for the patient when you listen to questions, show sincere concern, and state that you will pass any questions you can not answer on to the person who can provide answers.

As you gain experience in reading nonverbal behavior, you will detect many different indicators of patients' negative feelings. With increased skill in

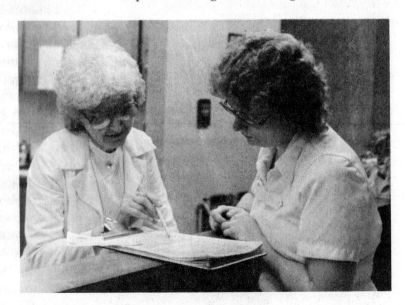

Without observing nonverbal behavior, how can you be sure someone understands what you have explained?

relating to others, you will be ready for the next challenge: encouraging others to express their feelings. You can do this while performing a procedure or otherwise serving a patient's needs by physical actions. You may lead off with a casual statement such as, "I suppose this visit to us is something of a nuisance to you," or "Most people find our agency a little frightening on their first visit." You might ask a direct question, but select your words carefully to avoid the appearance of prying. "Were you surprised that the doctor wanted you to have these studies done?" Or, "Have you had this type of test before?"

A *full exploration of feelings* is best left to professionals with counseling skills. However, you can encourage *expression of feelings* and still remain within your role as a health care provider. Be aware that your patient is a human being going through a stressful experience, indicate your willingness to listen, and give your full attention to the patient. But, in order to recognize those who need an understanding listener, you must receive the message. A *message of need is most likely to be sent nonverbally.*

The purpose of observing nonverbal communication, then, is to become sensitive to—or aware of—the feelings of others as conveyed by small bits of behavior, rather than words. This sensitivity enables you to adapt your behavior to these feelings, to consciously select your response, either verbal or nonverbal, and thereby have a favorable effect on others. The favorable effect may consist of providing emotional support, conveying that you care, defusing the other's fear or anger, or providing an invitation to release pent-up feelings by talking about the situation that aroused the feelings.

SETTING THE STAGE FOR PRACTICING INTERPERSONAL SKILLS

It is difficult to develop human relations skills without assistance from others. You need guidance from someone who has already developed a high level of skill: your teachers, other health professionals, a member of the school staff who has specialized in interpersonal relations, or possibly someone from the community who is a specialist in human relations.

Early Practice

Your beginning efforts to develop skill are best conducted in association with your classmates. You are all striving for improved interpersonal skills. Through the common knowledge you have all gained from your course, you should now be able to accept one another's efforts without criticism, accept suggestions from one another about how to improve, and explore your own feelings in a situation where others are also exploring their feelings. Ideally, your class will have a regular time for practicing interpersonal skills throughout the remainder of your course.

Continuing Practice

When you leave the school setting, opportunities for group practice may not be readily available. If you wish to continue practicing in a group situation, find a course or workshop that will provide opportunities for continued practice of your communication skills.

When you are employed as a health care provider, you will have to rely primarily on your own assessment of outcomes. As you improve your observation skills, you will be more aware of the effect of your behavior on other people. As you interact over a period of time with co-workers and patients, you can test your interpretations of their behavior. You will never reach the point of always interpreting behavior correctly. There is the ever-present risk of being wrong. Keep an open mind and be ready to revise your interpretation as you make new observations.

Striving to improve communication skills begins with practice in noting behaviors that signal the inner feelings or thoughts of a person. An observer who is fairly accurate in noting and interpreting these signals can anticipate the type of behavior about to occur and encourage it, or possibly change it, by careful selection of words or actions. The following exercises are designed to help you practice recognizing and interpreting nonverbal communication.

EXERCISE I: OBSERVING NONVERBAL BEHAVIOR

Purpose

In this exercise you will observe the nonverbal behavior of other people and hear a report from an observer about your own nonverbal behavior.

Objective

Given an opportunity to observe two people in a potentially stressful situation, you will observe, record, and report the nonverbal cues exhibited by one person in response to words or actions of the other.

OR

Given an opportunity to receive a report from someone who observed you in a potentially stressful interaction with another person, you will become aware of your nonverbal responses to the behavior of another person or to the stress of the situation.

Instructions

1. Organize in groups of four. Two members of each group will serve as observers, and two members will serve as actors. (The roles will be reversed for Exercise II.)

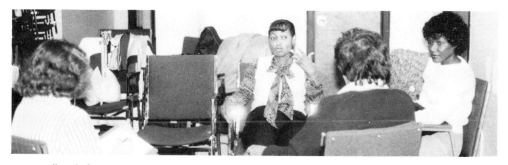

Feedback from an observer helps us to be aware of our own nonverbal behavior.

2. Read "The Incident to be Portrayed" on the following page.

3. Read the instructions that apply to your role (observer or actor).

4. The instructor will serve as timekeeper. You have the following time schedule for this exercise:
    a. Reading instructions and procedure for Exercise 1 ...... 2 minutes
    b. Preparation for the performance .... 5 minutes
        Actors: Read about the situation and the role you are to play.
        Observers: Review Unit 17.
    c. Performance .... 5 to 10 minutes
    d. Reports of observers to actors .... 3 minutes
    e. Interpretations of actors' nonverbal behavior .... 3 minutes
    f. Followup discussion (all four members participate) ..... 5 minutes
                                       Total ..... 28 to 33 minutes

Instructions for Observers

1. Decide which actor you will observe (Mrs. A. or Mr. M.).

2. Read all instructions for observers and study the chart for recording observations, page 312.

3. Observe one actor during the performance. On the chart, record (1) each act of nonverbal behavior by the actor you are observing and (2) what the other actor said or did just *before* the nonverbal behavior occurred.

4. When the performance has been completed, report the nonverbal behavior of your actor, together with the act or words of the other actor that preceded the nonverbal behavior.

5. Listen while the other observer reports to the other actor.

6. Listen while one actor (Mr. M.) interprets the meaning of the other actor's (Mrs. A.) nonverbal behavior and Mrs. A. describes feelings or thoughts at that point in the performance.

7. Listen as the other actor (Mrs. A.) interprets and Mr. M. responds.

Instructions for Actors

1. Decide which role (Mrs. A. or Mr. M.) each of you is to play in the performance.

2. Read about the role you are to play, but *do not read the description of the other role.* (This is important.)

3. After reading about the person you are to play, do the suggested activities at the end of the descriptive paragraphs. These are intended to help you identify with that person's feelings about self, the other person in the situation, job setting, and the problem situation around which the performance is built.

4. Role play the scene between Mrs. A. and Mr. M., behaving as though you were actually that person in that situation.

5. When the performance is finished, listen as your observer reports the nonverbal behavior you demonstrated during the performance.

6. Listen as the other actor describes the effect of your nonverbal behavior.

7. Try to recall your feelings and/or thoughts at the time each nonverbal communication occurred.

8. Listen while the other actor interprets each nonverbal behavior reported in your performance, then respond to this interpretation. You may agree with the other actor's interpretation; you may find it is partly correct; you may disagree completely. Describe your thinking and feeling at the time of the nonverbal communication and explain the "true meaning" of your nonverbal behavior.

9. Listen while the other observer reports to the other actor and then proceed through steps 5–8.

Instructions for Follow-up Discussion

1. Consider whether or not the nonverbal behavior demonstrated by each actor during the performance is typical of that person's "real-life" behavior when relating to others, especially in stressful situations.

2. Consider the examples of misinterpretation that occurred: which nonverbal behaviors were incorrectly interpreted by the other actor.

3. Actors: prepare a list of your nonverbal behaviors and the interpretation of each by the other actor. Ask your observer to check this summary report for accuracy and completeness.

THE INCIDENT TO BE PORTRAYED

Mrs. A. is supervisor of the clinical laboratory in a large medical center. She is always on duty at least fifteen minutes early and is very efficient in the performance of her duties. Mrs. A.'s responsibilities include preparing work schedules two weeks in advance, daily assignments for the staff, supervising all procedures performed in the laboratory, assisting the pathologist with complex procedures as necessary, and carrying out a variety of administrative duties.

The older employees remember all too well the disorganization and favoritism the existed when another person was supervisor. When Mrs. A. first became laboratory supervisor, she developed job descriptions and written personnel policies. These were discussed thoroughly with the staff, and each person was given a copy. In these personnel policies it states that employees of the laboratory should submit any special requests about schedules at least two weeks in advance.

Mrs. A. is always courteous to the staff, but does not confide in them or encourage friendships. She usually grants special requests for time off, but can be very firm in refusing such requests. In general, Mrs. A. maintains distance between herself and others, including the staff of the laboratory and the medical staff of the center.

Mr. M. is a member of the staff who completed his course of study a month ago and immediately started working in the laboratory where Mrs. A. is supervisor. He has taken the certification examination but has not received the results. His employee status is "provisional," and he is supposed to work directly under the supervision of a professional member of the staff.

Mrs. A. always spot-checks the day's tests; that is, she selects at **random** certain tests performed by laboratory staff and runs a second test herself to see whether or not she gets the same result as that obtained by the staff member. When she does find an error, the person who made the error can expect a call to her office and a stern lecture on the importance of accuracy.

During Mr. M.'s first week on the job, Mrs. A. frequently stood behind him as he performed a test, but always moved on without comment. On Wednesday of the fourth week of Mr. M.'s employment, Mrs. A.'s spot-checking included two laboratory procedures Mr. M. had run during the morning. Just before he was to go off duty, Mr. M. received word that Mrs. A. wanted to see him in her office immediately.

Observers: Study the Observation Record provided at the end of the unit for recording your observations. Review Unit 17 while waiting for the actors to finish their preparation.

Actors: You have five minutes to prepare for the performance. First, read about the role you are to act out. ("The Private Life of Mrs. A.," below or "The Private Life of Mr. M.," page 309.) It is very important that you *do not read the description* of the other role. Then, do the thought exercises at the end of the description. These exercises are designed to help you identify with the character you are to portray and "get in the mood" for a realistic performance.

THE PRIVATE LIFE OF MRS. A.

Mrs. A. is a divorcee with responsibility for two school-age children. Her husband deserted the family when the second child was one year old. At that time, she had been a homemaker for six years and had given up all plans for a career. When she found herself alone and responsible for providing for herself and the children, she immediately looked for employment. To her surprise, she found that she had the choice of several positions, for well-prepared personnel were in great demand. She chose the position that appeared to offer a chance for advancement. Then, she entered night school to improve her qualifications.

Mrs. A. has had a difficult time making ends meet, but sees to it that her children have opportunities for camping experiences, scouts, and music lessons. Although her own social life is limited, she is poised and self-assured in a social situation.

When Mrs. A. assumed the supervisory position at the medical center, the director of laboratories stated that she would be fully responsible for **quality control**—for seeing that high standards of accuracy were maintained at all times. The director also stated that her job would be in **jeopardy** if at any time a high percentage of errors should occur. The director also indicated that Mrs. A. had been offered the supervisory position because she seemed to have the potential for assuming responsibility: "The last supervisor was always running to me with little problems. I want a supervisor who can manage the lab and not bother me with a lot of details." Mrs. A. found that the lab needed many improvements, but proceeded slowly with these changes. After several years, the lab has become a well-organized department in which the work is done systematically and with a remarkable record for accuracy and efficiency.

At the time of the incident to be enacted, Mrs. A. has just received a telephone message that the regular employee for the weekend has been called out of town by a family emergency. She is faced with finding a way to cover the laboratory. The time schedule provides for minimal coverage because of several requests to have this weekend off. These requests were submitted on time and Mrs. A. felt safe in granting all these requests. Mrs. A. reflects that Mr. M., though a new staff member, has shown himself to be quite reliable. She decides to ask him to fill in on Saturday and Sunday, with the option of extra pay or compensatory time off. She asks a staff member to tell Mr. M. that she wants to see him before he leaves today.

Soon after sending the message to Mr. M., Mrs. A. receives a note from the director, requesting that she complete a questionnaire and return it immediately. She starts working on the report while waiting for Mr. M., and is almost finished when he knocks on the door.

Performance

Initiate the performance by greeting Mr. M. when he arrives at the door of your office. Let this greeting be rather abrupt, but pleasant. Indicate that he is to have a seat, then resume working on the report for the director. Take about one minute to finish it, then take it to the director's office. When you return, sit down behind your desk and look directly at Mr. M. for the first time since he entered your office. Chat casually about the weather, the medical center, some current event in the news, or something of interest in the laboratory. Ask how he is getting along, whether there are any problems, and similar "small talk." Do not rush through this; take at least three to five minutes. After about five minutes of casual conversation, tell Mr. M. that you are pleased with his work and that you have a favor to ask: Is he willing to work 8 to 4 P.M. Saturday and Sunday?

Preparation for the Role of Mrs. A.

> **NOTE:**   For the next 20 minutes, you *are* Mrs. A.

1. How do you feel about having to ask Mr. M. to work this weekend? (The employment agreement specifies a forty-hour week, scheduled Monday through Saturday between the hours of 7 A.M. and 10 P.M. for the stated salary.)

2. Think about your outstanding characteristics, as given in the description.

3. Consider how you feel about your new staff member, Mr. M.

THE PRIVATE LIFE OF MR. M.

Mr. M. served in the military for several years, rising to the rank of sergeant. After discharge he worked for several years in a small hospital, learning a number of laboratory procedures from personnel there. The physicians had found him trustworthy. They frequently delegated a test procedure to him and accepted his report without question. Eventually, Mr. M. realized that he must obtain educational preparation and appropriate credentials in order to progress in his career. For this reason, he enrolled in a laboratory course. There, he found that he was about fifteen years older than most of the people in the class. Also, he could already do many of the procedures studied, but he found the theory part of the course difficult. Mr. M. was considered to be an average student; he was careful not to let other students or the teacher know what long hours he put in trying to understand the material in the textbook and references. Mr. M. felt fortunate to have a teacher who tried to help students. The teacher had also served in the military; Mr. M. always felt comfortable going to the teacher for additional explanations or with specific questions.

Mr. M. completed his course one month ago and took the examination last week. He was very nervous about the examinations. Tests have always affected him adversely, making him unable to sleep or eat well as the day of the test approaches.

Mr. M. was interviewed by the male director of the laboratory when he applied for the position at the center. He assumed that he would be working directly under this man. He did not know that Mrs. A. was fully responsible for the laboratory until he met her the first day on the job.

This is the first time Mr. M. has ever been in a situation where he receives directions from a woman. At times, he finds himself wishing that the teacher from his course could be the supervisor of the laboratory. Then, he feels, this job would be great!

On the day of the incident to be enacted, Mr. M. has plans for the evening. He wants to get a haircut before the barbershop closes at 5:30, so it is necessary to leave the center promptly when he gets off duty at 4:30. He has worked rapidly during the day to be sure of finishing his assignments on time.

At 4 o'clock, Mr. M. receives a message to come to Mrs. A.'s office immediately. The staff member who delivers the message is wearing a half-smile that seems to say, "Oh, Boy! Now it's your turn to get it!" As he walks toward the office, Mr. M. is very much aware that two of his procedures were checked by Mrs. A. this morning. He just cannot believe he made an error on either procedure. He arrives at her office.

Performance

Begin by knocking on Mrs. A's office door. Continue as you think Mr. M. would react.

Preparation for the Role of Mr. M.

NOTE: For the next 20 minutes, you *are* Mr. M.

1. Why do you think Mrs. A. has sent for you?
2. How do you feel about Mrs. A.?
3. Should you find a position where there is a male supervisor?
4. Would you prefer to work directly under a physician?
5. How do you feel about your own competence?
6. What are you going to say if Mrs. A. claims that you made an error in one of your procedures?

EXERCISE II: INTERPRETING NONVERBAL BEHAVIOR

> **NOTE:** The same situation and characters will be used for Exercise II, but those who were observers in Exercise I will be actors in Exercise II, and those who were actors in Exercise I will be observers in Exercise II. Also, the learnings from Exercise II should be different, as indicated by the objective.

Purpose

In this exercise you will observe and interpret nonverbal communication and test your interpretation against the person's explanation of the feelings or thoughts that accompanied the nonverbal behavior.

Objective

Given an opportunity to observe two persons interacting in a stressful situation, you will observe and record nonverbal behavior, prepare a tentative interpretation of the nonverbal behavior, report your interpretation to the person, and revise the interpretation according to that person's description of his or her feeling state or thoughts at the time the nonverbal behavior occurred.

Instructions

1. Organize into groups of four. The members of the group who served as actors in Exercise I will serve as observers, and those who served as observers in Exercise I will serve as actors.

2. Refer to the instructions and procedures for Exercise I, according to your role in this exercise.

3. When you have completed the procedure outlined for Exercise I, discuss the following:
   a. Implications of consistent signaling to other persons, without realizing that you are communicating
   b. Implications of being "easy to read" in situations where you are competing with another person
   c. Implications of being "hard to read" if you want others to know that you are sincerely concerned about them, you care, and you want to help
   d. Possible uses for nonverbal behavior by health care providers to improve interpersonal relations

4. Following the group discussion, prepare a brief plan to guide you in using nonverbal behavior to improve relationships with (a) the clients of your health agency, (b) your co-workers, and (c) your supervisor.

OBSERVATION RECORD FOR EXERCISES I AND II: OBSERVING NONVERBAL BEHAVIOR

Actor being observed: _____ Role portrayed: Mrs. A. __ Mr. M. __

Observer: _____ Total number of observations: _____

Nonverbal behaviors exhibited by the actor:	Words or actions of the <u>other</u> <u>actor</u> that occurred just <u>before</u> the observed nonverbal behavior:

NOTE: Enter only enough words to provide the necessary information. Do not try to write complete sentences, as you may miss other observations while writing. In the column on the left, enter what you see as a nonverbal communication, not what you think it means. In the column on the right, enter the other actor's exact words or action (example "shook head from side to side").

References and Suggested Readings

Fast, Julius. *Body Language.* New York, NY: M. Evans, 1970. (This was one of the earliest books to call attention to the importance of nonverbal communication.)

Steere, Leo. *How to Read People: All the Secrets People Reveal through their Behavior, their Bodies, and their Handwriting.* New York, NY: Vantage Books, 1993.

Wolfgang, Aaron. *Everybody's Guide to People Watching.* Yarmouth, ME: Intercultural Press, 1995.

REVIEW AND SELF-CHECK

Complete each statement below, using information from Unit 17.

1. The expression "skill in interpersonal relations" refers to one's ability to _____

   _____ .

2. Selective observing means that _____ .

3. Some examples of nonverbal behavior that may signal a message are:

   1. _____

   2. _____

   3. _____

   4. _____

   5. _____

   6. _____

4. Steps for improving one's use of nonverbal communication are:

   1. _____

   2. _____

   3. _____

   4. _____

   5. _____

5. The purpose of observing nonverbal behavior is to _____

_____ .

ASSIGNMENT

1. The next time you watch a situation comedy on TV, concentrate your attention on one of the lead actors and note examples of nonverbal communication. Did the other characters react to or ignore the nonverbal communication? Did any specific example lead to a misunderstanding or conflict between two of the characters?

2. The next time you watch a comedian who does imitations (i.e., Rich Little or Dana Carvey), note the various mannerisms and facial expressions the comedian portrays. Comedians are keen observers of human behavior, and imitators are especially observant of small bits of behavior that characterize an individual. Note the specific mannerisms portrayed in the actor's imitation of a certain person.

3. Use your next movie or TV evening to study the communication styles of the actors. Especially note examples of the following:
    a. An actor who has a frozen countenance (facial expression does not change) most of the time. What nonverbal behaviors does this actor use to communicate?
    b. An actor who uses subtle changes in facial expression. What "body language" does this actor use to supplement facial expression?
    c. An actor who conveys feelings primarily through facial expression. Does this actor also make use of body language to communicate feelings and/or reactions to the action occurring?

Unit 18

Verbal Communication

OBJECTIVES

Upon completion of this unit, you should be able to:

- List three sources of communication breakdown.
- Define ambiguity.
- List three reasons why it is difficult to avoid ambiguity in verbal communication.
- List three ways to minimize ambiguity.
- State the meaning of "message discrepancy."
- List four sender-related causes of message discrepancy.
- List four receiver-related causes of message discrepancy.
- List two reasons why assumptions are a source of communication breakdown.
- Explain why expectations may cause a communication breakdown.
- Name one way you may assist others to clarify their communications to you.
- List five ways to send a clear message.
- List four ways to "hear" a message correctly.

KEY TERMS

Ambiguity	Assumptions	Clarification
Clarity	Enunciation	Inconsistency
Message discrepancy	Paraphrase	Reprimand
Unambiguous		

Workers in the health field spend much time communicating with others: patients and their families, visitors to the health agency, other members of the health team, and supervisors. As a health care provider, you need a high level of communication skill. Whenever and wherever people talk to one another, communication problems may occur.

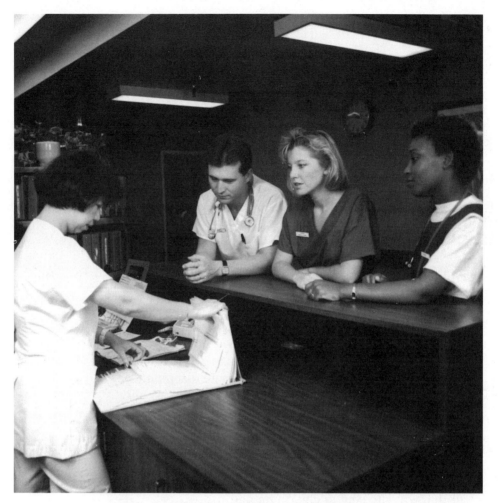

Any ambiguity should be clarified before concluding the team conference

It is tempting to assume that whatever you say to another person is understood—that your listener gets the meaning you intend to convey. In reality, there are numerous sources of communication breakdown: our language permits different meanings for many words, speech and hearing factors may distort what is heard, and nonverbal messages may differ from the spoken message. Many examples of misunderstanding, noncooperation, criticism, and other forms of conflict between people can be traced to a communication problem. Your preparation for working in the health field includes practice in improving your communication skills so you will have a minimum of communication problems.

AMBIGUITY

Ambiguity means vague, unclear. The opposite of ambiguity is **clarity.** The word **unambiguous** is sometimes used to mean completely clear or free of ambiguity.

It is difficult to avoid ambiguity in verbal communication for a number of reasons.

- A word may have several different meanings.

- The word used by the speaker may not be the best word for expressing the desired meaning.

- A pronoun may not clearly indicate who or what it represents.

For example, the word smart is used by some people to mean very intelligent; another person uses smart to mean sassy or disrespectful. Can you think of other meanings for this one word?

Some words or phrases have double meanings. They can be interpreted literally, or they may be used to mean something entirely different. The following illustrates this type of ambiguity:

> A: *"This cat is really good for mice."*
> B: *"How can you say that? He is afraid of mice. He even runs from them."*
> C: *"That's just what I mean. He is very good for the mice."*

A pronoun that may refer to more than one noun is another source of ambiguity. Suppose a patient tells the nurse, "Dr. Brown and Dr. White (both males) both came by to see me last night. They think I'm doing fine. He even said I may go home today." Does "he" refer to Dr. Brown or to Dr. White?

In attempting to avoid ambiguous statements, you should:

- Use words that have a single, precise meaning whenever possible.

- Use the best word for what you want to say.

- Use a noun to indicate who or what; if you use a pronoun (he, she, it, they), it should clearly refer to *one specific noun* used in the same sentence.

DISCREPANCIES IN A MESSAGE

Most of us are careless about verbal communication, especially when we are trying to attend to many things at once. In haste, we say *approximately* what we mean, then assume that the message received by the listener is the same as the message we intended to send. Also, we sometimes send one message nonverbally and state a different message verbally. Which message is the listener to believe?

Message discrepancy means that the message sent and the message received differ in meaning. The difficulty may be with the sender of the message or the receiver. When the problem is with the sender, it may be caused by:

•   Ambiguity in the message.

•   **Inconsistency** in the verbal and nonverbal messages.

•   Poor **enunciation,** causing some words to sound like other words with a different meaning.

•   Use of language the listener does not understand. (This is likely to occur if the listener is a child, a person from a different culture, or an elderly person who may not be familiar with newer meanings of a word.)

If the problem of message discrepancy lies with the receiver, it may be caused by:

•   Poor hearing

•   Selective listening (the individual listens only to certain parts of a statement)

•   Inability to understand the words used by the speaker, such as medical terminology

•   Acceptance of the wrong message when there is inconsistency in the sender's verbal and nonverbal communication

An example of inconsistency in verbal and nonverbal messages is the crying patient who says, "I'm all right. I feel fine." Sometimes the health care provider who is alert to nonverbal messages can pick up the true situation, as when a patient says, "There is nothing really wrong with me. The doctor says these are just routine tests." At the same time, the patient's countenance reflects a high level of anxiety. Whenever there is inconsistency in verbal and nonverbal messages, the listener must decide which message to believe.

In your endeavors to convey messages that are received (interpreted) as you intend:

•   Avoid ambiguous statements.

•   Select words and phrases the listener will understand.

- Speak clearly.

- Control your nonverbal signals to avoid sending a message that is different from your verbal message.

- Face the person to whom you are speaking.

In trying to "hear" others accurately:

- Give your full attention to anyone who is speaking to you.

- Listen to the words and observe nonverbal behavior in an effort to get the "real message."

- Use questions to clarify the speaker's intended meaning, especially (1) if the speaker uses ambiguous or unfamiliar words and (2) if the verbal and nonverbal messages are inconsistent.

ASSUMPTIONS AND EXPECTATIONS

Underlying many communication problems are **assumptions** and expectations held by the speaker or by the listener. *To assume is to accept as fact without any evidence or proof.* Sometimes we assume that another person "knows" how we feel or what we are thinking, even though we did not verbally express our thoughts or feelings. Actually, the person to whom we are speaking may be completely unaware of how we feel or what we are thinking. Or, the other person may make assumptions about how we think or feel and the assumptions are completely wrong! Making assumptions is certain to create misunderstandings and communication breakdowns.

Another frequent cause of communication problems is the expectation of a person, either the sender or receiver of the message. An **expectation** means thinking that something will occur. An expectation can cause the receiver to "read into" a message something that the sender did not intend. For example, suppose your supervisor walks in while you are taking a shortcut on a task, then later the supervisor sends for you. Having been "caught" taking an unauthorized shortcut, your expectation is that the supervisor is going to **reprimand** you. You are probably set to defend yourself or to accept blame and say you will not do it again. But perhaps, instead of reprimanding you, the supervisor says, "I noticed you were not following procedure. Let's take a close look at the method you were using. It may be more efficient than our present procedure." Let us hope you did not misinterpret the supervisor's opening statement before you found out that your expectation was wrong! Sometimes an expectation can even lead the listener to "hear" a message that is quite different from the words spoken. This takes the speaker by surprise, since the speaker is unaware of the other person's expectations.

IMPROVING COMMUNICATION SKILLS

Improving your communication skills requires that you test your habits as a sender-of-messages and as a receiver-of-messages. Fortunately, the same practice that helps you become more precise in your sending can also contribute to your skill in listening. As you become sensitive to ambiguities, inconsistencies, assumptions, and expectations, you will ask for **clarification** rather than risk a misunderstanding.

The following exercises are structured to provide practice in speaking, listening, and interpreting messages. After each exercise, an observer will report to you on your behavior as you interacted with another person. Your opportunity to serve as an observer will alert you to additional examples of ambiguous messages. Essentially, in these exercises, you will increase your skills in:

• Selecting and using words that clearly express your intended meaning in terms the listener is able to understand

• Testing your listener's interpretation of what you have said, then clarifying the meaning if there is a discrepancy

• Listening to others and consciously trying to get the "real" message, by screening out assumptions and expectations

• Questioning to obtain clarification from the speaker

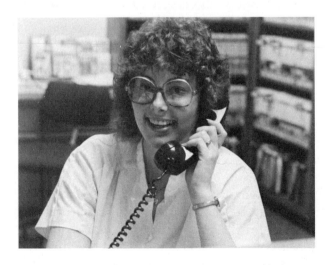

Telephone communication is almost entirely verbal, without the benefit of observing nonverbal behavior.

When you have made progress on each of these skills, the probability of you having a communication breakdown is less. As an effective communicator, you will also be more effective in establishing good relationships.

EXERCISE III: EXPRESSING IDEAS CLEARLY

The complete exercise consists of two rounds, each lasting about twenty minutes. Each member of the group will serve as observer for one round and communicator (participant in the discussion) for one round. The exercise may be repeated as many times as the class schedule permits, so that all members of the class can make definite progress toward achieving the objectives.

Purpose

In this exercise, you will practice making statements that convey your intended meaning to another person, with minimal chance of misinterpretation by the listener.

Objectives

In this exercise you will:

•   Express your intended meaning clearly.

•   Use your listener's nonverbal response to determine whether or not you conveyed your intended meaning.

•   Listen to the listener's restatement of your ideas and correct any misinterpretation by revising your original statement.

Instructions

1.   Organize into groups of four.

2.   Two members of the group will serve as observers and two members will participate in a discussion.

3.   The discussion will last ten minutes, then each observer will report what was heard and observed.

4.   The entire group will discuss the original statement that served as a basis for the discussion and list any obstacles to clear communication that occurred.

Procedure for Observers

Your task is to observe the communicators and report to the group at the conclusion of the ten-minute discussion. Then, assist in revising the statement that provided the basis for the discussion.

1. Decide which communicator each of you will observe.

2. Sit where you can observe your subject without distraction.

3. Use the Observation Record for Exercise III (page 327) to record your observations.

4. When the ten-minute time limit is called, report your observations. Then, listen while the other observer reports.

5. Discuss these reports as a group, with each member challenging others as necessary to clarify the meaning of any statement made.

6. Write a revised statement clearly reflecting the true meaning of the original statement.

7. Exchange roles for the second round. Read Procedure for Communicators and select a different topic from that used in the first round.

Procedure for Communicators

1. Your task is to help one another improve communication skills by giving special attention to the following:
    a. Ways to clarify ambiguous statements.
    b. Words that are unclear or have double meanings.
    c. Nonverbal behavior that may indicate confusion, doubt, misinterpretation, understanding, misunderstanding, agreement, or disagreement on the part of the listener.
    d. Your own assumptions about the meaning another person is trying to convey.

2. From the list of ten statements that follows, select one statement to use as the basis for your discussion.

3. One communicator will open the discussion by making the statement.

4. The other will challenge the speaker by saying, "What do you mean by that?"

5. The discussion will consist of efforts by each speaker to clarify the intended meaning of the statement. (If you wish, explore possible hidden meanings in the statement.)

6. Whenever you are in doubt about the other's meaning (a) ask specific questions in an effort to get clarification, or (b) restate the speaker's

meaning as you interpret it, and ask whether or not your interpretation is correct.

7. When you think the meaning is clear but disagree with the statement, you should (a) test your understanding by restating it in your own words and getting approval of your interpretation; then (b) state your own point of view (your disagreement).

8. Following the discussion, listen to the observers' reports, then discuss the reports as a group. Challenge any unclear statements, and require clarification from the one who made the statement.

9. Discuss the original statement. Revise it to provide a clear statement that will shed light on the problem between Mrs. A. and Mr. M. as outlined in Exercise I.

10. Exchange roles with the observers. In preparation for the second round, read Procedure for Observers.

STATEMENTS TO SERVE AS THE BASIS FOR DISCUSSION BY COMMUNICATORS

1. With all her personal problems, Mrs. A. should not be a supervisor.

2. Mrs. A. did not handle this situation very well.

3. Mrs. A. is a good supervisor.

4. Mrs. A. needs a course in supervisory techniques.

5. Mrs. A. needs professional help to work out her problems.

6. Mr. M. has a chip on his shoulder.

7. Mr. M. is hard to get along with.

8. Mr. M. is bucking for Mrs. A.'s job.

9. These two people will never be able to work well together.

10. There would not be a problem if Mr. M. would just shape up.

EXERCISE IV: PARAPHRASING IDEAS EXPRESSED BY OTHERS

Purpose

In this exercise, you will practice paraphrasing statements made by others as a means of testing your interpretation of the speaker's intended meaning.

Objectives

In this exercise you will:

- Restate the idea expressed by another person to reflect your interpretation of the intended meaning.

- Observe the nonverbal behavior of another person and interpret it to mean agreement or disagreement with what you are saying.

- Use questions to obtain clarification of a speaker's intended meaning, continuing the questioning process until the speaker approves your statement of the original intended meaning.

Instructions

1. Organize into groups of four, preferably with classmates who were not in your group during the other exercises.

2. Follow the same general procedure used in Exercise III.

3. Time limits are the same:
   a. A total of about twenty minutes for each round
   b. About ten minutes to discuss the topic
   c. Seven minutes for observers to report and the group to talk about any communication problems
   d. Three minutes to prepare a revised statement acceptable to all members of the group

Procedure for Observers

1. Your task is to observe the communicators and report to them at the conclusion of the ten-minute discussion. Then, assist in revising the discussion topic to provide an unambiguous statement—all members of the group must agree on its meaning.

2. Decide which communicator each will observe.

3. Use the Observation Record for Exercise IV (page 328) to record your observations.

4. When the ten-minute time limit is called, report your observations.

5. Discuss the communications, particularly examples of ambiguous statements and ways they could have been avoided.

6. Assist in revising the original statement.

7. Assume the role of communicator for the second round.

Procedure for Communicators

1. Your task is to test your ability to interpret correctly your partner's meaning. Your partner must approve your interpretation of what he or she just said, before you may state your own ideas.

2. With your partner, select a topic from the opinion statements listed in the next heading. (These are controversial topics. Some people will agree with one, while others will disagree. There is no "right" or "wrong" for any of these topics; they simply provide a basis for practice in communicating ideas to others.)

3. One communicator will open the discussion by making the chosen statement, somewhat emphatically, as though it is a personal opinion.

4. The partner must interpret what was said, using his or her own words. The first communicator must accept this interpretation as correct before the second communicator is free to react to the initial statement. The second communicator can react by:

    a. Agreeing and offering support to the statement
    b. Disagreeing and arguing against it
    c. Suggesting an alternative

5. Each communicator must first **paraphrase** the partner's last statement and obtain approval of the interpretation of the intended meaning before expressing *personal* ideas. Essentially, you *earn permission to offer your idea* by getting the partner's approval of how you interpreted his or her last statement.

6. If you think your partner's statement is ambiguous, seek clarification by asking questions, then try to paraphrase.

7. When time is called, listen to the observers' reports, then discuss their observations. Identify factors (assumptions, ambiguous words, etc.) that influenced the discussion, especially if you and your partner had difficulty interpreting each other correctly. Try to understand any difficulty you had in listening to your partner. Did your feelings interfere with listening? Did you experience feelings of resentment or anger when your partner misinterpreted you? Did your feelings interfere with efforts to clarify?

8. Use the last three minutes to revise the original statement. You do not have to agree with the statement, but all members of the group must agree on the meaning of the statement in its final form.

9. Assume the role of observer for the second round. Read Procedure for Observers.

OPINION STATEMENTS TO SERVE AS A BASIS FOR DISCUSSION

1. Health care providers should be allowed to go to classes during duty hours if they want to work on a higher certificate.

2. A health care provider should prepare for one role and remain in it throughout his or her career.

3. Advanced courses should be open to all health care providers who want to become professional practitioners.

4. Most people entering a health career want to help the sick.

5. Women make better health care providers than men.

6. Every health care provider wants to stay up-to-date.

7. People should be required to carry health insurance; then, when they need health care they will be able to afford it.

8. Patients should not expect health care providers to listen to their problems.

9. The government should take over the costs of health care.

10. Women are more suited to the role of an auxiliary worker than to the role of a professional.

11. Health maintenance organizations are preferable to the fee-for-service system for the delivery of health services.

12. A woman who is pregnant has the right to decide whether or not she will continue the pregnancy.

13. Everyone who has AIDS should be quarantined.

14. Sex education should not be allowed in the public schools. Sex education is for adults, not children.

15. Managed Care is the best system for providing health services.

CLASS CHALLENGE

Some of the *Opinion Statements for Discussion* are related to one or more trends or issues in the health field. Are you informed about these trends and issues? Do you know what changes are being proposed? What are the pros and cons for each issue?

OBSERVATION RECORD FOR EXERCISE III

Communicator being observed: _____

Observer: _____

Statement used as basis for the discussion: _____

Group's revision of the statement (enter after the final discussion involving communicators and observers): _____

Type of Observation	Observed Behavior
1. How does your subject show that he/she is listening?	
2. How does your subject ask the speaker to clarify meanings?	
3. How does your subject help the speaker clarify meanings?	
4. How does your subject indicate not understanding what the speaker means?	
5. How does your subject indicate understanding?	
6. Does your subject indicate understanding when there actually is misunderstanding? What was the evidence that a misinterpretation had occurred?	

OBSERVATION RECORD FOR EXERCISE IV

Communicator being observed: _____

Observer: _____

Statement used as basis for the discussion: _____

_____

Revised statement: _____

_____

Type of Observation	Observed Behavior
1. Is your subject making an effort to be clear?	
2. Is your subject using illustrations to clarify meanings?	
3. Is your subject using words and phrases with one precise meaning?	
4. As a listener, is your subject trying to restate the speaker's meaning accurately?	
5. Is your subject trying to follow the other's meaning or jumping from one idea to the next?	
6. Is your subject using nonverbal behavior to indicate need for clarification? What was the evidence that a misinterpretation had occurred?	
7. Is your subject's verbal and nonverbal behavior consistent?	

You may wish to continue your work on communication skills by studying an issue, then preparing an oral report, one side of a debate, or a written report. Thus, you will learn about important trends that may affect your work situation in the future and, at the same time, improve your ability to communicate ideas clearly.

References and Suggested Readings

Anderson, Carolyn. *Patient Teaching and Communication in an Information Age.* Albany, NY: Delmar Publishers Inc., 1990. Chapter 1, "The Communication Process," pp. 3–25.

Burley-Allen, Madelyn. *Listening: The Forgotten Skill.* New York, NY: John Wiley & Sons Inc., 1995. Chapter 3, "Barriers between Listener and Speaker," pp. 46–78.

Tamparo, Carol D. & Lindh, Wilburta Q. *Therapeutic Communications for Allied Health Professions.* Albany, NY: Delmar Publishers Inc., 1992. Unit 2, "Basic Communication Skills," pp. 24–48.

REVIEW AND SELF-CHECK

Complete each statement below, using information from Unit 18.

1. Three sources of communication breakdown are:

   1. _____

   2. _____

   3. _____

2. An ambiguous message is one that is _____ .

3. Some reasons for ambiguous verbal communication are:

   1. _____

   2. _____

   3. _____

4. Some ways to avoid ambiguous statements are:

   1. _____

   2. _____

   3. _____

5.   Message discrepancy means that _____ .

6.   The sender may contribute to message discrepancy in such ways as:

    1. _____

    2. _____

    3. _____

    4. _____

7.   The listener may contribute to message discrepancy in such ways as:

    1. _____

    2. _____

    3. _____

    4. _____

8.   As a sender, you can minimize message discrepancy by:

    1. _____

    2. _____

    3. _____

    4. _____

9.   As a listener, you can minimize message discrepancy by:

    1. _____

    2. _____

    3. _____

10. To assume means to _____ .

11. An expectation is _____ .

ASSIGNMENT

Complete the following exercises during the next month.

1.   As you watch television or attend a movie, note examples of:
   a.   Communication breakdown

    b. Poor listening skills on the part of one or more characters

    c. Message discrepancy

    d. Nonverbal communication unnoticed by other characters.

2   In a class discussion:

    a. List movies or TV programs in which a communication breakdown is a major basis for the plot.

    b. Share examples noted in Activity #1. Discuss the apparent cause(s) (i.e., faulty assumptions, message discrepancy, poor listening skills, etc.) of the communication problems in each example that was observed.

Section VI

Coping with Loss

You have now learned about human behavior, ways people react to threat, and how to communicate effectively. These learnings will prove invaluable as you work with people who are struggling to cope with loss. The ultimate losses are death (loss of one's own life) and bereavement (loss of a loved one).

In order to provide effective care to a terminally ill patient or to help those who are facing the loss of a loved one, the health care provider must have arrived at full acceptance of his or her own mortality and must have completely resolved any "unfinished business" related to past losses. Section VI is designed to help you learn about the relationship of loss and the grief process to physical and mental/emotional health.

The purpose of Section VI is to help you deal with your own mortality, clarify your beliefs about death, and become sensitive to the needs of terminally ill patients and their families.

Unit 19

Gains and Losses throughout the Life Span

OBJECTIVES

Upon completion of this unit, you should be able to:

- State one reason why a happy life event may be accompanied by sadness or depression.
- State three reasons why it is important to learn to cope with the small losses of life.
- List four steps for learning to cope with loss.
- Explain the significance of a loss.
- List three examples of loss that occur during each period of the life span: infancy, early childhood, the school-age years, adolescence, the young adult years, middle and late adult years, and senescence.
- State seven guidelines for using loss and grief as a growth experience.
- State one definition of euthanasia.

KEY TERMS

Amputation	Detachment	Euthanasia
Intangible	Invulnerable	Macabre
Mastectomy	Menopause	Mortality
Omnipotent	Stamina	Survivor guilt
Thanatology		

LIFE CHANGES AS GAINS AND LOSSES

Life involves a continuous succession of changes that require us to adjust and readjust. Some of these changes represent a gain of some type—new home, new member of the family, graduation, new job, or a promotion. Some changes represent a loss—being fired, losing an important object, losing a spouse through divorce, losing a loved one through death.

334

Many events involve both gains and losses. Moving to a new home is exciting, but it involves certain losses, including the familiarity of the old home and relationships in the old neighborhood. Graduation is usually a happy event—it symbolizes moving on to bigger and better things. But, graduation also means giving up a favorite teacher, no longer spending much of the school day with your classmates, giving up a familiar role for a new role and new responsibilities. You expect the big events of life to have a happy effect, so it is confusing to find that, instead of being happy, you are sad or even depressed. These negative feelings are due to an awareness (perhaps at the unconscious level) of losses that will result from an otherwise happy event.

Most people do not need to learn how to be happy about a gain, but many people do not know how to cope with loss. How to deal with losses may be one of life's most difficult lessons. It definitely is one of life's most important lessons, because unexpressed grief is a powerful influence on behavior and on emotional/mental health. There is also a relationship between significant loss and the occurrence of a serious illness or accident, usually within eighteen months following the loss.

LEARNING TO COPE WITH LOSS

If we learn early in life to deal effectively with "small deaths" (the losses that are part of living), then we are better prepared to deal with those losses that cause a radical change in our life situation. If we do not learn to "let go" (of whatever was lost) and to grieve appropriately for each loss, then there is an accumulation of suppressed emotions—grief, anger, guilt, and fear. Suppressed emotions are eventually expressed in some form, such as uncontrolled outbursts, depression, or inability to cope with daily life problems. Inability (or failure) to express such feelings is characteristic of people who develop intense fears (phobias), commit suicide, or develop alcohol/drug dependency.

Actually, we have a choice. We can learn to accept the inevitable losses of life and express our grief appropriately, thereby maintaining control and emotional well-being. Or, we can go through life without learning how to deal with loss—reacting with anger about the "unfairness" of life or suppressing our grief, thereby risking loss of control when these feelings eventually erupt.

Dr. Elisabeth Kubler-Ross is a psychiatrist who has worked with dying patients for many years. She believes that the dying process extends throughout life and that we go through the stages of this process repeatedly as we experience significant changes in our lives. The best preparation for dealing with death, she maintains, is to learn to grieve appropriately for the "small deaths" (i.e., losses) that accompany any major life change. Once we have learned to grieve, we are able to cope better with the "big" losses that will, inevitably, occur in each of our lives.

Learning to cope with loss involves several distinct steps:

1. Recognize the losses involved in a life event.

2. Grant yourself the right to grieve for each loss.

3. Recognize and accept the various emotions involved in your reaction to each loss.

4. Allow yourself time to grieve; accept that grief is a process that extends over a period of time.

SIGNIFICANCE OF LOSS

Losses are of many types: objects, people, relationships, jobs, money, body image (i.e., **amputation,** radical **mastectomy**), or **intangibles** such as beliefs, faith, one's sense of security, self-esteem. The significance of a loss is very personal. A person's reaction to a loss *reflects its meaning to that person,* rather than its value as perceived by others.

Some types of loss may be experienced at any time throughout life: moving, personal relationships, death of a loved one, personal property, health. Reactions to such losses are influenced by the period of life in which they occur. Children often do not understand the reasons for a loss, and adults may fail to note or accept the child's emotional reaction. Adults have the advantage

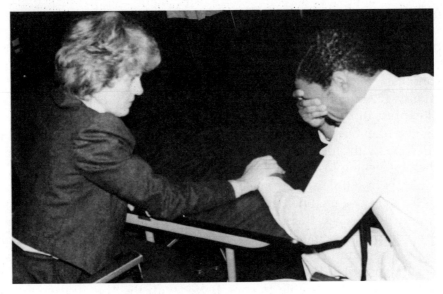

The significance of a loss is very personal.

of being involved in some decisions that result in a loss, such as moving, so their emotional reaction is tempered by an understanding of reasons for the decision. For many elderly people, the greatest loss of all is losing control over decisions that affect the remainder of their lives. Moving into a child's home or into a nursing home results in at least partial loss of control over one's daily activities. The reaction to such a change often includes hopelessness and resignation. The most devastating loss is the loss of life—one's own or that of a loved one.

LOSSES DUE TO DEATH

The impact of a death on each survivor is influenced by numerous factors, including age of the survivor, relationship to the deceased, the survivor's past experience in coping with significant losses, age of the deceased, and circumstances surrounding the death.

- Was the death expected? Did it follow a lengthy terminal illness?

- Does the death represent a release from pain and suffering?

- Was the death sudden and unexpected? In this situation, the survivors must cope with shock initially, then with their loss.

- What was the age of the deceased? If the deceased was elderly and the survivors believe that he or she had "lived a good life," the loss is easier to accept. If the deceased was young, grief is likely to be accompanied by anger and a sense of injustice.

Certain circumstances surrounding a death have an especially powerful impact on survivors.

- **The death was accidental.** Was the accident due to someone's negligence or carelessness? If so, anger and blaming may delay the beginning of a healthful grieving process. If a survivor was involved in the accident, that person may feel that he or she was responsible for the death. Or, that person may experience **survivor guilt,** wondering "What right did I have to survive?" or believing "I should have been the one who died." Anyone who is experiencing survivor guilt needs professional counseling.

- **The death was related to violence or criminal activity (mugging, burglary, or drive-by shooting).** Survivors of this type of death must deal with anger, perhaps a desire for revenge, as well as grief.

- **The death was a murder or homicide.** Survivors must deal with shock initially, then questions of "Why?" and "Who?" If the killer was a member of the family, survivors may divide into two groups. Some will refuse to believe the perpetrator's guilt and will loyally support his or her defense. Others will direct anger at the accused and seek "justice" for the deceased. In both cases, these emotions are likely to interfere with the grief process.

- **The deceased was on life support.** Who made the decision to discontinue it? Even when a Living Will and Advance Directives exist, the decision to discontinue life support is difficult for family members. If some family members disagree with the decision, then the decision-maker has to cope with their criticism in addition to personal feelings about making that fateful decision. Unfortunately, there are still some physicians who do not respect Advance Directives, believing they must use all available measures to sustain life, in spite of the dying person's expressed wishes and hopeless condition. In those situations, the decision-maker has to be very assertive about having the provisions of the Advance Directive carried out. The emotional impact of the loss may be delayed by the activities required for allowing the person to die and by the emotions aroused by that difficult situation—anger, perhaps guilt, loyalty and love for the dying person, and a sense of mission to ensure that his or her wishes are respected.

- **The death was due to self-inflicted injury—suicide.** This type of death is especially difficult for survivors. Because suicide is widely misunderstood, it is important that health care providers have a broad view of this type of death.

SUICIDE

Any death by suicide places family members and associates of the deceased in a soul-searching position:

Why did I not recognize the signs that he or she was in such distress?
Why was I not more sensitive to his or her unhappiness?
What did I do that caused this terrible act?
Why did I not express my love?
Why was I so critical?
Why did I not insist that he or she seek help?
What could I have done to prevent this act?

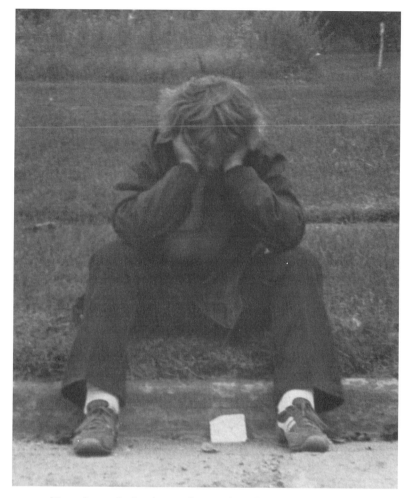

The impact of loss through death is influenced by factors surrounding the death. (From Barbara A. Backer, Natalie R. Hannon, and Noreen A. Russell, *Death and Dying: Understanding and Care,* 2nd Edition, p. 228. Albany, NY: Delmar Publishers Inc., 1994.)

For a child, the immediate reaction is usually rage: "How could Mommy (or Daddy) leave me?" There may also be powerful feelings of guilt:

"When she (he) sent me to my room I wished she (he) was dead. It's all my fault."

"If I had been a better daughter (son), Mommy (Daddy) would not have done this."

"If only I had said, 'I love you' more often."

For parents there may be many questions, most pertaining to "how could I have been a better parent?" For siblings, the entire range of emotions is possible, depending upon the relationship with the deceased. For surviving spouses, the emotional impact may range from relief to a devastating sense of loss, depending upon the quality of the marital relationship. Friends and associates may be affected differently by suicide than by a death due to accident or illness. Some of the questions above may haunt those who associated with the deceased on a daily basis, especially the question, "What could I have done to help?"

Suicide is considered an honorable death in some cultures. In certain Asian societies, someone who has lost honor, for whatever reason, is *expected* to commit suicide. Japanese pilots were trained during World War II for suicide missions, to sacrifice their lives for the honor of their country. But in America today suicide is regarded by many people as a dishonorable act; in fact, most states have laws that treat suicide as a crime. Some insurance companies do not pay if a death is due to suicide. Most life insurance policies exclude suicide for a specific period of time, usually two years.

Some suicides are accidental. It is well-known among adolescent males that constriction of the throat can increase orgasm when masturbating. When a male is found hanging with a rope or belt around the throat, it is sometimes because his effort to enhance a sexual experience did not go as planned. Perhaps a chair or stool turned over or his foot slipped, and an accidental hanging occurred. Though a coroner's report may indicate whether or not this was the case, such information would not be made public. If this type of accident occurred but the victim was still found alive, he may be admitted to the hospital in an unconscious condition.

A more common hospital admission is the person who has ingested a poison, taken an overdose of some drug, shot himself, or attempted to cut a blood vessel. These are "incomplete suicides."

> **NOTE:**   Do not describe a suicide as "successful" or "unsuccessful." A suicide is either "complete" or "incomplete."

One who completes a suicide by any means is found dead, and therefore will not come under your care. Most people who complete a suicide have a history of suicide attempts. Who is to know when a person who survived one suicide attempt will make another attempt that becomes a completed suicide? As a health care provider, avoid thinking that any suicide attempt is "just trying to get attention." The attempt may be a call for help, but "attention" is not the motive.

Why would anyone ingest a poison or take a lethal dose of a drug? Why would someone cut themselves? Why put a bullet through one's head? (Guns

PROGRESS

Ring

      Ring

            Ring

Hello. You have reached the Fulton County suicide prevention hotline.

    If you have just slashed your wrists, press 1.

    If you have just swallowed poison, press 2.

    If you are playing Russian roulette, press 3.

    For all other methods, press 4.

If you are merely contemplating suicide, or would like to speak to a counselor, please stay on the line.

We're sorry. All counselors are busy now. Please stay on the line. You'll be placed in sequential hold, and your call will be answered in the order in which it was received. Thank you for your patience.

    (Insert seven minutes of doctor's office type music.)

New voice: Hello. Hello? This is the counselor. May I help you?

Hello?

    (Fade to black.)

LSM, 1993

A Bipolar patient pokes fun at the Helpline. Manic-Depressive humor often has a **macabre** *tone, reflecting hopelessness and suicidal ideation.*

are used more often by males than females.) The only logical answer is that the individual is desperately trying to escape an intolerable life situation, a painful or debilitating physical condition, or the hopelessness that accompanies deep depression. Dr. Kay Redmon Jamison is the author of several books on depression and manic-depressive illness and coauthor of a comprehensive review of research and clinical findings related to mood disorders. She has found that persons with manic-depressive illness (MDI) or clinical depression have an overwhelming need to escape the hopelessness of the depressive state. Some people use drugs, alcohol, or both as a means of escape for months or years. Some people cut themselves because the pain of cutting provides escape from "feeling nothing."

These victims of a biological illness (disruption of one or more neurotransmitters in the brain) are considered mental patients, but most are highly intelligent and capable of productive work when not in the depressed state. In fact, many creative people—composers, musicians, writers, poets, actors—are manic depressive and do their best work when in the hypomanic state, but are incapable of productive activity when depressed.

The greatest danger of suicide is when the person is coming out of a depressed state. Many depressed persons do not have the energy to carry out a suicide. As they recover from depression, they not only have the energy but also know that sooner or later they will again experience the hopelessness of depression. Two months stand out as the time of year when suicide rates peak: May and October.

One journalist spoke of her depressed periods as a "bottomless hole" or a "black abyss" of hopelessness and despair. After two attempts, she completed a suicide just when her physician and family believed she was recovering from her latest bout of depression.

According to Dr. Jamison, the suicide of a person who is depressed *is not an act of will*; it is a desperate effort to escape from the effects of depression. Approximately forty-five percent of MDI victims commit suicide by the age of forty. Dr. Jamison also estimates that only two out of five persons with MDI have been diagnosed and are under treatment. That leaves three out of five who may be using alcohol and drugs to escape their severe mood swings and who may eventually commit suicide, never having been diagnosed or given the opportunity for treatment.

It is likely that you will encounter a hospitalized patient who has attempted suicide. It is especially important for care-givers to keep in mind that they do not know the circumstances of that patient's life-situation. Any one of us may at some time in our lives experience emotionally overwhelming circumstances. Without having experienced such conditions, we do not know how we would react. Only those who have experienced hopelessness, depression, or mood swings over a period of time can understand the distress of a person who attempts suicide.

The implications for you as a health care provider are clear. Do not judge the patient who has attempted suicide. Know that this person needs emotional support and respect. Keep in mind your philosophy of individual worth, be a compassionate caregiver, demonstrate caring, and *listen*. Anyone who has attempted suicide should be evaluated by a psychiatrist and, according to the diagnosis, given appropriate treatment. Long-term counseling is needed by most survivors of a suicide attempt, to learn effective ways of coping with depression, mood swings, and life problems.

EUTHANASIA

The word **euthanasia** is derived from two Greek words: eu (good) and thanatos (death). Euthanasia is a complex and controversial subject that involves philosophical views of life and death, ethical considerations, religious beliefs, and legal questions. Before taking a position for or against euthanasia, become informed about each of these aspects. With increasing knowledge and exposure to a variety of viewpoints, you will be prepared to formulate an opinion based on information, rather than value judgments alone.

The discussion below is limited to basic information that you, as a health care provider, should know and understand. For that reason, the definition that forms the basis of this discussion is more restricted than that used by authors who present a comprehensive discussion. As used below, euthanasia is any action, requested by the patient but performed by someone else, that accelerates the dying process. The request may be made because of intractable pain, loss of bodily control, or a deteriorating condition that will inevitably result in helplessness. Modern writers differentiate active and passive euthanasia, based on how the death occurs. *Active euthanasia* involves an *intentional intervention* (usually, administration of medication) for the purpose of causing death. *Passive euthanasia* consists of *withholding* and/or *withdrawing treatment,* with the intention of allowing the person to die of the underlying disease process. This definition of passive euthanasia includes withholding or discontinuing life support procedures, such as artificial ventilation, cardiopulmonary resuscitation, and tube feedings. This will be discussed further in relation to patients' rights to refuse treatment, in Unit 20.

In some European countries, euthanasia is an accepted practice. A 1991 survey in Holland, commissioned by the government, revealed that 2,300 Dutch patients receive euthanasia every year. In 1994, the Dutch parliament passed a law that specifies the conditions under which a physician may perform euthanasia without the risk of prosecution. This law requires that doctors follow a 28-step checklist and that all euthanasia incidents be reported to the government. In the United States, active euthanasia is illegal regardless of the patient's condition or expressed wishes.

Because some patients wish to accelerate the dying process, rather than live out their days under intolerable conditions, existing laws are being challenged. The well-publicized actions of Dr. Jack Kevorkian are labeled "physician-assisted suicide" (PAS), rather than euthanasia. (Some writers present "assisted suicide" as a type of euthanasia.) Dr. Kevorkian helps to set up a lethal situation, but the patient commits the act that results in death. The first person assisted in suicide by Dr. Kevorkian was Janet Adkins, a 54-year-old woman with Alzheimer's Disease. Dr. Kevorkian was present, set up the mechanism for administering a lethal dose of potassium chloride, and Mrs. Adkins pushed the button that caused the injection to occur.

Even though he does not personally administer a fatal dose, Dr. Kevorkian has been brought to trial repeatedly under a Michigan state law that prohibits "assisted suicide." Each time, he has been acquitted by the jury. The Michigan State Supreme Court has ruled the state law to be unconstitutional.

In August, 1996 Dr. Kevorkian assisted Judith Curren, a nurse with a painful, debilitating illness, to commit suicide. Because this person did not have a terminal illness, her case is especially controversial and will probably receive much publicity. Ms. Curren is the thirty-fifth assisted-suicide by

Dr. Kevorkian. Within a month, Dr. Kevorkian participated in the assisted-suicides of two other patients.

Dr. Kevorkian is trying to force the medical profession, law-makers, and the public to reconsider the rights of patients and their doctors to decide appropriate treatment under special circumstances. He believes these rights should include the right to escape an intolerable condition by choosing to die, either through euthanasia or assisted suicide. Since both "euthanasia" and "assisted suicide" tend to arouse strong emotions, the phrase "facilitation of the dying process" would help to maintain an objective focus during discussion of this topic.

The danger of both euthanasia and assisted-suicide is misuse; someone other than the patient may benefit from the death. Obviously, beneficiaries of a patient's estate should not be allowed to influence the decision. Every effort should be made to ensure that the patient has not been coerced into requesting death. Most supporters believe that only under clearly defined conditions and with the expressed wish of the patient should either procedure be carried out. The decision should not be left to one doctor and one patient. Rather, a panel of experts should review each case and conduct a face-to-face interview with the patient.

Dr. Edwin Shneidman, a professor of **thanatology,** speaks of the increasingly humanistic approach to death as "one of the most refreshing currents" in thanatology. In regard to euthanasia, he questions:

"Should a weakened citizen, too ill to kill himself, have the right to say, 'Enough!' And, consider what we read and know of occasional heinous derelictions in some nursing homes, what are the chances, without any opportunity for redress, of abuses in the practice of voluntary euthanasia?" (Shneidman, 1984)

Another writer has stated, in regard to suicide and rights of the dying, "The Christian inhibition against suicide applies *a fortiori* to giving incurably and painfully ailing human beings the merciful release that human Christians give, as a matter of course, to animals when these are in the same plight." (Toynbee, in Shneidman, 1984) In the decade since those words were written, there have been many books, articles, movies and television programs that focus on questions related to the rights of dying patients and their families.

At present, increased public awareness and challenges to existing laws suggest that additional significant changes probably will occur over the next several years. It remains to be seen if those changes will include legalization of euthanasia or assisted suicide.

DEATH OF A PARENT

The death of one's parent is a unique type of loss, regardless of one's age and the age of the parent. For each of us, parents provide a link to our ancestry, our own life history, and most of what we learned as children. In *Motherless Daughters,* author Hope Edelman states that loss of a parent is one of life's most stressful events. A young child is likely to experience rage, perceiving the death as abandonment. Loss of a parent during childhood also means the loss of parental guidance through current and future developmental tasks. The deceased parent will be missing from important life events: graduations, recitals, athletic performances, the wedding, the birth of one's own children. It also means the loss of a grandparent to one's future children.

The death of a same-gender parent means the loss of a parental role model. This loss is especially significant during adolescence, a time of struggling to establish one's own identity. Although adolescence is characterized by some degree of rebellion, this period of life involves developmental tasks that are best accomplished under parental guidance. Sometimes the death of a parent forces a child into an adult role. The oldest girl may assume maternal responsibilities for care of younger siblings and for managing the household. An adolescent boy may become "the man of the house" and seek work to help support the family.

Regardless of the ages of surviving children, the age of the parent at the time of death may become the age at which the child expects to die. Thus, a man whose father died of a heart attack at age 52 may develop high levels of anxiety when he approaches that age. Reaching the age of the deceased parent is known as the "parental trigger," a time when one becomes especially aware of one's own **mortality.**

There is special significance to the loss of one's mother, since "mother" represents nurturing, caring, comfort, a sense of security, trust. The need to be mothered extends into adulthood. There are certain special times when mothering, or the help of one's mother, is needed, such as preparations for a wedding or the birth of one's first baby. Becoming motherless can lead to a longing that continues for years

The loss of a father also has special significance, especially during childhood. "Father" to most people means protection and security. If the mother has been a homemaker, death of her husband may mean a financial crisis. If it becomes necessary that she seek employment, then the children experience two losses: Daddy abandoned us, now Mommy is abandoning us every day to go to work. The family's standard of living may be lower without the father's income.

Regardless of which parent died, surviving children may be profoundly affected psychologically, especially if they do not grieve appropriately for their loss. *Displacement* may occur if feelings were not fully expressed during the mourning period; they may emerge, greatly magnified, later in life when some other loss occurs. *Transference* is manifested by persistent seeking of fulfillment from others, placing them in the position of parental substitute. It is also possible to become "stuck" emotionally. While maturing in other respects, the individual remains emotionally immature in relation to death, authority figures, abandonment or any other aspect associated with the parent's death. For example, Harry died of a sudden heart attack when his son was twelve years old. Numerous relatives pointed out to the twelve-year-old son that he was now the man of the house. In his new role, Harry, Jr. did not feel free to cry or express his grief, but in fact he was emotionally devastated. Many years later, any talk about sickness or dying would result in an angry outburst or he would leave the room. The son was emotionally "stuck." As an adult, he still could not express the grief he felt at the loss of his father. Any of these psychological effects can seriously interfere with future relationships.

LOSSES IN SPECIFIC PERIODS OF THE LIFE SPAN

Preparation for coping with a significant loss comes from experiencing a variety of losses throughout life. The individual who learns during childhood that certain life experiences are "small losses" for which one should grieve appropriately is better prepared to cope with a major loss than someone who has not learned to recognize and grieve for a loss. Learning to cope with loss begins in infancy; the types of losses and their significance vary according to the period of life.

Losses of Infancy and Early Childhood

The prenatal period is a very special time for both mother and fetus. If there are no complications or difficult circumstances, the pregnant woman experiences very positive feelings during most of the pregnancy. For the fetus, life in the womb is the ultimate in security and safety. At the time of delivery, the family gains a new member—one of life's happiest events. But birth is the end of pregnancy—the loss of a once-only relationship between mother and infant. If the baby is breast-fed, the mother and infant establish another very special relationship. Weaning is a "small death" because it requires both mother and infant to "let go" of this special relationship forever.

During infancy and early childhood, any separation from the parents (or other caregivers) is perceived as loss. The child, not knowing that the parents will return, feels deserted. Sadness is a natural reaction to separation; but separation from those who represent security and belonging can also arouse fear, anger, and even guilt. When a young child is hospitalized and no member of the family remains with the child, the child's emotional reaction may be manifested as withdrawal. Early separation experiences may be the source of fears and anxieties in later life about the loss of a relationship.

Judith Viorst, in her book *Necessary Losses*, describes the effect of being hospitalized for three months at the age of four:

". . . three virtually motherless months because the hospitals of that time rigidly restricted visiting hours. Years after I had recovered from the illness for which I'd been hospitalized, I suffered from the effects of the hospitalization. And among the manifestations of my separation anxiety was my newly acquired habit—which continued until my middle teens—of sleepwalking."

She goes on to describe one of her sleepwalking experiences at the age of six, in which she left her home late at night and crossed a busy intersection. Arriving at a fire station, still asleep, she told an astonished fireman, "I want the firemen to find my mommy." Her comment: "A six-year-old can desperately want her mommy. A six-month-old can desperately want mommy too."

Viorst states that separation anxiety manifests in three stages: protest, when the child cries and screams; despair, a deep sorrowful yearning for the missing mother; then, **detachment,** in which the child greets the returning mother with coldness, even tries to distance himself or herself from the parent. *Detachment,* a shutdown of loving feelings, deals with loss by punishing the mother for having left, by masking the rage that is felt, and by putting up a defense against the pain of being abandoned. The effects of detachment may last for a day or a lifetime, seriously interfering with the ability to love and trust others. Viorst reasons that the emotional scars of frequent or prolonged separations from the mother are due to an innate need of every infant:

"The mother-child bond which teaches us that we are lovable. The mother-child bond which teaches us how to love. We cannot be whole human beings—indeed we may find it hard to be human—without the sustenance of this first attachment." (Viorst, 1986)

The importance of parental attachments, especially during infancy and childhood, should be understood by parents who must leave their children at frequent intervals. Special efforts should be made to establish a loving relationship and minimize the child's distress at being left in day-care or with a baby-sitter. A good daycare center offers a loving and supportive atmosphere for the child, in recognition of the distress felt by an infant/child as a normal reaction to separation from mother.

Health care providers need to understand desertion reaction, spend as much time as possible with a child whose parents have left, and provide emotional support as needed. Above all, do not subscribe to the value judgment that a crying child is "just spoiled." Be aware that the crying child may believe he or she has been abandoned.

Many changes in relationships occur during early childhood. The child achieves more independence (and less dependence) as growth and development occur. Dependency is another type of special relationship, so the child's achievements also involve changes in relationships. Entering kindergarten or school is an exciting, sometimes frightening experience. The child loses the comfort, safety, and security of home, but gains new experiences, a peer group, and new adult contacts. The mother loses her dependent "knee baby" and gains a school child who is increasingly independent.

Losses During the School-Age Period

Throughout the school-age years a child repeatedly experiences losses and gains. Each promotion means leaving a familiar teacher and gaining a new one. There may be a loss of some classmates, although new children may come into the class at intervals. Friendships may break up, with any grief over the loss obscured by anger or guilt about the cause of the break-up. A change of school during this period includes numerous losses, which may or may not be offset by gains available in the new school. Completion of the elementary grades includes loss of some relationships and also loss of a familiar role. Promotion to middle school or high school usually means giving up many childhood activities upon entering the world of adolescence.

Losses During Adolescence

Gains and losses related to growth and development, dependence vs. independence, and promotion from one grade to another continue through adolescence. For the most part, emotional effects of these types of loss or gain are manageable. A person with adequate adjustment copes with these changes reasonably well. But some life events of adolescence have the potential for arousing very strong emotional reactions: establishing a boy/girl relationship, getting a job, and graduating. During this period social relationships are established with members of the opposite sex. When such a relationship ends, one or both parties may experience intense emotional reactions to the loss, regardless of whether or not the couple became sexually active and even if the break-up was agreed on by both. If the break-up resulted from parental interference, then the grief is complicated by anger and resentment that may have long-term effects on family relationships.

Adolescence is also the time when many young people obtain their first job, which requires learning a new role and includes a significant gain—one's own income. If the job is terminated, both role and income are lost; the circumstances may even include loss of self-esteem.

Graduation from high school is perceived by students and their families as a happy event. The losses involved are seldom talked about. A high school graduation results in the breaking up of many relationships. It also represents the beginning of passage into adulthood and many new responsibilities. Although some students maintain their dependence on parents through additional years of education, for many the relatively carefree life of childhood and adolescence ends forever with graduation from high school.

Losses of the Young Adult Years

The adult period of life is characterized by vocational choices, the struggle for financial independence, establishing adult coping strategies, affirming one's sexuality through marriage or a relationship, starting a family, setting up a home, and developing a satisfying life-style. Each of these activities may provide much satisfaction and happiness. Each is also fraught with the possibility of loss: getting fired from a job; ending a marriage through divorce; losing property through theft, fire, or natural disaster; losing friends or family members through death; moving, which often includes a loss of a support network of friends, family, or both.

The adult period of life involves a continuous sequence of gains and losses, both large and small. Accepting the joy that life may bring and also learning to cope with the pain of loss leads to continued growth and a full life. Trying to escape pain by avoiding life experiences that include the risk of loss, such as marriage or a loving relationship, does not lead to growth and precludes living a full life. Part of the adult life experience is accepting the risk of losing some of what we have gained.

Losses of Middle Age

Ideally, middle adulthood is a period for enjoying rewards of one's labors during the early adult years. For many, however, this is a period of continued struggle for financial survival. The expenses of a family peak as children reach high school and college. If the family's income has increased through the years, then these expenses may be manageable. Otherwise, adolescent members of the family may have to become wage-earners.

The struggle for financial security involves relatively frequent gains and losses. For example, a promotion may mean additional salary and prestige, but result in the loss of free time if new responsibilities require longer hours or taking work home at night. Any unexpected expense may result in loss. For example, a long-awaited vacation at the beach may be lost because the car has to have a new transmission.

Parents usually welcome the growing independence of their children. There may also be some sadness at loss of the child/parent dependent relationship. As children leave home to attend school, set up their own apartments, or marry, parents may experience a real sense of loss. A woman who has been a homemaker for many years is prone to experience a loss of life purpose as the children leave home. Departure of the youngest child is especially difficult. "Empty nest syndrome" is a well-known depressive reaction to this event.

A loss of purpose is not limited to the middle-aged homemaker. Most young adults have goals—for achievement, recognition, making the world a better place, proving themselves in one way or another. During the middle adult years, these goals may still inspire a worker to strive harder. At some point, however, many people begin to realize that they will not be able to achieve some of their goals. As this realization reaches full consciousness, the individual may experience a profound sense of loss. Attitudes toward the job may change, the quality of work may be lower, there may be expressions of hopelessness. These negative feelings can be diffused by setting goals that are realistic for diminishing levels of energy.

Recognition of a very significant loss—namely, the loss of one's youth—occurs sometime during the middle years. This may occur on a fortieth or fiftieth birthday, or it may develop gradually as physical **stamina** diminishes, physical proportions change, baldness develops, wrinkles appear, or once-firm tissues become flabby. Many people accept the effects of time and adapt their life-styles to accommodate physical changes. Some people, however, experience a "midlife crisis" and set out to prove to the world (and to themselves) that they are still young. A long-term marriage may break up during this period, as one partner seeks younger companions to bolster the belief, "I am still young and attractive." Loss of youth is very painful to those who subscribe to the current emphasis on youth and sex appeal in the mass media. **Menopause** represents a very significant change for a woman—namely, loss of the ability to reproduce. For a man, occasional periods of impotence threaten self-esteem.

Middle age is a period when some loss of sensory capacity begins. This period of life is sometimes spoken of as the time of the five Bs: baldness, bifocals, bridges, bulges, and bunions. But this is also the time of life when potentially serious health problems may develop. As life span has increased during the past fifty years, the incidence of chronic diseases has risen markedly. Loss of health is so significant that many people, upon being told that they have a particular disease, react with "I don't believe it."

Denying a newly diagnosed disorder is not limited to serious illness. An adult who is told that recurrent sore throats are due to allergy may refuse to have allergy studies performed. This person's self-concept may not include "I am a person with an intolerance for certain foods and other substances in my life situation." A person who is diagnosed as having early arthritis may think immediately of people with deformed hands or those who complain constantly of their "arthritis pain." The initial reaction is "I will not become deformed, and I will not accept continuous pain in my life." Denial eventually gives way to acceptance of the diagnosis, after the individual has had time to adjust to symptoms and changes in body function.

Losses During Senescence

The senescent period of life—old age—is now considered to consist of three periods: the young-old period, ages 65 to 74; the middle-old period, ages 75 to 84; and the old-old period, age 85 and above. The fastest growing population segment in the United States is the 85 and older group. Because of this increased life span, we are seeing a relatively new phenomenon—elderly persons caring for their even more elderly parents. For these care-givers, death of a parent is a loss that is experienced during old age.

The senescent period of life includes more losses than gains. Physical losses eventually include diminished vision, hearing, taste, mobility, and memory. These losses usually develop gradually, but may be accelerated by any serious illness. Any chronic condition, such as arthritis, increases awareness of losses. When buttoning a shirt or tying a shoe becomes increasingly difficult, the individual is reminded daily of lost mobility and dexterity.

Psychological losses are also numerous during senescence. Retirement is a serious threat to mental health. For people who have not developed interests and activities outside of their work, there is no longer a daily routine of meaningful activity. A reason for getting up in the morning is lost. One's work-related identity is lost. Daily interaction with co-workers is lost. Since retirement benefits seldom equal work-related income, financial loss may be significant. All of these losses are a serious threat to self-esteem, so serious that a period of depression following retirement is relatively common. In fact, some retirees develop a life-threatening illness within two years following retirement. This emphasizes the importance of having a purpose in life and being actively involved in meaningful activities.

Social losses affect the elderly more than other age groups. Friends and close family members move or die. The loss of a specific friend may also mean the loss of a social activity shared with that person. The loss of a spouse may mean being left out of social activities in which the couple has participated for years. A son or daughter moving to another town means the loss of daily contact with immediate family, especially grandchildren. For many elderly persons, social life gradually diminishes. Loneliness and aloneness may characterize the daily life of an elderly person.

The loss that is feared by most elderly people is loss of independence. When an elderly person is deemed unable to live alone, the result is loss of one's home, loss of a familiar bed, loss of choices in what to eat and when. Loss of independence is accompanied by loss of self-esteem. Moving to a retirement home or confinement in a nursing home involves so many losses for the individual that there is often an immediate decline in health. All too often the emotional reactions of elderly people to these radical changes in life style go unrecognized and unacknowledged.

STRIVING FOR READJUSTMENT FOLLOWING SIGNIFICANT LOSS

Loss involves pain. The intensity of the pain depends upon the degree of commitment to that which is lost. Coping with the pain of loss is a life-skill that is essential to mental and emotional health.

Loss, although painful, can be an opportunity for growth. In order to grow, we must acknowledge that we are not **invulnerable,** that we are not **omnipotent.** Growth includes learning what we can and cannot control. Once we accept that these are limits on what we can control, it is easier to deal with the fears, guilt, and anger related to loss over which we had no control.

Loss requires saying "good-bye" to someone or something that has been an important part of our life. Letting go of the past does not mean forgetting, nor does it diminish the value of what was lost. Letting go is necessary for closing the door on what has been and opening the door to a new chapter of life—a life without that which has been lost.

A loss, then, is more than just a loss. It is a threat to our belief system and, therefore, to our reality. And because we tend to cling to our beliefs and what we perceive as reality, the first reaction to loss is disbelief, or denial. So, in addition to adjusting to a void created by the loss, we must also restructure our reality and our belief system. It is not uncommon to hear one who is grieving state, "I just don't know what I can believe in anymore."

Throughout life, each significant loss requires that we restructure our belief system and also work through the feelings involved in our reaction to the loss. Until the belief system has been restructured, a person may be disorganized and unable to function effectively in personal life or on the job. It is essential, therefore, that each of us learn about losses, reactions to loss, and the grief process. Such learnings enable us to provide emotional support to others who are grieving, prepare us for coping with the loss of loved ones through death, and help us accept the ultimate loss of our own being. It is especially important that health care providers understand the significance of loss, recognize reactions to loss, and encourage those who have experienced loss to grieve. There are many opportunities in health care agencies for a sensitive caregiver to recognize someone's need for emotional support as they deal with significant loss.

GUIDELINES FOR USING LOSS AND GRIEF AS A GROWTH EXPERIENCE

The following guidelines may appear simple. They are relatively easy to accept—intellectually. Accepting them at the *emotional level,* however, requires dealing honestly with one's feelings and beliefs. The result should be an increase in readiness to cope with the reality of loss and to help others who have experienced a significant loss.

1. Learn to recognize the small losses that occur in your life and allow yourself time to grieve appropriately for each.

2. Accept anger, fear, and guilt feelings as part of many grief reactions.

3. Allow time for grieving.

4. Acknowledge your own vulnerability to losses and pain.

5. Acknowledge your lack of total control. You may control some aspects of your life, but some events are beyond your control.

6. Acknowledge your own mortality—the fact that your life will end at some time.

7. Accept that life involves change, including losses. Some changes require that we modify our belief systems to fit the new reality.

8. Following a loss, work through the feelings. When you are ready, "let go" of the past (which includes the loss).

9. Believe that you can learn to cope with whatever loss you may experience.

10. Be supportive of those who have suffered a loss.

References and Suggested Readings

Backer, Barbara A., Hannon, Natalie R. and Russell, Noreen A. *Death and Dying: Understanding and Care;* Second Edition. Albany, NY: Delmar Publishers Inc., 1994. Chapter 8, "Ethical Issues," pp. 203–223; Chapter 9, "Suicide," pp. 229–253.

Choice in Dying. *Choices,* Fall 1996 (5:3). New York, NY: Choice in Dying.

Edelman, Hope. *Motherless Daughters: The Legacy of Loss.* New York, NY: Dell Publishing, 1994.

Goodwin, Frederick K. & Jamison, Kay Redfield. *Manic-Depressive Illness.* New York, NY: Oxford University Press, 1990.

Humphrey, Derek. *Final Exit: The Practicality of Self-Deliverance and Assisted Suicide for the Dying.* Eugene, OR: The Hemlock Society, 1991.

Jamison, Kay Redfield. *Touched with Fire: Manic-Depressive Illness and the Artistic Temperament.* New York, NY: The Free Press, 1993.

Shneidman, Edwin S., Ph.D. (Ed.) *Death: Current Perspectives;* Third Edition. Palo Alto, CA: Mayfield Publishing Company, 1984.

Shneidman, Edwin S., Ph.D. *The Suicidal Mind.* New York, NY: Oxford University Press, 1996.

Toynbee, Arnold. "Various Ways in Which Human Beings Have Sought to Reconcile Themselves to the Fact of Death." Chapter 8 in Shneidman, 1984.

Viorst, Judith. *Necessary Losses: The Loves, Illusions, Dependencies and Impossible Expectations That All of Us Have to Give Up in Order to Grow.* New York, NY: Simon & Schuster, 1986. Chapter 1, "The High Cost of Separation," pp 21–33.

Sources of Information on the Internet

Choice in Dying
Internet e-mail address: cid@choices.org
Web site: http://www.choices.org

Euthanasia Research and Guidance Organization (ERGO)
ergo@efn.org To subscribe to their mail-list, send e-mail to majordomo@efn.org
with the message, "subscribe ergo (your own e-mail address)" but do not
enter quotation marks in the body of the message; ignore the subject line.
Subscription is immediate.
Web sites: http://www.efn.org/~ergo and
http://www.rights.org/~deathnet/ergo.html

The Hemlock Society
Web sites: http://www.hemlock.org.hemlock
http://www.finalexit.org
http://www.finalexit.org/world.fed.html

The Voluntary Euthanasia Society of Scotland (VESS)
Web site: http://www.euthanasia.org/fastaccs.html

REVIEW AND SELF-CHECK

Complete each statement below, using information from Unit 19.

1. When a person is sad or depressed at the time of a "happy" event, it is
   because _____ .

2. Reasons for learning to cope with loss are:

   1. _____

   2. _____

   3. _____

3. Four steps for learning to cope with loss are:

   1. _____

   2. _____

   3. _____

   4. _____

4. A person's reaction to loss can be understood only in terms of _____

   _____

   _____ .

5. Losses of infancy and early childhood include:

   1. _____

   2. _____

   3. _____

6. Losses during the school-age period include:

   1. _____

   2. _____

   3. _____

7. Losses during adolescence include:

   1. _____

   2. _____

   3. _____

8. Losses during young adulthood may include:

   1. _____

   2. _____

   3. _____

9. Losses of middle age may include:

   1. _____

   2. _____

   3. _____

10. Losses during senescence include:

   1. _____

   2. _____

   3. _____

11. Loss can be perceived only as a painful experience, or as _____

   _____ .

12. Loss and grief can lead to personal growth if the individual

    1. _____

    2. _____

    3. _____

    4. _____

    5. _____

    6. _____

    7. _____

ASSIGNMENT

1. List significant changes that have occurred in your life, starting with your earliest memories and continuing to the present.

2. Set up a worksheet with three columns with the following headings: EVENTS, GAINS, LOSSES. In Column I, list significant events in the past two years of your life. Beside each event, list in Column II what you gained and in Column III what you lost as a result of that event.

3. List three of your possessions that are important to you. How do you think you would react if you learned that these items had been destroyed in a fire?

4. What is your usual pattern of behavior following a loss?
   a. Write a description of this pattern in terms of your feelings, how you express these feelings, the people with whom you share your feelings, and your behavior.
   b. Prepare a set of guidelines to help you improve your ways of coping with loss. Be prepared to share these guidelines during a class discussion.

5. Participate in a small group activity.
   a. Describe reactions to a significant loss that you have experienced or observed.
   b. Which of these examples are healthy reactions to loss?
   c. Which represent an unhealthy reaction to loss?

6. Compare the items below with your list of significant life changes (developed in Activity #1). Add any of these events that have occurred in your life, so that your list is relatively complete.
   a. Death of a grandparent, parent, brother, or sister
   b. Death of a spouse, son, or daughter
   c. Death of any other relative who was very important to you
   d. Death of a friend or classmate when you were a child
   e. Separation, divorce, or end of a long-term sexual relationship
   f. Marriage or establishment of a sexual relationship
   g. Any move—from one neighborhood to another, one city to another, or one state to another
   h. Change of school
   i. Major purchase—house, car, other
   j. Loss of personal possession—theft, foreclosure, fire, other
   k. New family member
   l. Pregnancy
   m. Serious illness of a family member
   n. Diagnosis of a serious or chronic illness (yours)
   o. Obtaining a new job; being fired from a job
   p. Change in job responsibilities or work schedule
   q. Radical change in financial situation
   r. Moving out of parents' home
   s. Your child moves out of your home
   t. Loss of freedom—confined to your room, not allowed to date or use the car, jail
   u. Radical change in life-style
   v. Entered military service, college, other educational program

   NOTE: Continue to add to your list as you think of other changes that have occurred in your life.

7. Review your list of changes. Place a checkmark beside each change that involved a significant loss.

8. List your significant losses.

9. Read one or more articles on "euthanasia." Take notes and be prepared to participate in a class discussion on "Why euthanasia and assisted suicide should be legalized."

   NOTE: Your instructor may choose to change the topic to ". . . *should not* be legalized."

10. Obtain a recent article (1997 or later) about Dr. Jack Kevorkian to share with the class.
    a. As a group, list the diagnoses of patients Dr. Kevorkian has assisted to commit suicide.
    b. Describe the effects Dr. Kevorkian has had on public attitudes, medical practices in care of patients with terminal illness or conditions perceived by the patient as intolerable, and state legislation.

Unit 20

Death: Changing Attitudes and Practices

OBJECTIVES

Upon completion of this unit, you should be able to:

- List three contrasts between past and current practices related to death and dying.
- Define "thanatology."
- List five examples of beliefs about death.
- List three reasons death education can allay fears about death.
- State five conditions that contribute to "death with dignity."
- Name five issues related to end-of-life care.
- Name four reasons the courts are sometimes involved in end-of-life decisions.
- Define "advance medical directive."
- State one purpose of the Living Will.
- State one purpose of the medical Durable Power of Attorney.
- List four provisions of the Patient Self-Determination Act.
- Develop a personal philosophy about death and end-of-life care.

KEY TERMS

Brain death	Bereavement	Conservator
Forgo	Ethical	Immortal
Litigation	Medicalize	Moral
Proxy	Quality of life	Surrogate

DEATH AND DYING

Many people view death as the ultimate loss—the absolute end of life. Thus death is an enemy to be feared and avoided at all costs. A totally different view is reflected in the writings of Dr. Elisabeth Kubler-Ross, who titled one of her books *Death: The Final Stage of Growth.* As a result of her many years of attending dying patients, Dr. Kubler-Ross proposed that the dying process involves a series of emotional/spiritual changes that, ideally, terminate with feelings of peace and tranquility prior to death. The dying process, then, can be an opportunity for spiritual growth. Some dying people need help to move through this process. Others seem to undergo this growth through their own beliefs, values, and inner resources.

Between these two extreme views of death, there is a wide range of beliefs. These differences are due in part to cultural attitudes and practices in care of the dying, which have undergone a marked change in modern cultures during the past half-century. This unit reviews those historical changes, examines some influences on beliefs about death, and discusses current and emerging attitudes and practices related to death and dying as reflected in a variety of issues and legal involvement in health care decisions.

Past Attitudes and Practices

In 1789, Benjamin Franklin wrote, "In this world nothing is certain except death and taxes." His comment reflects an awareness and acceptance of death that was common until the era of modern medicine. Prior to this century, the leading cause of death was infection. Infant and child mortality rates were high; few families escaped the loss of a child. Death was familiar—a common experience that was highly visible to people of all ages. Illness and death were most likely to occur in the home, with family members and friends gathered around. It was the custom for each member of the family to bid the dying person farewell. In return, the dying person gave his or her blessing to favored relatives. The deathbed scene often included advice and charges to the survivors—to develop certain virtues, care for other survivors, gain honor for the family name.

Death was viewed as a reunion with deceased loved ones. The joyful anticipation of this reunion overshadowed any sadness at leaving the survivors. In some cultures, death was (or still is) celebrated as a release from the troubles of this life and a welcome passage to a happy and trouble-free existence in "the hereafter."

Mourning was public, as well as private. A widow was expected to wear black for at least a year following the death of her husband. Men wore a black band on the left sleeve as a public display of mourning for the deceased. The survivors did not participate in social events for many months. Women, in particular, were expected to remain in seclusion during the mourning period. There were frequent visits to the cemetery. The gravemarker and subsequent care of the grave symbolized respect for the deceased and devotion of the survivors. In many other ways survivors demonstrated to relatives and the community their love and respect for the deceased. Until recently, both illness and death were a family affair.

Changing Attitudes and Practices

Beginning in the early 1900s, infection was brought under control through improved sanitation and immunization. During the late 1930s and 1940s, the sulfa drugs and penicillin were discovered. These changes in the prevention and treatment of infection resulted in dramatic decrease in deaths due to infection, especially among infants and children. As the life span increased, the primary causes of death became cancer, heart disease, degenerative disorders, and accidents. Care of the sick and injured shifted from the home to the hospital. Responsibility for care of the sick was delegated to health care personnel, with family members relegated to the role of bystanders. This trend resulted in isolation of the patient from family members, who were "protected" from personal experience with serious illness and death. Children, especially, were excluded from contact with the hospitalized patient. Illness and death ceased to be a family affair.

As a result of this trend, many people today have never been personally involved with serious illness or the dying process. They have been deprived of the opportunity to learn to accept death as a part of the natural order of things. Death is now perceived by many people as a terrible tragedy that "ought not to happen, especially to me and my family."

These changes of the past fifty years have great significance for emotional and mental health. Due to the invisibility of the dying process and abandonment of many mourning rituals, there is a growing tendency to deny death. In American society, it is almost as though there is a conspiracy of silence. One just does not talk, or even think, about death until it strikes within one's circle of relatives or friends.

When death does touch a family, there may be a tendency to deny the grief process. Today, the community generally does not provide for bereaved people the kind of long-term support that can facilitate the grief process. Instead, survivors are expected to "pick up the pieces and get on with their lives" soon after the funeral.

In the work setting, life may go on as usual the day after a colleague's funeral, with no one willing to introduce the subject of death into the informal communication channels. The formal communication channel may acknowledge this loss of a member of the organization with a memorandum or floral offering. Otherwise, the work routine continues with minimal recognition that a member is missing, unless the deceased held an important position. Thus, death is kept out of sight and out of consciousness as much as possible.

Current Attitudes and Practices

Changes in infant and child mortality have had a particular effect on societal attitudes toward death as it relates to age. Whereas death is acceptable for older people (generally age sixty and above), it is viewed as inappropriate for someone under the age of thirty to die. Yet, less than a hundred years ago, parents felt blessed if half of their children survived to age twelve. Today, we find it especially tragic—unacceptable and terribly unfair—when a child dies. This attitude is especially prevalent among teenagers and young adults, who tend to think of themselves as **immortal** because "death is for old people." This attitude tends to modify with the passing years and accumulated life experiences. By middle age, most people begin to accept the reality of death, even if they are not yet able to acknowledge the inevitability of their own death.

Changes in the health care system have contributed to changes in societal attitudes toward death. In fact, a highly significant change in attitudes toward death has occurred *within* the health care system. Instead of accepting death as an inevitable outcome of some diseases, death is perceived as an enemy to be conquered with whatever resources the system can offer: new and better drugs, life-support systems, surgical replacement of body parts, heroic measures to restore vital functions. Some physicians believe they have a responsibility to maintain life in the physical body as long as possible, regardless of the patient's potential for recovery or a meaningful existence. Concern for the *quantity* of life has replaced concern for the *quality* **of life.** When all measures available prove inadequate to keep a patient alive, some personnel view the death as a personal failure. ("If only I had made rounds thirty minutes sooner!") or as a failure of the system ("If we had been able to use such-and-such, we could have saved that patient.")

Modern practices in care of the dying deprive the patient and family members of the opportunity to share in the dying process. Many Intensive Care Units and Cardiac Care Units allow visitors only for brief periods a few times a day. Many hospitals do not permit children to visit, even if a patient requests one last opportunity to see them.

Recently, however, there is increasing awareness of a need to examine societal attitudes toward death and care of the dying. Some hospitals have modified their policies regarding visitors, some even permitting small children to visit a dying grandparent, parent, or sibling. Hospice and home care of a dying person are increasingly recognized as alternatives to hospitalization. More families now participate in the dying process, thereby permitting the dying person to retain a sense of family membership until the end. These recent trends recognize and respect the *human needs* of the dying person.

THE EMERGENCE OF THANATOLOGY

During the 1950s a new interest and concern about death and dying emerged, largely due to the work of Dr. Elisabeth Kubler-Ross, sociologists, social workers, and pastoral counselors. Many professionals who were working with dying patients recognized that their educational programs had not prepared them for this role. The concern of these professional workers to meet the needs of patients with terminal illness led to the emergence of *thanatology,* the study of death and dying, and to death education for health care providers and for the public.

Thanatology involves people from a variety of disciplines: sociology, theology, psychology, counseling, social work, nursing, and medicine. Their work has led to increased awareness of the needs of dying persons, the importance of the grief process, techniques for helping patients and their families cope with death and **bereavement,** and the need for death education.

THE MEANING OF DEATH

An important aspect of death education is learning to accept one's own mortality. In the past, this important lesson was learned early in life through direct experience with serious illness and death itself, usually in the home. Current practices that isolate dying patients prevent this direct involvement. But death education can help people think through the meaning of death, resolve their fears, reach some level of personal acceptance and come to terms with their own mortality. In addition, death education can prepare people to accept their feelings as legitimate reactions when they do have to cope with a death crisis. It is especially important that health care providers who care for dying patients resolve their fears about dying, since subconscious fears about death influence how one interacts with a person who is dying.

The meaning of death for each person is influenced by cultural background, religious beliefs, and life experiences. Following are examples of beliefs about death:

- Death is the end of existence.

- Death is only the end of physical existence.

- Death is a natural, biological event that concludes life.

- Death is the loss of everything—life itself, the future, loved ones, possessions.

- Death means separation from loved ones.

- Death means a reunion with loved ones who have already died.

- Death is the enemy. It should be fought with all available resources up to the end.

- What follows death is unknown, therefore it is a fearsome event.

- Death is a test of one's faith, therefore it must be faced with courage and a willingness to accept pain and suffering.

- Death is a change to another form of existence.

- Death is a transition, the soul moves to another plane of existence.

- Death is the beginning of a new life—perpetual existence in Heaven or Hell, depending upon Divine judgment of one's deeds on earth.

Some of these beliefs perpetuate fear of death. Others reflect acceptance of death as natural or as a transition.

Fear of death is, in part, the result of **medicalizing** and **institutionalizing** death. The result is that most people today have not had the opportunity to participate in the dying process. According to Dr. Kubler-Ross, "Any child who has experienced the death of a brother or sister, mother or father, grandfather or grandmother, in his own home, surrounded by peace and love, will not be afraid of death or dying anymore . . ." (Kubler-Ross, 1969)

Death education can help people deal with their fears about death and clarify their own beliefs about death. It can help them understand that preparing oneself for dying includes grieving for what must be given up: relationships with family members and friends; ambitions, goals, purposes, and dreams for the future; material possessions; and, finally, one's own physical body. Thinking through these losses while in a state of good health usually results in a new perspective on what is important in life. The survivors of Near Death Experiences (NDE) report a peaceful interlude that left them with no fear of death and with new attitudes toward the value of each life experience.

DEATH WITH DIGNITY

Increased attention to death and dying has resulted in several trends: the hospice movement, preparation of personnel to provide counseling for dying patients, and Advance Directives for end-of-life care. The right to die with dignity is inherent in the philosophy of hospice. Death with dignity embodies at least the following:

- The dying person is permitted to retain some control.

- The dying person has the freedom to choose his or her style of dying.

- The dying person is allowed to openly discuss death.

- The dying person is allowed to prepare for dying in his or her own way.

- Human mortality is a biological fact.

- The dying patient's care focuses on maintaining *quality of life*, rather than quantity of life.

- Intervention in the dying process, when the prognosis is hopeless, is inappropriate if such intervention violates the patient's wishes.

- Some interventions prolong dying.

Death with dignity, then, implies that the highest possible quality of life is maintained and that the dying person's rights and wishes are respected by caregivers. By participating in decisions and being allowed to make choices, the dying person maintains self-esteem and a sense of integrity as a worthwhile human being. Familiar surroundings help the patient maintain a sense of identity. Those who die at home have the advantage of familiar surroundings and the presence of family members, friends, and even pets. Arrangements that permit the person to die at home can also benefit survivors, though some families are not able to cope with full-time care of a dying person. In any case, dying at home is now recognized as an alternative to dying in the institutional setting.

SOCIETAL ISSUES RELATED TO CARE OF THE DYING

The availability of life-support technology has given rise to ethical, moral, and legal questions previously unknown to any society. New types of decisions face the physician, the patient, and next-of-kin—decisions that can contribute to guilt feelings, inappropriate procedures, and medical practices based on fear of litigation. It is important that health care providers are aware of issues pertaining to the care of dying patients.

Issues that concern society as a whole are those that establish medical and legal precedent for future decisions. Issues that concern the patient and family are largely those that involve constitutional rights. Some of these issues are currently being argued in the courts; others are appearing in the medical literature and at conferences as **ethical, moral,** and legal questions. Issues of particular concern to everyone participating in care of the dying are (1) the definition of death, (2) quality of life versus quantity of life, and (3) rights of patients and their families.

The Definition of Death

What indicates that a person is dead? This question is especially important now that donor organs are needed for transplants. The *legal definition* of death in forty-six states and the District of Columbia uses **brain death** as the primary criterion; other states accept *cessation* of cardiopulmonary functions as the primary criterion. The *medical definition* is based on cessation of respiratory or circulatory functions or irreversible coma. In some hospitals brain death is measured in terms of (1) cerebral functions (consciousness, responsiveness to stimuli) and (2) brain stem functions (control of vital processes). Where both measurements are made, the patient is not declared brain dead unless at least two physicians agree that brain stem function is absent.

The definition of death is especially relevant to the care of young accident victims. It is indeed difficult to give up hope for a young person whose body appears normal, even though tests indicate that there is no brain activity.

Determination of the moment of death is a pressing decision when other patients are waiting for a donor organ. A surgeon waiting to perform an organ transplant is understandably impatient about any delay in pronouncing a potential donor dead. The Uniform Anatomical Gift Act specifies that the physician who declares a patient dead must not be involved with a patient who is awaiting a donor organ. A proposed Uniform Determination of Death Act specifies that both cardiopulmonary and brain function criteria must be met before body organs may be removed. (Shneidman, p. 131) Any state that adopts these statutes, or develops its own statute with clearly stated criteria for determination of death, is providing legal protection for a dying person who is a potential organ donor.

Quality of Life versus Quantity of Life

Which is more important, the *quality* of life or the *quantity* of life? When the current state of medical practice offers no hope for a patient's recovery, to what extent should life-extending procedures be used? Intravenous fluids, blood transfusion, and tube feedings may be used to maintain life, rather than to cure disease. Often such procedures are continued even when a patient's condition is hopeless. Life can be maintained for days, or even weeks, until the body refuses to continue to function. Is the physician or family obligated to "do everything possible" to *extend* life? Or, should life-maintenance procedures be discontinued when there is no hope of recovery and the quality of life is nil? Who should make such a decision—the patient (if mentally competent)? the next-of-kin? or the physician? Who should make such a decision if the patient is *not* mentally competent or is comatose?

Rights of Patients and Their Families

When the recommended medical treatment of a condition has extreme side effects, causes more pain than the disease itself, or involves radical surgery that permanently alters body appearance, does the patient (or the parents, if the patient is a minor) have the right to refuse treatment? Medical opinion is that *any medically approved treatment should be used.* But some patients reject surgery or such treatments as chemotherapy, choosing instead to *let the disease run its natural course.* Although a physician cannot force surgery or chemotherapy on an adult, there have been court judgments that required a child's parents to allow physicians to administer chemotherapy to a child.

Does a patient who is mentally sound have the right to refuse extreme measures for maintaining life? This issue, also, has been before the courts. Judges generally use brain death as the criterion for authorizing a physician to

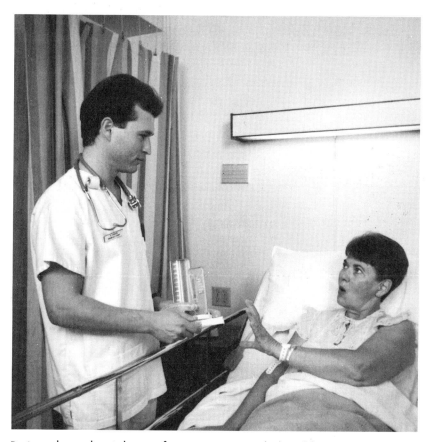

Patients have the right to refuse treatment, including life-support measures and resuscitation.

discontinue treatment of a comatose patient. The question is far more complex when a patient is conscious and mentally competent. If the patient has no hope of recovery and does not want to continue to suffer, does that person have the right to say "pull the plug"? Medical personnel tend to label such a decision "suicide." Others maintain that discontinuing artificial life-support is "allowing nature to take its course." Some people view the use of life-support procedures for dying patients as prolonging death, rather than extending life. The concept of death with dignity includes the patient's right to reject life-support and resuscitation procedures.

Do Not Resuscitate Orders

After the technique for cardiopulmonary resuscitation (CPR) became an integral part of the curriculum for all health care personnel, it became common practice to "call a code" for any patient who stopped breathing, even if the person was terminally ill. This was especially true in teaching hospitals, where numerous medical students and interns were expected to learn resuscitation procedures, including open-heart massage. When it was recognized that resuscitation is inappropriate for some patients, a new type of physician's order came into being: Do Not Resuscitate (DNR). This order is written by the attending physician for patients who are expected to die and for whom no further treatment is feasible.

With the development of hospice and a growing trend toward care of a dying person in the home setting, there was need for end-of-life procedures for patients outside the hospital setting. If care-givers called emergency services after the patient died, the paramedics who responded were legally obligated to begin CPR, unless there was a written DNR. By the end of 1995, twenty-four states had enacted laws regarding Nonhospital DNRs. Each of these laws requires that the DNR order be written on the specific state's Department of Health form. Neither a Living Will nor a physician's order on letterhead stationary or prescription pad is valid.

Third-Party Interventions

Changes in the care of persons in a comatose, brain-dead state began during the 1970s and 1980s. Several cases (i.e., Karen Ann Quinlan) aroused public interest in the rights of next-of-kin to discontinue life-support measures for patients who were brain-dead. Then there were cases (i.e., Nancy Cruzan) that challenged the use of tube feedings to maintain a comatose patient. Law suits, appealed all the way to the U.S. Supreme Court, pitted hospitals, nursing homes, and some religious groups against relatives of a comatose patient. These lawsuits laid the foundation for passage of state laws related to Living Wills and Durable Power of Attorney, the passage of a federal law specifying that patients have the right to refuse treatment, and the development of guidelines for Do Not Resuscitate (DNR) orders.

If an advance directive exists, the law almost always supports the rights of families to make end-of-life decisions for a patient who is no longer conscious or competent to make decisions. This is based on a rule of law known as "standing," which means that only those with a "real interest" are involved in the **litigation.** When there is no advance directive and the health care agency refuses to discontinue life-support measures for a brain-dead patient, then the family has to seek a court order requiring that life-support be discontinued.

In the Nancy Cruzan case, such an order was obtained. Then, a *third party who did not know Nancy Cruzan or her family* filed for an injunction, arguing that artificial feedings should continue. This action was based on the third party's beliefs about "doing everything possible" to prolong life. The result was that the legal process was extended, adding to the family's emotional ordeal and financial burdens. Eventually, the court found that the third party did not have "standing." Only then could the earlier court ruling be carried out. The *four years* of legal proceedings that followed the family's request to discontinue tube feedings were extended several months by the third-party intervention. The best protection against having a third party attempt to influence end-of-life medical decisions is to have a valid Advance Directive and discuss it with the physician, family, and friends.

LEGAL ASPECTS OF THE RIGHT TO DIE

A number of right-to-die issues have now been addressed by the U.S. Supreme Court, the U.S. Congress, and most state legislatures. In the Mary Beth Cruzan case the Supreme Court ruled that there is a constitutional right to die, but that it is up to the states to define those rights. Later Congress passed the Patient Self-Determination Act (PSDA), which mandates that patients be informed about the right to participate in medical decisions regarding their treatment. Living Will laws have now been passed by forty-seven states and the District of Columbia. In addition, forty-eight states have a medical Durable Power of Attorney (DPA) law. The Living Will and medical DPA laws are the result of widespread consumer resistance to indiscriminate use of medical technology that can prolong life indefinitely. Both documents pertain to *self-determination—* the right of a patient to participate in medical decisions and, specifically, the right to refuse medical treatment. Medical Durable Power of Attorney and the Living Will are both included in "Advance Medical Directive."

The Living Will

The Living Will permits individuals to indicate their wishes regarding medical care. It is especially valuable if the individual becomes incapable of conveying

FLORIDA LIVING WILL

INSTRUCTIONS

PRINT THE DATE

PRINT YOUR NAME

Declaration made this _____ day of _____ , 19 ___ .

I, _____ , willfully and voluntarily make known my desire that my dying not be artificially prolonged under the circumstances set forth below, and I do hereby declare:

If at any time I have a terminal condition and if my attending or treating physician and another consulting physician have determined that there is no medical probability of my recovery from such condition, I direct that life-prolonging procedures be withheld or withdrawn when the application of such procedures would serve only to prolong artificially the process of dying, and that I be permitted to die naturally with only the administration of medication or the performance of any medical procedure deemed necessary to provide me with comfort care or to alleviate pain.

It is my intention that this declaration be honored by my family and physician as the final expression of my legal right to refuse medical or surgical treatment and to accept the consequences for such refusal.

In the event that I have been determined to be unable to provide express and informed consent regarding the withholding, withdrawal, or continuation of life-prolonging procedures, I wish to designate, as my surrogate to carry out the provisions of this delcaration:

PRINT THE NAME, HOME ADDRESS, AND TELEPHONE NUMBER OF YOUR SURROGATE

Name: _____

Address: _____

_____ Zip Code: _____

Phone: _____

An example of an advance directive that includes a living will and a health care proxy. (Reprinted by permission of Choice in Dying, 200 Varick Street, New York, NY 10014, 212–366–5540.)

FLORIDA LIVING WILL—PAGE 2 OF 2

I wish to designate the following person as my alternate surrogate, to carry out the provisions of this declaration should my surrogate be unwilling or unable to act on my behalf:

PRINT NAME, HOME ADDRESS, AND TELEPHONE NUMBER OF YOUR ALTERNATE SURROGATE

Name: _____

Address: _____

_____ Zip Code: _____

Phone: _____

ADD PERSONAL INSTRUCTIONS (IF ANY)

Additional instructions (optional):

I understand the full import of this declaration, and I am emotionally and mentally competent to make this declaration.

SIGN THE DOCUMENT

Signed: _____

WITNESSING PROCEDURE

Witness 1:

Signed: _____

Address: _____

TWO WITNESSES MUST SIGN AND PRINT THEIR ADDRESSES

Witness 2:

Signed: _____

Address: _____

© 1996
CHOICE IN DYING, INC.

Courtesy of Choice In Dying, Inc.
200 Varick Street, New York, NY 10014 212-366-5540

6/96

An example of an advance directive that includes a living will and a health care proxy. (Continued)

INSTRUCTIONS

FLORIDA DESIGNATION OF HEALTH CARE SURROGATE

PRINT YOUR NAME

Name: _____

         (Last)   *(First)*   *(Middle Initial)*

In the event that I have been determined to be incapacitated to provide informed consent for medical treatment and surgical and diagnostic procedures, I wish to designate as my surrogate for health care decisions:

PRINT THE NAME, HOME ADDRESS, AND TELEPHONE NUMBER OF YOUR SURROGATE

Name: _____

Address: _____

_____ Zip Code: _____

Phone: _____

If my surrogate is unwilling or unable to perform his or her duties, I wish to designate as my alternate surrogate:

PRINT THE NAME, HOME ADDRESS, AND TELEPHONE NUMBER OF YOUR ALTERNATE SURROGATE

Name: _____

Address: _____

_____ Zip Code: _____

Phone: _____

I fully understand that this designation will permit my designee to make health care decisions and to provide, withhold, or withdraw consent on my behalf; to apply for public benefits to defray the cost of health care; and to authorize my admission to or transfer from a health care facility.

Additional instructions (optional):

I further affirm that this designation is not being made as a condition of treatment or admission to a health care facility. I will notify and send a copy of

© 1996
CHOICE IN DYING, INC.

An example of an advance directive that includes a living will and a health care proxy. (Continued)

FLORIDA DESIGNATION OF HEALTH CARE SURROGATE—PAGE 2 OF 2

this document to the following persons other than my surrogate, so they may know whom my surrogate is:

PRINT THE NAMES AND ADDRESS OF THOSE WHOM YOU WANT TO KEEP COPIES OF THIS DOCUMENT

Name: _____

Address: _____

Name: _____

Address: _____

SIGN AND DATE THE DOCUMENT

Signed: _____

Date: _____

WITNESSING PROCEDURE

TWO WITNESSES MUST SIGN AND PRINT THEIR ADDRESSES

Witness 1:

    Signed: _____

    Address: _____

Witness 2:

    Signed: _____

    Address: _____

SAMPLE

© 1996
CHOICE IN DYING, INC.

Courtesy of Choice In Dying, Inc.
200 Varick Street, New York, NY 10014 212-366-5540

6/96

An example of an advance directive that includes a living will and a health care proxy. (Continued)

such wishes to the doctor and family. People who have foresight to prepare a Living Will protect their families from having to make painful decisions regarding medical treatment if there appears to be no chance of recovery. Living Wills also provide guidance for the physician regarding extreme measures such as life support and resuscitation.

The Living Will is especially useful in cases of coma or prolonged dying when there is no hope of recovery. Ideally, the Living Will should be prepared and signed *before* the onset of illness or accident. If a patient wants to sign a Living Will after being admitted to a health care facility, additional witnesses and safeguards are required. The Living Will presents the patient's wishes in writing. Many recent court cases have been based on statements the patient made to family and friends indicating that he or she would not want to be kept alive in a vegetative state. In the absence of a Living Will or other written instructions, lengthy legal proceedings may be required before the patient is allowed to die a natural death (i.e., life support and/or artificial nutrition may be discontinued).

Everyone who completes a Living Will and/or a medical Durable Power of Attorney should discuss their advance directive(s) with the physician, their families, and especially the **proxy** (i.e., person named as decision-maker in the medical Durable Power of Attorney). The discussion should be specific about one's beliefs and wishes regarding the kind of end-of-life care desired, and about any medical interventions that are not wanted. Without such meaningful discussions at intervals, there is risk that one's wishes will be ignored, even if an advance directive has been completed.

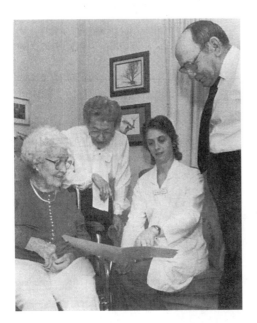

A patient should discuss advance medical directives with the physician, nursing staff, family, and especially with the proxy named in a Medical Durable Power of Attorney. (From Carolyn Anderson, *Patient Teaching and Communication in an Information Age.* NY: Delmar Publishers Inc., 1990.)

It is not necessary to involve a lawyer in preparing a Living Will. Each state has a specific form, available from the office of any state legislator and from most hospitals. Choice in Dying, Inc. (CID) is a nonprofit organization dedicated to education of the public and health professionals about the rights of persons to be involved in health care decisions at the end of life. CID provides state-specific forms and guidelines free through its web-site, free to anyone who makes a tax-deductible contribution, and for a nominal fee to others. A Living Will form should be filled out according to the instructions, signed in the presence of witnesses who are not family members or beneficiaries, and then signed by the witnesses. The original should be filed in a safe place; copies should be provided to members of the family. Upon admission to a hospital, a copy should be added to the patient's chart; *a family member should obtain a receipt from a hospital representative, acknowledging that an Advance Directive for that patient is on file.*

The Durable Power of Attorney

The medical Durable Power of Attorney is a document that designates a specific person to make medical decisions if the patient is unable to do so. The desires of the individual should be made clear to the **surrogate** decision-maker at the time the document is prepared. When illness or accident occurs, the decision-maker is responsible for seeing that the patient's wishes are carried out. Some DPA forms include statements pertaining to life-support, resuscitation, and artificial feeding, so that specific instructions are included in the legal document.

The Patient Self-Determination Act (PSDA)

Effective December 1, 1991 any hospital, nursing home, hospice or health maintenance organization (HMO) that receives federal funding (Medicare and Medicaid) must inform patients about their rights, specifically the right to refuse certain types of treatment. This federal law also prohibits health care providers from discriminating against a patient who elects to **forgo** life-sustaining procedures. The Patient Self-Determination Act specifies that any patient who enters a hospital or nursing home must be informed about:

- The right to make decisions about medical treatments
- The right to refuse a treatment (medical or surgical)
- The right to prepare an Advance Medical Directive (AMD) if the patient does not already have a Living Will or medical DPA
- The procedure in that institution for preparing an AMD
- The right to have an AMD made part of his or her medical record

This law resulted from the proliferation of court cases regarding the use of life-support procedures for patients who were in a vegetative state. A number of families have experienced great emotional trauma and incurred tremendous legal expense in the effort to allow their loved one, in a state of irreversible coma, to die. There was also a court case in which an eighty-four-year-old man was resuscitated even though his chart had a Do Not Resuscitate (DNR) order signed by the physician. Health care providers, regardless of their own opinions, must respect the wishes of patients if those wishes have been stated in an AMD.

PSDA will serve the needs of many patients, especially those with terminal illnesses and those who choose to forgo certain medical procedures. But it does not solve the problem of a comatose person who does not have an AMD. Who knows when an accident, or sudden life-threatening illness will result in brain damage and a vegetative state? The only sure protection against the use of undesired measures, when there is no hope of recovery, is to have an AMD prepared *before* illness or accident occurs.

Table 20–1 shows some of the requirements of the Patient Self-Determination Act.

TABLE 20–1
The Patient Self-Determination Act

Provisions of the PSDA apply to all health care agencies that receive federal funds (Medicare and Medicaid reimbursement).

Each health care institution will—

- Provide written information to each patient regarding
  a. The right to make decisions regarding medical care, including the right to refuse medical or surgical treatment,
  b. The right to prepare advance medical directives,
  c. A copy of the institution's written policies regarding the implementation of such rights.

- Document in the patient's medical record whether or not the individual has completed an advance directive.

- Provide care without discrimination against the patient who has completed an advance directive.

- Establish policies and procedures to ensure compliance with state law regarding advance directives.

- Provide educational activities for staff and the public on the matter of advance directives.

The Department of Health and Human Services will—

- Provide a national public education campaign.

- Develop written materials explaining patients' rights, to be distributed by health care facilities.

The Law and Assisted Suicide

Laws related to assisted suicide have been proposed in various state legislatures. When the Iowa legislature passed a law that established penalties for assisting with a suicide, it became the thirty-fourth state to criminalize this act. The state laws that criminalize assisted-suicide in two states, New York and Washington, were found to be unconstitutional by two federal circuit courts. The rulings of the circuit courts were appealed by the two states. The U.S. Supreme Court heard arguments for and against the constitutionality of these two state laws in January, 1997 and, on June 26, 1997 reversed the lower courts and upheld these two state laws. In spite of the Supreme Court's ruling, the right-to-die controversy probably will continue for some time.

The Michigan law under which Dr. Kevorkian was charged and tried has already been challenged and found to be unconstitutional. The District Attorney who charged Dr. Kevorkian with murder was not reelected. His successor has now dismissed the pending charges against Dr. Kevorkian.

In 1994 the Oregon state legislature authorized a referendum that resulted in passage of the Death with Dignity Act. This law permits any resident of Oregon who is suffering from a terminal illness to request that the physician provide medication for the express purpose of ending his or her life. The Oregon law has been challenged and is now on hold until a federal court rules on its constitutionality. Two other states—Washington and California, have held similar referendums that failed to pass by a small margin. The fact that three states have put the question of assisted suicide to a public vote reflects a growing momentum of public support for assisted suicide.

Involvement of the Courts in Health Care Decisions

Increasingly, the legal system is becoming involved in health care decisions. This is most likely to occur when (1) relatives of a comatose person believe life support should be discontinued, but there is no Advance Directive, (2) an Advance Directive is ignored by health care personnel, or (3) the family wants to do "everything possible" for their loved one, even though the physician and hospital believe life support/nutrition should be discontinued.

In the first type of situation, the courts use one of two standards for determining whether or not life support may be discontinued. The "substituted judgment" standard recognizes that most individuals have not prepared Advance Directives and that their loved ones can best decide that individual's preference for end-of-life care. The "clear and convincing evidence" standard requires that the patient's preferences have been clearly stated to relatives or friends prior to becoming unable to make medical decisions personally. The presentation of "clear and convincing evidence" by her former co-workers led to the court ruling that life support could be discontinued for Nancy Cruzan, who remained in a persistent vegetative state for eight years before a court ruling permitted the discontinuance of tube feedings. The family's legal battle lasted for four years, with tremendous emotional trauma and overwhelming financial burdens, legal and medical. The tragedy of this situation is still being played out; the toll became unbearable for Nancy's father, who committed suicide in 1996.

The second type of situation is discussed under the topic "A Dilemma for Health Care Providers." The third situation is less common, in that most families of a comatose patient accept the recommendation of the physician. If a family does demand that treatment continue, even though there is no hope of improvement in the patient's condition, the hospital or physician may request that the court appoint a **conservator.** The responsibility of the conservator would be to evaluate the situation and recommend a course of action based on what the patient probably would want, if able to speak for him or herself.

A DILEMMA FOR HEALTH CARE PROVIDERS

Sometimes health care personnel choose to ignore Advance Directives, believing that they are obligated to do everything possible to keep a patient alive. This behavior involves conflict between the health care provider's philosophy of health care and the legal rights of patients. The conflict may extend beyond the staff, involving hospital policy and established procedures.

Liability for Performing Unwanted Treatment

Performing heroic measures to restore breathing or a heartbeat can be enormously satisfying. As conveyed on television, it is an exciting part of being a health care provider. But resuscitating someone who has a DNR order violates that patient's rights and is illegal. Keeping alive someone who has provided written instructions that prohibit life-support measures for end-of-life care not only violates the patient's rights, but is also illegal. Either approach can result in prolongation of suffering, further medical expenses for the patient and family, and possibly litigation against health care providers and the hospital.

The Ohio Court of Appeals has found that there is valid cause for action if a patient's wishes to forgo specific medical procedures are ignored. If it can be shown that the patient suffered adverse effects from treatment administered over the patient's objections, damages may be awarded. Every health care provider should be informed about the legal aspects of Advance Directives; knowing which patients have advance directives is the responsibility of each care-giver.

Preparation for Death and Dying Situations

You may or may not be preparing for a role in health care that includes the care of dying patients. Regardless of your expected role, you should be prepared for participation in a life-or-death situation, either in your career or in your personal life. Know the provisions of federal laws and the laws of your state pertaining to the rights of patients and their families; know the policies of your employing health care agency, and be aware of your own beliefs about death and dying. The concept of death with dignity, knowledge about Advance Directives, and awareness of the provisions of the Patient Self-Determination Act should help you to accept the rights of patients to participate in decisions about end-of-life care. You should also learn to accept the inevitability of death, the limitations of medical science, and the inappropriateness of heroic measures in some situations. It is especially important that you develop your own philosophy about death, which includes facing your own fears about death and accepting your own mortality.

Thoughtful consideration of the following questions will help you clarify your beliefs and develop your own philosophy of death.

- What do I believe about death?

- What do I believe about my own death?

- What fears do I have about dying?

- What would I have to give up if I were dying?

- What work do I want to complete before I die?

- What relationships do I want to mend before I die?

- What do I want to say to my loved ones before I die?

- What do I want to say to a loved one before he or she dies?

- Who should dispose of my possessions following my death? Who is to receive what?

By developing a personal philosophy of death, you will have clearer beliefs about the care of a dying patient. If the health care provider role you expect to assume does not involve caring for dying patients, you may be tempted to ignore this exercise. But you cannot be sure what the future holds—in your career or in your personal life. So, consider the following items in terms of "What do I believe about the care of a patient who . . .":

- Does not want to be resuscitated if a cardiac arrest occurs?

- Refuses intravenous fluids or tube feedings during the final stages of an illness?

- Refuses dialysis, even though the kidneys are not functioning?

- Refuses chemotherapy, even though the oncologist insists there is a 20 percent chance it will help?

- Begs the doctor, "Just let me die."

- Begs the doctor, "Just put me out of my misery."

Inadequate management of pain is the reason some patients wish for death or consider suicide. The expression of a wish for death, then, may mean that the patient needs additional attention and improved management of pain. However, many dying patients have accepted death and are ready—mentally, emotionally, and spiritually—even before the physical body ceases to function. Be sensitive to the needs of such patients, and especially to a patient's readiness for death.

Ethics Committees

The Karen Ann Quinlan court decision included a recommendation that ethics committees, rather than the courts, should handle controversial patient care situations. In 1995, the Joint Commission on Accreditation of Health Care Organizations began requiring that health care facilities set up a code of ethical behavior. As a result, most hospitals are establishing ethics committees to review patient care conflicts. Some ethics committees involve patients' families in hearings, thereby ensuring that all viewpoints will be heard and increasing the probability of a decision that will be acceptable to the hospital, the physician, and the family. In other hospitals, the ethics committees exclude families from the hearing, relying on reports of the medical staff for rendering a decision. The latter approach carries the risk of having the patient's end-of-life choices ignored in favor of aggressive medical treatment. A professor of health law has stated, "A poorly run committee threatens to become, quite literally, a form of secret law." (*Choices,* Summer 1996)

Ideally, ethics committees would always protect the patient's well-being, while also respecting the expressed wishes of the patient and family for end-of-life care. Also, ethics committees can and should encourage staff training in the legal and ethical issues most often involved in patient care/institutional conflict.

SUMMARY

Unit 20 has addressed the concept of death with dignity, the rights of patients and their families to participate in decisions related to end-of-life care, the definition of death, Advance Medical Directives, and laws pertaining to rights of patients. A number of issues are being addressed in the medical community, the mass media, and the courts: definition of death, when life support may be discontinued, when artificial feedings for persons in a persistent vegetative state may be discontinued, the right of a patient to choose suicide, culpability of a person who assists a patient to commit suicide, and the moral/ethical/legal aspects of euthanasia. Some of the legal issues may be resolved within the next several years. In the meantime, everyone involved in end-of-life decisions and all health care providers must resolve for themselves the ethical and moral issues related to end-of-life care and intentional acceleration of the dying process.

References and Suggested Readings

Backer, Barbara A., Hannon, Natalie R., & Russell, Noreen A. *Death and Dying: Understanding and Care;* Second Edition. Albany, NY: Delmar Publishers Inc., 1994. Chapter 1, "Death in American Society," pp. 1–16; Chapter 8, "Ethical Issues," pp. 203–223.

Choice in Dying, Inc. *Choices: The Newsletter of Choice in Dying.* New York, NY: CID, Summer, 1995 (4:2); Spring, 1996 (5:1); Summer, 1996 (5:2).
Advance Directives: State Document with Guidebook
Artificial Nutrition/Hydration, 1994
Medical Treatments & Your Living Will, 1996.

Choice in Dying, Inc. *Advance Directives and End-of-Life Decisions.*
Cardiopulmonary Resuscitation, Do-Not-Resuscitate Orders and End-of-Life Decisions, 1995
You & Your Choices, Advance Medical Directives.

Colen, B.D. *The Essential Guide to a Living Will.* New York, NY: Prentice Hall Press, 1991.

Kubler-Ross, Elisabeth, M.D. *On Death and Dying.* New York, NY: MacMillan Publishing Co., Inc., 1969. *Death: The Final Stage of Growth.* Englewood Cliffs, NJ: Prentice-Hall, Inc., 1975; *To Live Until We Say Good-Bye.* Englewood Cliffs, NJ: Prentice-Hall, Inc., 1978.

Seguin, Marilynne, R.N. and Smith, Cheryl K., J.D. *A Gentle Death.* Toronto, Ontario: Key Porter Books,

Shneidman, Edwin S. *Death: Current Perspectives.* Palo Alto, CA: Mayfield Publishing Co., 1984.

Videotape: "WHOSE Death Is It, Anyway?" Available from Choice in Dying, 1–800–521–3044.

Sources of Additional Information

Choice in Dying, Inc. (CID), 200 Varick St., New York, NY 10014-4810.
Advance Directive packages, including legal forms with instructions for each of the 50 states, can be ordered by telephone or can be downloaded from CID's web site.

For information about living wills: 1–800–989–WILL
e-mail: general inquiries   cid@choices.org
            membership/publications   services@choices.org
web site: http://www.choices.org

REVIEW AND SELF-CHECK

Complete each statement below, using information from Unit 20.

1. Use the chart below to contrast past and current practices related to death and dying.

Past Practices	Current Practices
1. _____	_____
2. _____	_____
3. _____	_____

2. The field of thanatology is devoted to the study of _____ .

3. List five examples of beliefs about death.

   1. _____

   2. _____

   3. _____

   4. _____

   5. _____

4. List three reasons death education may allay fears about death.

   1. _____

   2. _____

   3. _____

5. State five conditions that contribute to "death with dignity."

   1. _____

   2. _____

   3. _____

4. _____

5. _____

6. Name five issues related to end-of-life care.

    1. _____

    2. _____

    3. _____

    4. _____

    5. _____

7. Four reasons the courts may be involved in end-of-life decisions are:

    1. _____

    2. _____

    3. _____

    4. _____

8. Advance Medical Directive refers to _____ or

    _____ .

9. The purpose of a Living Will is _____ .

10. The purpose of the Medical Durable Power of Attorney is _____

    _____ .

11. The Patient Self-Determination Act includes the following provisions:

    1. _____

    2. _____

    3. _____

    4. _____

12. Write out the meaning of each acronym below:

    AMD _____

    DPA _____

    PSDA _____

    DNR _____

    HMO _____

13. The purpose of the PSDA is _____ .

14. Use this textbook or a dictionary to define the following words:

Ethical	Mortality	Proxy
Moral	Immortality	Surrogate
Culpability	Liability	Conservator

ASSIGNMENT

1. Draw a line that represents your life span. It can be any shape or length. The beginning represents birth; the end, death. Mark several significant events at points along the line.

2. Study your life line. Does it make you uncomfortable? If so, consider possible reasons for this effect.

3. Think about death for 15 seconds, then write down five to ten adjectives that immediately come to mind.

4. Think about your own death for five seconds. Write down two words that describe your feelings.

5. Consider your losses if you were to die in an accident tomorrow.
   a. List the relationships you would lose.
   b. List the possessions you would be giving up.
   c. List any uncompleted tasks you would leave behind.

6. Refer to your list of relationships and your list of possessions. Decide how you would want your property distributed. Prepare instructions to guide your survivors in carrying out your wishes:
   a. disposition of your body
   b. a funeral or memorial service
   c. disposition of your property
   d. care of your survivors, if you have dependents

7. Write your obituary, including age at time of death, the cause of death, the achievements or affiliations for which you will be remembered, your survivors, the final arrangements.

8. Now that you have thought about your death, list tasks you will complete as soon as possible.

9. Participate in a class discussion about the following topics:
    - Withholding artificial feedings from a patient who is in an irreversible coma
    - Withholding artificial feedings from a patient who is conscious but approaching death
    - "Do not resuscitate" orders
    - A patient's right to refuse a treatment the doctor wants to administer
    - Discontinuing life-support for a patient in a persistent vegetative state
    - Discontinuing life-support for a conscious patient who requests that it be discontinued
    - Discontinuing dialysis for a patient who does not want to live as a quadriplegic

10. At the top of a blank sheet of paper, write "What I believe about death." List your present beliefs.

11. At the top of a blank sheet, write "What I believe about care of a dying patient." List your present beliefs.

12. Participate in a class discussion about the responsibilities of health care providers to help patients understand their rights and the use of Advance Medical Directives.

13. Use library or Internet resources to obtain information (the facts) on the following cases:
    Nancy Cruzan
    Karen Ann Quinlan

14. Obtain a copy of the procedure followed in your affiliated health care agency to inform newly admitted patients about Advance Medical Directives. Consider your future role as a health care provider; what will be your responsibilities in regard to AMDs?

15. Obtain a copy of the legal document used in your state for Advance Medical Directives. Read through the document. It is a Living Will? a Medical Durable Power of Attorney? What rights does it give the patient? What rights does it give the family?

16. Interview each member of your immediate family to find out what they know about Advance Medical Directives. Provide information and encourage them to develop the appropriate Advance Medical Directives.

17. Using the appropriate form for your state, prepare your own Advance Medical Directive, sign it (with the necessary number of witnesses), and inform your family that you have an Advance Medical Directive.

18. Discuss the specific choices you have indicated in your AMD with your family, the proxy named in your Medical Durable Power of Attorney, and your physician.

Unit 21

Grief and Bereavement

OBJECTIVES

Upon completion of this unit, you should be able to:

- Define grief, anticipatory grief, and bereavement
- List four influences on reactions to loss.
- List five emotional components of grief.
- List physical effects of grief—five immediate effects and four delayed effects.
- List five mental/emotional effects of grief.
- List five behavior effects of grief.
- List two needs of a bereaved person.
- List five conditions that facilitate the grief process.
- List six conditions that inhibit the grief process.
- Name the five stages of the grief process as described by Dr. Kubler-Ross.
- List five indications of unresolved grief.
- State five guidelines for assisting the family of a dying patient.

KEY TERMS

Anticipatory grief   Condolences   Cremation
Grief   Grief work   Interment

MEANINGS

Grief is a normal and natural reaction to loss. The emotion is one extreme of a continuum that ranges from mild disappointment, through various degrees of sadness, up to the intense and painful state that we call grief or sorrow. **Anticipatory grief** is grieving that occurs prior to the actual loss, usually during a terminal illness. *Bereavement* is separation from or loss of someone who is very significant in one's life. Grief is the predominant emotional response to

387

bereavement. **Grief work** is a process of working through the emotional reaction to loss, reorganizing one's life patterns, and achieving some degree of adjustment. Grief work is important to future emotional and mental health. Uncompleted grief work is like a time bomb ticking away.

REACTIONS TO LOSS AND BEREAVEMENT

Each person reacts in his or her own way to each of life's losses. Some people react mildly for a short period of time to a specific loss. Another person may experience intense feelings for days, weeks, or months following a similar loss. Dr. Kubler-Ross has noted that many people experience a grief reaction similar to the five stages of dying, even if a loss is relatively small. For example, Mr. B. lost a set of keys that include the house key, several office keys, and the car keys. He went through the following stages during a period of ten days:

- I just don't believe I would lose my keys. (Denial)

- I am furious that those keys haven't been found. (Anger)

- If those keys turn up, I will always put them on the refrigerator as soon as I get home. (Bargaining)

- I'm not worth very much if I can't even keep up with my keys. (Depression)

- The keys are definitely lost. I may as well have some additional keys made. (Acceptance)

The reaction to loss of an object may be relatively mild and of short duration, depending on the meaning of the object to its owner. Losses that are related to one's self-esteem, such as loss of a job or the end of a relationship, tend to produce emotional reactions that are more intense and of longer duration than losses that do not threaten self-esteem. A sudden or unexpected loss produces an intense reaction that begins with shock and disbelief.

Some grief reactions include not only sadness, but also some degree of anger, hate, guilt, anxiety, or even panic. *Anger* is usually a major component in grief when the age of the deceased is "inappropriate" for dying, such as infancy and childhood, adolescence, young adulthood, or "the prime of life." A survivor may actually feel anger toward the deceased for "going away and leaving me." This reaction is especially likely in a child whose parent has died. *Anxiety* is related to the future: "How can I live without . . . (that which was lost)?" or "How can I make certain this never happens to me again?" *Panic* is related to recognition that one does not have the power to control the loss of a loved one. *Guilt* may be concerned with control: "Could I have prevented this from happening?" or blame: "If I had been more loving, this wouldn't have happened." Children who are not old enough to understand terminal illness or death are especially prone to guilt, because a child's anger toward a family member or playmate is likely to be expressed as an explosive "I hate you!" or possibly, "I wish you were dead!" A child may recall past actions, words, or thoughts and perceive that behavior and the death or illness as having a cause/effect relationship.

Grief is painful. Grief related to loss of a loved one through death usually results in a profound grief reaction. The remainder of this unit limits discussion of grief to this type of loss.

EFFECTS OF GRIEF

The death of a loved one has both physical and psychological effects. Shock is the immediate reaction. Profound shock is likely if a death is sudden or unexpected, the result of an accident or act of violence, or a suicide. In contrast to sudden bereavement, a lengthy illness provides time for anticipatory grieving prior to the actual death. Intensity of the immediate grief reaction, then, is determined by whether the death was expected or unexpected, a sudden or slow process, violent or nonviolent. If shock is severe, the survivor cannot begin grief work until the physical effects of shock have subsided.

In the absence of severe shock, a grief reaction can range from little or no visible reaction to uncontrolled, destructive behavior. The immediate physical effects include tightness in the throat, a choking sensation, shortness of breath, weakness, a feeling of emptiness or a knot in the stomach, nausea. These effects

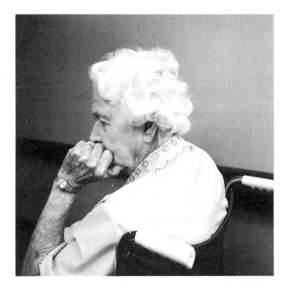

Grief has both physical and psychological effects.

may subside within a few hours, to be replaced by loss of appetite and/or digestive problems, disturbed sleep patterns, restlessness, frequent sighing, and crying that may continue intermittently for days, weeks, or months.

The mental/emotional effects of bereavement include preoccupation with thoughts of the deceased, lack of interest in other people, irritability, difficulty in organizing thoughts or making decisions, difficulty in concentrating or remembering, feelings of hopelessness, feelings of guilt, and possibly a tendency toward blaming self or others for the loss. Some behavioral effects of grief are lack of interest in grooming, refusal to participate in previous activities or hobbies, poor performance of tasks at home or on the job, reminiscing about the deceased, idealizing the deceased (forgetting negative aspects of the deceased), and clinging to personal reminders.

These effects of grief vary in intensity and duration according to a survivor's relationship to the deceased, personal ways of dealing with strong emotion, and patterns of behavior learned in previous life crises. How a survivor deals with grief determines future adjustment.

IMPORTANCE OF THE GRIEF PROCESS

Grief may be a period of pain from which one strives to recover as quickly as possible. It may also be a growth experience in which one learns to accept certain realities:

- We are vulnerable to certain life experiences, including losses.

- We are not all-powerful. We only have control over *some* aspects of our lives.

- We are mortal, not immortal.

- There will be a time when life for each of us comes to an end.

- Loss requires saying "good-bye" to some aspect of life, but loss can also mean a new beginning.

- "Letting go" does not diminish the importance of what was lost, but it does free the survivor to make the necessary adjustments for continuing to live without the deceased.

The bereaved should make his or her own decisions about involvement with other people and participation in activities. Some people need a period of time for withdrawal or denial before accepting the finality of the loss. If the grief process is delayed too long, however, the person's adjustment deteriorates, and a delayed grief reaction eventually occurs, possibly with destructive effects. Because grieving leads eventually to adjustment and denying grief leads to deterioration in life adjustment, anyone who has suffered a loss, should (1) be encouraged to grieve and (2) continue to have emotional support until grief work has been completed.

INFLUENCES ON THE GRIEF PROCESS

Any person who has experienced a significant loss has the right to grieve. A person's grieving tends to be consistent with the personality and usual coping styles. The intensity and duration of grieving are influenced by the relationship to the deceased and past experiences with loss. Friends and family should grant each survivor the right to grieve in his or her own way.

Working through the stages of denial, anger, and bargaining prior to the actual death seems to facilitate grief work during the bereavement period. Spending quality time with the dying person—sharing memories, expressing feelings, touching and holding—facilitates **anticipatory grieving** and also eases the dying process.

Emotional Support

Grieving is facilitated if family members share their feelings and if relatives and friends are supportive throughout the process. It is especially important that this emotional support come from those with whom the bereaved must restructure his or her life—resume the daily routine of old responsibilities,

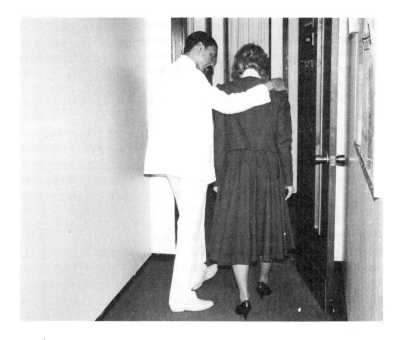

A survivor may need encouragement to express the feelings that accompany loss.

assume new responsibilities, and restructure relationships that no longer include the deceased. This support network is especially important on significant dates—anniversaries, birthdays, and holidays—throughout the first year of bereavement.

Acceptance of Loss

Grief work begins with acceptance of the loss—the finality of death. Sometimes there is intellectual acceptance without emotional acceptance. Only when the finality of the loss is accepted at the emotional level can grief work begin. The survivor needs encouragement to "be with" his or her feelings by expressing the sadness and pain, rather than denying the feelings or hiding them from others.

Making Final Arrangements

Participating in the tasks related to death seems to facilitate acceptance. Before or immediately after the death, someone must notify relatives, friends, coworkers, the minister, and the family lawyer; prepare an obituary; care for and remove the body; plan for the disposal of the body (burial, **cremation**); plan a service (funeral, memorial); purchase a cemetery lot (or decide how to dispose of the ashes if cremation is chosen); complete paperwork (death certificate, notices to insurance and annuity companies, government agencies, banks). Insofar as possible, the tasks that involve decision-making should be completed prior to the actual death, because one who is experiencing powerful emotions should not make important decisions. The closest survivors should make certain decisions. Some people, however, are unable or unwilling to make funeral plans while the patient is still living.

Some people want to be involved in the final stages of the dying process, and some want to assist with final care of the body. Being present at the final moments of life is beneficial to survivors and also to the patient. Many dying patients state that dying alone is their greatest fear. For survivors, being with the patient in those last moments is preparation for emotional release. Bathing, dressing, and grooming the body provides an opportunity for saying "good-bye" in the most loving and caring way possible. This is especially appropriate if the deceased is a child. Sometimes the survivors participate in closing the grave with handfuls of dirt. This, too, is a way of saying "good-bye" and moving toward emotional acceptance of the loss.

The body of the deceased and the final service both play a role in acceptance of death. The body is a stimulus to the release of feelings. The funeral service and **interment** provide opportunities to express the intense feelings that immediately follow the death and help prepare the survivors for grief work. The alternative to a traditional funeral, such as a memorial service, can also facilitate the grief process.

Grief Inhibitors

In the belief that people need to be protected, someone may try to keep those closest to the deceased from participating in these tasks. Friends or relatives may encourage survivors-to-be to withdraw from the death scene and to delegate final tasks to others. The survivors may even be deprived of time with the loved one, either during the final moments or immediately after death, in the mistaken belief that witnessing the death or being with the body would be traumatic. No matter how good their intentions, people who influence the family to withdraw from the death scene deprive the family members of an experience that facilitates "letting go" and beginning the grief process.

Children, especially, are likely to be excluded. As they observe atypical adult behavior and disruption of the family's normal routine, they may be confused, frightened, or angry. They need careful explanations about what is happening, much comforting, and a chance to say "good-bye" to the dying person *if they wish to do so.*

Numerous conditions, in addition to those already discussed, can inhibit the grief process: a sudden death, an untimely death, the mode of death (accident, suicide, violence), unresolved grief from past losses, past tendency to suppress anger and grief, ambivalent feelings toward the deceased, the use of drugs or alcohol to suppress feelings, resuming normal activities too early, isolation from a death (war in a foreign country), or uncertainty about a death (a plane crash or fire in which the remains are difficult or impossible to identify). The uncertainty created when the body cannot be viewed makes it especially difficult for survivors to accept the death. There is, instead, a tendency to cling to the belief that "(name of the victim) will come back home some day."

Condolences

Most people find it difficult to express their **condolences** to the bereaved. All too often, statements that are offered as words of comfort or as reassurance actually deny the importance of grief or imply that the person has no right to grieve. The following are examples of such statements:

- "You must be strong" implies that showing one's grief is a sign of weakness.

- "You must be a little man" when said to a young boy, denies that child the right to grieve and also implies that, as a male, he is not allowed to cry.

- "It's time to get on with your life" is a way of saying, "I do not grant you any more time for grieving."

If a year has passed, the person may need professional counselling to facilitate the completion of grief work. But the last statement above would be totally inappropriate a month, or even several months, after the death of a loved one. An inappropriate statement may indicate that the speaker does not understand the grief process or its importance to a survivor's future adjustment.

GRIEF WORK

The grief process does not flow smoothly, nor is it effortless. Management of grief requires time and energy and involves much psychological pain. The grief process requires at least a year for completion. If the deceased was close (parent, spouse, child), this process may extend over a period of several years.

Stages of Grief

Wayne Oates, a well-known pastoral counselor and author who has worked with dying patients and their families for many years, describes the grieving process as consisting of six stages:

- **Stage 1:** The survivor is in a state of shock. If the death was sudden or unexpected, the shock may be severe enough to require medical care. Anticipatory grief can minimize the intensity of shock when the death actually occurs, but cannot fully prepare one for the actual event of death.

- **Stage 2:** The survivor is able to interact with others and perform some tasks but does so as though in a daze.

- **Stage 3:** The survivor is caught in a struggle between reality and fantasy, behaving at times as though the deceased is alive but, at other times, being well aware of the loss. During this period there is a tendency to dream about the deceased.

- **Stage 4:** The survivor expresses intense grief in various ways as the reality of the loss is accepted.

- **Stage 5:** Certain people, objects, events, or dates evoke memories of the deceased, resulting in brief periods of sadness or depression.

- **Stage 6:** Readjustment is achieved as a purpose in living emerges, and satisfaction is found in various life activities.

Both the Kubler-Ross model and the Oates model emphasize that *grief is a process that must run its course.* In both models, the bereaved experiences a sequence of emotional states over a period of time. The expression *grief work* is used to describe these experiences. Grief work is not accomplished if the individual denies grief.

Ideally, grief work should begin within a few days of the death. Following the initial stage of shock and denial, there is a release of feelings, which may be followed by a period of confusion. There may be recurrent dreams about the deceased. Memories may crowd the mind, making it difficult to concentrate or even to sleep. This is a time when talking about the final days of the deceased has a therapeutic effect. There is a need to remember and to review the relationship with the loved one—the good memories and the bad memories. The survivor must work through not only the sadness, but also any anger, hate, and feelings of guilt. This "working through" is best accomplished through talking with others about one's loss and expressing the feelings of the moment. For some people, there is a need to talk *to* the deceased—say what was left unsaid during their time together, ask for forgiveness, or express regrets. Crying is effective for expressing both sadness and anger, but verbalizing is especially effective for diffusing sadness and anger and resolving guilt feelings. Those with creative talent may express their feelings through music, art, or writing. Each mourner must work through these feelings in his or her own way, sometimes in private and sometimes with the help and support of others.

Eventually, the sadness is replaced by loneliness—an intense loneliness that is not relieved by the presence of others. The bereaved is beginning to realize that the void left by the deceased cannot be filled by anyone else. The unique relationship with the deceased is lost forever. This is a period of freeing oneself from the deceased; with time, the loneliness gives way to hopefulness. When talk begins to focus less on the loss and more on changes needed to adjust to life without the deceased, the grief process is nearing completion.

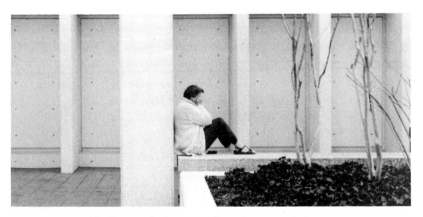

Grief often includes a profound sense of aloneness.

With additional time, the survivor resumes some former activities, establishes new relationships or modifies old relationships to exclude the deceased, and begins to find satisfaction in daily activities. At that point, the survivor is "getting on" with his or her life. Successful completion of grief work leads to a greater understanding of life, greater compassion for the suffering of others, and higher levels of sensitivity to the needs of others who have suffered loss.

Uncompleted Grief Work

Some survivors fail to complete the grief process, either because feelings are suppressed or because certain conditions inhibit the grief process. Grief that is not resolved may be indicated by hyperactivity, inappropriate feelings, physical illness (possibly with the symptoms of the deceased), changes in relationships with others, hostility, depression, or a lack of feeling. Sometimes the grief reaction becomes chronic; that is, the bereaved becomes locked into the early stages of the process and does not progress toward readjustment. Denial of grief at the time of the loss may result in a delayed grief reaction after weeks, months, or even years, usually at the time of another death or when a close friend is grieving.

Supportive friends and relatives can contribute greatly to successful grief work. Professional counselling is needed, however, when a survivor manifests denial or evidence of uncompleted grief work.

ROLES OF HEALTH CARE PROVIDERS

The health care provider is likely to be in contact with relatives of a dying patient when they are survivors-to-be, rather than throughout the bereavement period. Since the physician has primary responsibility for providing information about a patient's condition, health workers must know what the patient, as well as the family, has been told. This can be determined by carefully worded questions and by observation of nonverbal behavior. Active listening is effective for learning what the physician has told the patient and family and identifying where the other person is emotionally. Sometimes it is appropriate to use open and honest communication, such as "I feel sad that your husband is so sick."

The health care provider's goal is to help the family, not by giving information or expressing personal opinions, but by helping the other to express feelings and work toward acceptance of the loss at his or her own pace. There are now various professional workers who are prepared to provide skilled counselling for patients and their families. Large hospitals have chaplains and social workers, some of whom have this special preparation for helping others cope with a life crisis. Smaller hospitals and most nursing homes rely on community resources to provide this specialized service.

Nurses have the advantage of providing care throughout the day and night. Other personnel visit the patient or stay with families for a relatively brief period of time. Each death/bereavement situation is unique, so there cannot be a single procedure to guide the health care provider. But, there are guidelines that may help the caregiver adapt to each situation.

GUIDELINES FOR ASSISTING THE FAMILY OF A DYING PATIENT

1. Be available to the family as much as possible. (Do *not* use the Nurses' Station as a refuge to avoid interacting with the family.)

2. Use active listening to encourage the expression of feelings.

3. Interact with the patient as you provide physical care. Model for family members the expression of caring, even if the patient is not responsive.

4. Be tolerant of what you see and hear. Various members of the family are at different stages of grieving, and each is reacting to a life crisis in his or her own way.

5. Encourage close family members to stay with the patient, to talk and touch as much as possible throughout the dying process. This is important, even if the patient is comatose.

   NOTE: Be aware that the hospital has an intimidating effect on many people. To "stay out of the way," they may miss their final opportunity to be with the loved one who is dying, unless you encourage them to stay close by.

6. As appropriate, offer to call the family minister, priest, or rabbi. If the family does not have a spiritual advisor, offer to call the hospital chaplain.

7. If you observe that a family needs assistance in dealing with their grief, contact the hospital chaplain or social worker.

8. Know the available sources of help in your community and share this information with a family as appropriate. For example, *Compassionate Friends* is a support group for parents who have lost a child.

9. Work on your own "unfinished business" related to past losses and on your own fears related to death. Until you have accepted you own mortality and completed your own grief work, you cannot be fully effective in helping others to cope with death and dying.

References and Suggested Readings

Backer, Barbara A., Hannon, Natalie R., & Gregg, Joan Young. *To Listen, To Comfort, To Care.* Albany, NY: Delmar Publishers Inc., 1994. Chapter 10, "Grief and Bereavement," pp. 151–166.

Crenshaw, David. *Bereavement: Counseling the Grieving throughout the Life Cycle.* New York, NY: The Crossroads Publishing Co., 1995.

Grollman, Earl A. *Bereaved Children and Teens: A Support-Guide for Parents and Professionals.* Boston, MA: Beacon Press, 1995.

James, John W. & Cherry, Frank. *The Grief Recovery Handbook: A Step-by-Step Program for Moving Beyond Loss.* New York, NY: Harper-Perennial, 1989. (The authors are co-founders of The Grief Recovery Institute.)

Jarrett, Claudia Jewett. *Helping Children Cope with Separation and Loss;* Revised Edition. Boston, MA: Harvard Common Press, 1994.

Jensen, Amy Hillyard. *Healing Grief.* Redmond, WA: Medic Publishing Co., 1980. (Twenty-two page booklet, available from the publisher: P.O. Box 89, Redmond, WA.)

Oates, Wayne E. *Your Particular Grief.* Philadelphia, PA: The Westminster Press, 1981.

Schatz, William H. *Healing a Father's Grief.* Redmond, WA: Medic Publishing Co., 1984. (Twenty-four page booklet, available from the publisher at P.O. Box 89, Redmond, WA.)

Tamparo, Carol D. & Lindh, Wilburta Q. *Therapeutic Communications for Allied Health Professionals.* Albany, NY: Delmar Publishers Inc., 1992. Unit 11, "The Therapeutic Response to Clients Experiencing Loss, Grief, Dying and Death," pp. 233–242.

Sources of Information

The Compassionate Friends, Inc., P.O. Box 1347, Oak Brook, IL 60521

The Grief Recovery Institute, 8306 Wilshire Blvd., Los Angeles, CA 90211.

REVIEW AND SELF-CHECK

Complete each statement below, using information from Unit 21.

1. Grief is _____ .

2. Anticipatory grief is _____ .

3. Bereavement is _____ .

4. Grief work is _____ .

5. Reactions to loss are variable, depending upon such factors as:

    1. _____

    2. _____

    3. _____

    4. _____

6. A grief reaction may include *various emotional components,* such as:

    _____ , _____ , _____

    _____ , and/or _____ .

7. The immediate *physical effects* of grief may include:

    1. _____

    2. _____

    3. _____

    4. _____

    5. _____

8. Some of the *delayed effects* of grief are:

    1. _____

    2. _____

    3. _____

    4. _____

9. Mental/emotional effects of grief may include:

    1. _____

    2. _____

    3. _____

    4. _____

    5. _____

10. Some behavior effects of grief are:

    1. _____

    2. _____

    3. _____

4. _____

5. _____

11. In view of the consequences of denying grief, it is important that bereaved people:

    1. _____

    2. _____

12. Conditions that facilitate the grief process:

    1. _____

    2. _____

    3. _____

    4. _____

    5. _____

13. Conditions that inhibit the grief process:

    1. _____

    2. _____

    3. _____

    4. _____

    5. _____

    6. _____

14. The five stages of grief, as described by Dr. Kubler-Ross:

    1. _____

    2. _____

    3. _____

    4. _____

    5. _____

15. Some indications of unresolved grief:

    1. _____

    2. _____

    3. _____

4. _____

5. _____

ASSIGNMENT

1. If you have lost a member of your immediate family, write a brief description of your reaction—immediate and throughout the first year. Evaluate your grief work: Was it effective? Or, do you have "unfinished business?"

2. If you have never experienced the loss of a loved one through death, prepare for the time when you will have such an experience by writing out a list of guidelines that would help you complete the grief process.

3. Participate in a small group discussion.
   a. Compare the stages of grief as described by Kubler-Ross and by Oates.
   b. Compare your own experiences with grief to each of these models.

4. Participate in a class project to identify your community resources for assisting bereaved people. Which of these provide immediate, but short-term assistance? Which ones provide long-term assistance?

5. Think about the following situations and be prepared to participate in a small group discussion about the (1) reactions reflected in each situation and (2) conditions that could have changed the reaction:
   a. A family of four adult children and one adolescent experienced a sudden death of their father. Sarah, being a nurse, took charge of the situation. She delegated tasks to each of her brothers and sisters. One sister was so overcome with grief that she could not perform her assignments, so Sarah took care of those tasks in addition to her own. Sarah was described by relatives as a "tower of strength for all of us." From the time when news of the death was received until the estate was settled, Sarah stayed busy "doing what has to be done." Approximately ten months following her father's death, Sarah was admitted to the hospital in critical condition. Although she recovered, her convalescence required almost a full year.

b. Melissa was a college graduate who had worked for six years to help her husband finish law school and set up his law practice. As soon as she became pregnant, 'Lissa quit her job to be a full-time homemaker. When her two children were two and four years old, Bob went to a distant city on business. He decided to fly so he could be home in time to spend the weekend with his family. On Friday evening, a plane crashed as it was landing at the local airport. News of the crash was broadcast within minutes. 'Lissa heard the newscast and knew that Bob was supposed to be on that flight. Her parents heard the newscast and rushed over to be with their daughter. They found her cheerfully setting the table for dinner. When they told her about the crash, she responded, "I heard that newscast. But I know Bob didn't get on that plane." After several weeks, workers at the crash site still had found nothing that could provide positive identification of Bob. Two years later, 'Lissa is still saying, "I know Bob is alive. Someday he will walk through the front door."

Unit 22

Caring for the Dying Person

OBJECTIVES

Upon completion of this unit, you should be able to:

- List five fears commonly expressed by a dying person.
- List and explain the five stages of dying, as proposed by Dr. Kubler-Ross.
- Explain dying as a growth process.
- State the requirements for a "healthy" reaction to dying, as proposed by Lindemann.
- List seven conditions that contribute to adjustment of dying patients, according to Carey.
- Discuss three personal and family issues related to care of a dying person.
- Discuss three medical issues related to care of a dying person.
- List five issues related to the rights of patients.
- Explain the role of health care providers in care of the dying.
- State five guidelines for meeting the needs of a dying patient.
- List five advantages of dying at home.
- State the primary focus of "palliative care."

KEY TERMS

Manifestations	Palliative	Humane
Taboo	Transformation	Plateau
Curative		

REACTIONS TO DIAGNOSIS OF A TERMINAL ILLNESS

As a result of current practices in the care of terminally ill patients, many middle-aged people today have had little or no personal contact with a dying person. Their experience with death is limited to occasional attendance at a funeral. There is a universal tendency to fear that which is unknown and foreign to one's own experience, so death and dying have been relegated to the closet. Death is **taboo** as a topic of conversation for most people. But, diagnosis of an illness for which there is currently no cure brings a patient and family members face to face with the reality of death. The reaction to such news includes fear—fear of the unknown and fear of death.

Counselors who work with dying patients have identified a number of fears expressed by many patients.

- What happens after death. What lies beyond death?

- Will I be forgotten?

- Will my loved ones be cared for adequately without me? If they can get along without me, does that mean I was not important to them?

- What will become of my work, my life-long efforts to accomplish something? Will my work be continued by someone else? Will someone else take credit for my work?

- What will happen to my property? Will my possessions be cared for? How will they be distributed?

- Will I become dependent on others?

- Will I be a burden?

- Will I lose my mind?

- Will I lose control of my life? Who will make important decision that affect me?

- Will I have more pain than I can bear?

- Will I be left to die alone?

A major responsibility of caregivers is to recognize **manifestations** of fear and encourage a patient to verbalize them. Expressing their fears about death to an understanding listener facilitates the dying process.

STAGES OF DYING

According to Dr. Elisabeth Kubler-Ross, a dying person goes through five stages, beginning with denial and ending with acceptance that death is approaching. At some point, the dying patient begins to grieve for all that must be given up: relationships with loved ones and friends, material possessions, ambitions, life goals and purposes, plans for the future, and ultimately, one's body.

Hope is important throughout the five stages. Without hope, the patient would lapse into despair. Fear, also, may be part of a patient's emotional state in any or all of the stages.

Although some thanatologists disagree with Dr. Kubler-Ross about the stages of dying, her model does provide a framework for understanding the feelings a dying person may experience. Naming these stages undoubtedly has helped nurses and other caregivers recognize the needs of dying patients and accept behaviors that represent a patient's progress in relation to the dying process.

Denial

The first stage of dying involves denial—"No, I am not dying. It just isn't true." This reaction seems to occur regardless of whether or not a person is told directly that he or she has a terminal illness. Denial may be manifested in many ways: changing doctors repeatedly, continuing one's daily routine as though nothing is wrong, refusing to talk about the illness, refusing treatment or embarking on a search for any and all treatments.

Denial serves a useful purpose. As a defense mechanism, it gives the patient time to deal with the shock of knowing that life is coming to an end. Denial may recur at intervals throughout the dying process.

Anger

The second stage of dying is characterized by anger. As the patient begins to face the reality of terminal illness, the reaction is, "Why me? Why not somebody else?" During this stage, the patient may direct anger at anyone and everyone. It is a difficult time for health care providers as well as the family. The caregivers, it seems, cannot do anything right during this period. The patient's behavior is easier to tolerate if one remembers that this patient is in the process of learning to face his or her death.

Bargaining

In the third stage of dying, the patient begins to bargain—with God, Fate, the doctor or nurses, or the family. This bargaining may be unknown to the caregivers, or it may be shared. Perhaps the patient prays to stay alive until some particular event—the birth of a grandchild, a wedding, a child's graduation. Perhaps the patient promises to change behavior or life-style, if he or she can have a second chance: "If only I can be well again, I'll never take another drink." Bargaining may take the form of being a "good" patient—cheerful and cooperative regardless of annoying treatments or pain.

Depression

The fourth stage is marked by depression. With increased symptoms, especially pain or weakness, the patient can no longer maintain denial; bargaining seems pointless; anger gives way to sorrow over impending losses. Dr. Kubler-Ross believes that this period involves two different types of depression: (1) a *reactive depression* to the impending losses faced by the patient and (2) a *preparatory depression* related to the impending separation.

Acceptance

The fifth stage is one of acceptance. Provided the patient has enough time and is helped to work through the previous stages, this stage represents several accomplishments.

- The patient is neither depressed nor angry.

- The patient has grieved for the many losses.

- The patient is tired and/or weak.

- The patient dozes frequently for short periods.

The stage of acceptance is not a happy stage. It is more likely to be, according to Dr. Kubler-Ross, devoid of feeling. But, the patient is at peace.

Health care providers should not expect a dying patient to move systematically through these five stages. One patient may appear to skip a stage; another may continue in denial up to the time of death; still another may appear to reach acceptance very quickly. The stages do, however, provide a useful framework for identifying a specific patient's needs. By responding appropriately according to a patient's current emotional state, each health care provider can contribute to a patient's progress toward acceptance.

DYING AS A GROWTH PROCESS

When death is viewed in light of the many losses involved, it is difficult to think of dying as an opportunity for growth. Viewed in terms of the emotional changes and the **transformation** that may occur as the dying process is completed, both spiritual and emotional growth become evident. According to Dr. Mwalinu Imara, author of "Dying as the last stage of growth" in Dr. Kubler-Ross' book, *Death: The Final State of Growth*, ". . . the dying stage of our life can be experienced as the most profound growth event of our total life's experience. . . . if we are fortunate enough to have time to live and experience our own process, our arrival at a **plateau** of creative acceptance will be worth it."

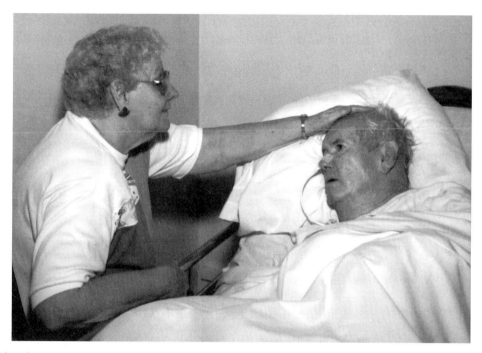

The dying person can withdraw in despair, suppress feelings about approaching death, or reach out to others.

The dying person has a choice: to withdraw in despair, to suppress negative emotions, or to reach out to others. It is through the third option that growth occurs. Growth requires commitment to experiencing self, becoming aware of one's own identity, communicating one's experience to others, and accepting that one's life has purpose and meaning. These changes are facilitated by a support network of loving and caring people, who also have the opportunity for growth as they share in the dying experience.

Many people need the help of a skilled counselor to work through the negative aspects of life experience. The goal of helping a dying person work through the dying process is to have him or her achieve emotional adjustment and live life to the fullest during whatever time remains. Arrival at the stage of acceptance with a sense of peace indicates successful resolution of the emotions of the dying process. Dr. Kubler-Ross states, "Anyone who has witnessed a patient in peace and not in resignation will never forget it. . . ."

Erich Lindemann, author of "Reactions to One's Own Fatal Illness" in Shneidman's *Death: Current Perspectives; Third Edition,* suggests that a "healthy" reaction (to dying) requires free expression and sharing of feelings with loved ones and close friends. Once the dying person can deal with the notion of having an illness for which there is no cure, he or she can enrich the time remaining through a series of activities.

- Review one's life—various experiences and relationships and the meanings of each.

- Visit places and people that are important.

- Review memories with friends and relatives.

- Make up for missed opportunities.

- Resolve old conflicts.

- Think through and talk over with loved ones such questions as "What will happen to my survivors?" and "How will my place be filled?"

Although these activities may be painful, there will also be much joy as these experiences are shared with others who have been a part of one's life experience. According to Lindemann, those who "do a good job of recalling their own lives and their own shared experiences" are most likely to serve as a positive model of the dying process.

Raymond G. Carey, author of "Living until death: A program of service and research for the terminally ill" in Dr. Kubler-Ross' *Death: The Final Stage of Growth,* reports a number of conditions that contribute to successful adjustment of dying patients.

- Interest and concern of relatives and family clergy

- Warm, supportive relationship with at least one person

- Relatively good adjustment and past patterns of successfully coping with problems

- Strong religious beliefs, especially if the person has truly tried to live according to these beliefs

- Belief that one's life has meaning

- Belief in life after death

- Willingness to talk about the illness and approaching death

- Previous contact with a dying person who achieved a state of inner peace

- Honesty combined with reassurance (not of cure, but of continued support and control of pain) from the physician

- Control of pain, because pain interferes with adjustment

In addition to striving for emotional adjustment, the patient must face a number of challenges. The illness and impending dependence on others necessitates changes in life-style and relationships. For those who have a high level of independence, certain changes in self-concept are difficult, but necessary.

- From "I am an independent person" to "Others must do some things for me"

- From "I am self-directing, capable, and in control of my life" to "I must let others have control over some aspects of my life"

In addition to these changes in self-concept, there must be a change in planning. Instead of thinking "Some day I will . . . ," a dying person must think, "Today I will. . . . " It is also important that the dying person continue to feel that life has meaning.

PERSONAL AND FAMILY ISSUES RELATED TO CARE OF THE DYING

When a person is diagnosed with an incurable illness, certain decisions must be made. What treatments should be used? Should drugs or treatments that are known to have serious side effects be used? Should experimental drugs or procedures whose effects are not fully known be used? Should the patient find another physician? Another clinic? Another medical center that may have "a new cure"?

If the patient's condition is deteriorating or the patient is in the terminal phase of illness, questions about care must be decided. Should the patient be in a hospital or nursing home? Should the patient be at home? Who will provide care? Can this responsibility be rotated among family members? Or will one person have to provide around-the-clock care? Is there a home health service that could provide skilled care as needed? Is there a hospice in the community? The most important questions are:

1. Where does the patient want to be during his or her final days?

2. If the patient wants to die at home, is the family willing and able to undertake the care of a dying person at home.

In *Coming Home: A Guide to Home Care for the Terminally Ill*, Deborah Duda states that dying at home is "the old, natural way which most of the world never questioned." She lists eighteen advantages of dying at home and seven conditions under which this decision would *not* be appropriate. Among the advantages she lists are that the dying person feels wanted, can influence surroundings, has more freedom and control, maintains respect and dignity, can enjoy home-cooked food, has the opportunity to express feelings to various relatives and friends, and the familiar setting is conducive to family support as the patient does the inner preparation for death. Another advantage, not included in Duda's list, is privacy; the patient's last days are family-centered, with minimal intrusion by outsiders. Also, the monetary cost of dying at home is minuscule, compared to the costs of intensive care and life-maintenance procedures commonly used in hospitals during the final days of a patient's life.

Dying at home is not appropriate, according to Duda, when either the patient or the family does not willingly choose this alternative to institutional care. Some families are not able to provide care, either because of their own limitations, or because the patient's needs cannot be met in the home setting. If family members cannot handle the emotional drain, the physical demands of caring for someone who is terminally ill, or the overall stress of such a situation, then choosing to die at home would not be appropriate. If the patient has arranged to be an organ donor and the specific terminal illness does not preclude use of the organs, then the patient's death should occur in the hospital setting with a surgical team on call to harvest any usable organs as soon as the patient is pronounced dead.

Arranging for someone to die at home requires careful planning. The family should contact hospice and home health services to arrange for assistance and consultation services as needed. Roles should be discussed and agreed upon; the primary care-giver should be selected, with others agreeing to assume care at specific times. This may draw a family closer together as they share the common goal of providing loving care for the person they will soon lose. Or, the family may become divided by disagreements and unequal division of responsibilities, with one or two persons carrying most of the burden. Careful advance planning may prevent the latter situation and allow the patient to spend his or her final days in a harmonious family setting.

PALLIATIVE CARE

"**Palliative** care" refers to the type of care that should be provided when a patient's illness is terminal, (i.e., cure or significant improvement is no longer possible). The primary focus of treatment is *comfort*, both physical and psychological, rather than *cure*. Effective palliative care provides relief from such physical symptoms as pain, shortness of breath, and nausea. Palliative care also includes emotional support to relieve anxiety, accept the dying process, grieve for impending losses (life itself, as well as loved ones left behind, and material possessions), and to say "Good-bye" to loved ones. The reason most often cited by patients who request euthanasia or assisted suicide is *intolerable* *pain;* this means that palliative care is *not* being provided, nor is the patient's pain being managed effectively.

Family and close friends are an important part of palliative care. Their presence may relieve a patient's fear of abandonment—of dying alone. Frequent visits by the person designated as "agent" in an Advance Medical Directive may provide reassurance that end-of-life decisions will be honored. Many patients who have prepared an Advance Medical Directive do not want "high-tech" interventions, believing that such measures prolong *dying,* rather than *living.* Many physicians, with a strong commitment to prolonging life, recommend such measures as additional chemotherapy, mechanical ventilation, artificial feeding (IV or tube), or dialysis, even when the patient is in the final stages of dying. The patient, if able, the family, and especially the "designated agent" should question the benefit of such recommendations and keep in mind the right to refuse treatment.

Palliative care is most easily provided in the home or in a residential hospice. Most hospices in the United States are home-based, however, and the time hospice personnel can spend in each patient's home is somewhat limited. It is more difficult to provide palliative care in hospitals, where policies require the use of heroic measures to prolong life and the transfer of dying patients to intensive care units. This may change, as the Health Care Financing Administration explores ways to reimburse hospitals for palliative care. Also, some nursing homes are now affiliating with hospices in order to offer palliative care, rather than transferring any dying resident to an acute care facility. Palliative care is not the prevailing modality for care of dying patients; it is currently a medical issue, a personal and family issue, and a "patients' rights" issue.

MEDICAL ISSUES RELATED TO CARE OF THE DYING

Diagnosis and prescription of therapy are responsibilities of the physician. When the diagnosis of a fatal disease is confirmed, the physician faces several difficult questions.

- Does an adult patient have a right to know the diagnosis?

- Does an adult patient have a right to decide who should be given information about his or her condition?

- Does a physician have a duty to inform a patient that he or she is dying?

- How much information should the patient be given?

- Should the patient be told that he or she is dying?

- How and when should the patient be told?

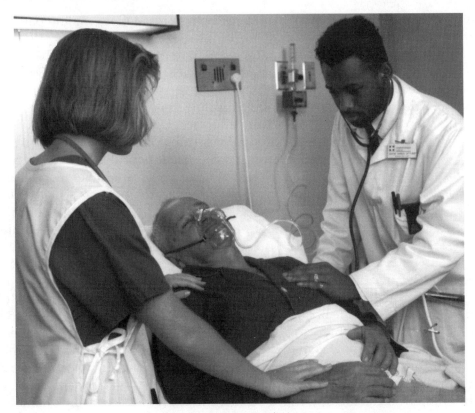

When diagnosis of a fatal illness has been confirmed, the physician must decide how and when, as well as how much, to tell the patient.

Past medical practice has been to tell the family that the patient is dying, but "protect" the patient by telling as little as possible. This is a departure from ethical practices related to confidentiality. Does a dying patient have less of a right to confidentiality than one who is not dying? Several studies have revealed that (1) the majority of physicians do not make a practice of telling patients that they are dying, and (2) that the majority of people believe they would want to be informed.

John Hinton suggests that *how* the information is given is important. It is possible to convey in a tactful and caring manner that the illness will be fatal. People listen selectively, so each patient is likely to deal consciously only with as much of the message as he or she is able to handle at that moment. Hinton offers several reasons why patients should be informed.

- A patient who is not told that he or she is dying is deprived of opportunities to talk about the illness and dying. This "conspiracy of silence" results in the patient feeling isolated.

- A dying patient needs to get his or her affairs in order. This pertains to everyone, not just the wage earner or a business person. Getting one's affairs in order includes personal as well as business and financial decisions.

- Many dying patients want to deal with spiritual matters in preparation for dying.

- Lack of correct information may lead the patient to seek help from one practitioner after another, until financial resources have been exhausted. A second opinion often is desirable, but a fruitless search for a nonexistent cure may be avoided by honest communication.

Some patients want to have full information about their disorder, the treatment options available, and probable course of the illness. In general, the defense mechanisms provide some protection against being overwhelmed. The patient focuses on some aspects of the illness and ignores others, according to the current capacity for coping. Other patients do not want to be told and are willing to delegate control and all treatment decisions to the physician. It would be destructive to try to force such a patient to "face the truth." On the other hand, such patients are likely to ask questions that indicate a need for reassurance. These patients usually suspect the truth, and their questions indicate a need to talk. Active listening may reveal underlying fears and anxieties for which the patient needs reassurance that he or she will be cared for and that pain will be alleviated.

Many physicians provide information to their patients gradually and try to balance bad news with something positive. Later, they give additional information according to the patient's readiness. How much to tell the dying patient must be decided by each physician, based in part on each patient's situation and emotional stability.

Health care providers involved in care of a dying patient should know what the physician has told the patient so they can respond appropriately to questions from the patient and family. Many patients find comfort in talking about their illness and dying with a sensitive caregiver. Frequent contact with caring people who *listen* results in the patient coming to terms with the illness. When there is good communication with family members, relationships improve. Good communication with health care personnel increases the patient's trust.

ISSUES RELATED TO RIGHTS OF THE DYING PERSON

Some issues discussed in Units 19 and 20 pertain to rights of patients. Rights issues are also concerned with truth, informed consent, control, choices, and protection of personal dignity. The issue of truth has already been discussed as

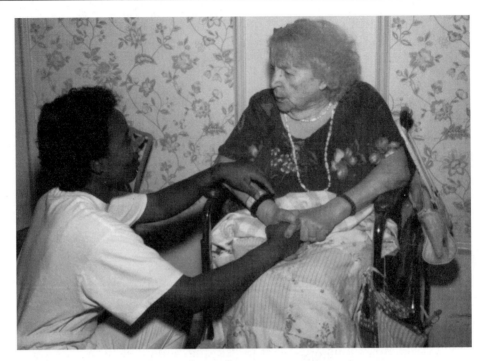

A warm, supportive relationship is important to a dying patient.

a medical question; but, truth is also related to informed consent. A patient who signs an agreement to undergo surgery or certain other treatments should do so only after being given full information.

- What is the probability that the surgery or treatment will help?

- What are the possible side effects?

- Will irreversible body changes result?

- Are alternative treatments available?

- What is the cost of the recommended treatment?

Some patients prefer to delegate decisions to others; that choice should be respected. Many patients wish to retain some degree of control and to participate in decisions; this, too, should be respected. Choices regarding life-maintenance procedures and Advance Medical Directives have already been discussed. Some other choices of patients, especially during the final days, include:

- Solitude versus being surrounded by significant others

- Remaining at home versus being in the hospital

- Remaining alert versus being sedated much of the time

Choices made by the patient or family members may conflict with what a health care provider considers to be "best" for the patient. This is a conflict of values. If the patient and family have arrived at acceptance of impending death, and if they are concerned about death with dignity, health care providers may feel frustrated that various available procedures are not being used to prolong life (or the dying process, depending upon one's view). It may help the health care provider to keep in mind that the Patient Self-Determination Act, Advance Directive legislation, and Informed Consent statutes are the result of practices that force unwanted procedures on dying patients.

ROLES OF HEALTH CARE PROVIDERS

Terminal illness by definition results in death. The goals of care for terminally ill patients, therefore, are different from the goals for patients who have the potential to regain physical well-being. It is difficult for many health care providers to accept as a goal anything other than "getting better." Working with dying patients requires that a health care provider be able to *substitute palliative goals for **curative** goals.* Palliative goals include keeping the patient comfortable, being available to listen, providing comforting touch as appropriate, accepting the patient's choices, and respecting the patient as a human being, even if comatose and nonresponsive.

The stages of dying proposed by Dr. Kubler-Ross can help health care providers to understand accept some of the behaviors manifested by a dying person. For example, anger directed at a caregiver is more easily accepted if viewed as one manifestation of a specific stage of the dying process. But attempting to "place" a patient in one stage or another does not serve the patient's needs. Rather, effective care demands the utmost in caring, always keeping in mind that this patient's emotional needs are paramount. Lindemann noted, " . . . one can be surprised at how little actual time expenditure is needed to say the right word at the right time, and not too much. . . . " The "right word" is any word or phrase that conveys acceptance—of the patient as a human being and of the patient's way of coping. Striving to cope with the approaching end of life is a most difficult psychological task. Perhaps the patient who is perceived by the staff as "difficult" is a patient who does not know how to accomplish this task.

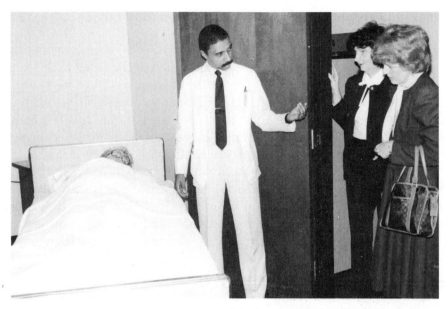

Working with dying patients requires substituting palliative goals for curative goals.

The health care provider can become the patient's accomplice in dealing with the process of dying, or the health care provider can ignore the process and relate to the dying person "as the target of our ministrations." (Lindemann, in Shneidmann, 1984) It is all too easy to ignore the basic humanity of a dying person if one becomes totally preoccupied with the technology used to maintain physical processes.

The tendency to ignore patients' end-of-life choices, including Living Wills and DNR orders, continues to characterize hospital care of dying patients. The Robert Wood Johnson Foundation funded a research project known as "Support," in which the care given to nine thousand critically ill patients in five different medical centers was monitored. The findings were disturbing: inadequate physician-patient communication, an excess of aggressive treatment, needlessly prolonged pain. The authors of an article in Newsweek state, " . . . despite two decades of right-to-die activism, vast numbers of Americans continue to die in intensive-care units, alone and in pain, after days or weeks of futile treatment—even if they have living wills."(Cowley & Hager, 1995) According to the physician who directed this study, " . . . the system doesn't know when to stop."

In an effort to sensitize physicians to the needs of dying patients, a Task Force on Quality Care at the End of Life has been set up by the American Medical Association. When aggressive-but-futile treatment is ordered by a physician, other care-givers find themselves in a difficult position as they care for patients whose Advance Medical Directive states that they do not wish to have life-maintenance procedures in their final days. If you accept a position that involves care of dying patients, be sure the policies and customary practices of that institution are compatible with your own philosophy regarding end-of-life care.

GUIDELINES FOR CARE OF A DYING PERSON

These guidelines can be useful as you strive to provide **humane** care consistent with the choices and needs of a dying patient.

- Reassure the patient as needed that you will be there and that you will do all possible to provide comfort. Then keep your word.

- Be aware of the patient's emotion state. Respect the patient's unique way of reacting to the illness and dying.

- Let the patient know that you care. Use touch as appropriate and be with the patient as much as your other duties permit.

- Listen—a patient provides clues to feelings and anxieties.

- Do not force your feelings or your beliefs on the patient.

- Whenever appropriate, allow the patient to express a preference about his or her care.

- Respond to a patient's request for prayer, a religious reading, ritual, or service. Call the hospital chaplain or the patient's spiritual advisor as appropriate.

References and Suggested Readings

Backer, Barbara A., Hannon, Natalie R., & Gregg, Joan Young. *To Listen, to Comfort, to Care.* Albany, NY: Delmar Publishers Inc., 1994. Chapter 2, "Death and the Process of Dying," pp. 13–26; Chapter 5, "Hospice Care and Pain Management," pp. 65–77.

Choice in Dying, *Choices: The Newsletter of Choice in Dying,* Winter, 1996 (5:4). New York, NY: Choice in Dying.

Cowley, Geoffrey & Hager, Mary. "Terminal Care: Too Painful, Too Prolonged," *Newsweek,* December 4, 1995, pp. 74–75.

Duda, Deborah. *Coming Home: A Guide to Home Care for the Terminally Ill.* Santa Fe, NM: John Muir Publications Inc., 1984.

Kubler-Ross, Elisabeth, M.D. *Death: The Final Stage of Growth.* Englewood, NJ: Prentice-Hall, 1975. Chapter 4, Carey, Raymond G. "Living Until Death: A Program of Service and Research for the Terminally Ill," pp. 75–86; Chapter 6, Imara, Mwalinu. "Dying as the Last Stage of Growth," pp. 149–163.

Kubler-Ross, Elisabeth, M.D. *On Death and Dying.* New York, NY: MacMillan, 1969.

Kubler-Ross, Elisabeth, M.D. *To Live Until We Say Good-Bye.* Englewood, NJ: Prentice-Hall, 1978.

Shneidman, Edwin S. *Death: Current Perspectives;* Third Edition. Palo Alto, CA: Mayfield Publishing Co., 1984. Chapter 15, Hinton, John. "Speaking of Death with the Dying," pp. 152–161; Chapter 17, Bok, Sissela. "Lies to the Sick and Dying," pp. 171–186; Chapter 23, Lindemann, Erich. "Reactions to One's Own Fatal Illness," pp. 257–265; Chapter 24, Saunders, Cicely. "St. Christopher's Hospice," pp. 266–271.

Tamparo, Carol D. & Lindh, Wilburta Q. *Therapeutic Communications for Allied Health Professionals.* Albany, NY: Delmar Publishers Inc., 1992.

Viorst, Judith. *Necessary Losses: The Loves, Illusions, Dependencies and Impossible Expectations That All of Us Have to Give Up in Order to Grow.* New York, NY: Simon & Schuster, 1986. Chapter 19, "The ABC of Dying," pp. 305–324.

REVIEW AND SELF CHECK

Complete each statement below, using information from Unit 22.

1. The usual reaction to diagnosis of a fatal illness includes _____ , _____ , _____ , and _____ .

2. Some of the fears commonly expressed by a dying person are _____ , _____ , _____ , _____ , and _____ .

3. The stages of dying, as described by Dr. Kubler-Ross, are:

   1. _____

   2. _____

   3. _____

   4. _____

   5. _____

4. Dr. Kubler-Ross maintains that the dying process can be a growth experience. Such growth requires commitment to:

   1. _____

   2. _____

   3. _____

5. The goal of helping a dying person work through the process is to

_____ and _____ .

6. According to Lindemann, a "healthy" reaction to dying requires

_____ .

7. Conditions that contribute to successful adjustment by a dying person:

1. _____

2. _____

3. _____

4. _____

5. _____

6. _____

7. _____

8. Some personal and family issues related to care of a dying person:

1. _____

2. _____

3. _____

9. Some medical issues related to care of a dying person:

1. _____

2. _____

3. _____

10. Issues related to the rights of patients include _____ ,

_____ , _____ ,

_____ , and _____ .

11. The goals of care for a dying patient are _____ ,

rather than _____ .

12. Providing palliative care requires that the caregiver:

1. _____ .

2. _____ .

3. _____ .

4. _____ .

5. _____ .

13.   Five advantages of dying at home:

1. _____ .

2. _____ .

3. _____ .

4. _____ .

5. _____ .

ASSIGNMENT

1.   Think about your first experience with death. How old were you? Was the deceased an important person to you? If you were a child, what were you told about death? Did you participate in or witness any part of the dying process? Were you involved in any rituals related to the death? Were you encouraged to grieve? Did those closest to the deceased display their grief to you? How was their grief manifested? Did this experience contribute to your fear of death? If it were possible to change that experience, what would you change so that the experience would help you (1) accept the reality of death as a part of life and (2) face your own mortality (that is, your own inevitable death) without fear?

2.   Participate in a class discussion to identify various ways health care providers could try to meet the following needs of a dying person:
   a.   Relative freedom from pain and discomfort.
   b.   Maintenance of independence, insofar as possible.
   c.   Satisfaction of any remaining wishes (things I wish I had done).
   d.   Maintenance of self-esteem when it becomes necessary to yield control to others.
   e.   Achievement of emotional adjustment, acceptance of impending death, and a state of inner peace.

3. In a class discussion, consider the following questions:
   a. How can the rights of a comatose patient be protected?
   b. What are the rights of a dying patient whose organs could be used as transplants for patients in the same hospital?

4. List things you have been wanting to do "some day." If you learned today that you have a terminal illness, which of these would you try to do before you die? Why not set dates and plan to do them?

5. List three people who are very close (either relatives or friends). Beside each name, write out two or more statements that you would want to make if that person were dying. When did you last tell each of these people how important he or she is to you? Plan what you will say to each of these people the next time you are together.

6. Write out a set of guidelines for your next of kin describing the care you wish to receive when you are terminally ill.

Section VII

Trends in Health Care

Health care in the United States is in a state of rapid change. As a health care provider you should be informed about current trends and issues, especially those that may affect roles and relationships of health care personnel.

Large segments of the public are now well-informed about health matters; with increasing knowledge, many people want to participate in health care decisions. Most states now have Living Will laws. By federal law any hospital that receives federal funds (such as Medicare and Medicaid) must inform patients about Living wills and the patient's right to refuse life-sustaining measures under certain conditions. Life-style and stress management are now widely recognized as major factors in both treatment and prevention of illness. And, more people are using alternative (nonmedical) approaches to health care.

Some patients enter the health care system with a passive attitude: "I'm sick. Fix me. You health care providers are supposed to make me well." These patients are not likely to refuse treatments or seek alternative therapies. But there is a new breed of patient who poses a different challenge to health care providers. This type of patient asks questions and expects answers, may refuse an invasive procedure or specific treatment, and may even question whether or not orthodox medicine can help with his or her health problem. Inadequate answers or a judgmental attitude on the part of a health care provider may interfere with establishing rapport or, worse, may alienate the patient. It is essential, then, that health care providers understand and accept those patients who wish to assume more responsibility for their own health and actively participate in decisions about their health care.

Section VII is designed to help you learn about selected trends in health care as a basis for working with this "new breed of patient" with a nonjudgmental attitude; to expand your understanding of holistic health, healing, and the role of stress management in health maintenance; and to provide you with a broad view of therapeutic alternatives, both medical and nonmedical, as a basis for functioning in the health care system of the future.

Unit 23

Health Care through the Ages

OBJECTIVES

Upon completion of this unit, you should be able to:

- Define terms related to health care practices, as used in this unit: allopathic medicine, orthodox, holistic, alternative therapy, psychosomatic, and quackery.
- State two reasons why some innovations in science and medicine are initially rejected or labeled as quackery.
- State one reason empirical data, rather than data obtained by scientific research methods, are often used to justify psychophysiological types of therapy.
- Name one current health care practice that has its roots in each of the following: ancient cultures, Greece and Rome, the early Judeo-Christian period, and China.
- Name five significant scientific or medical advances during the past 400 years that provided the foundation for today's orthodox health care practices.
- Name two beliefs about sickness (or the sick) that were common in early cultures and are still prevalent today.
- Name three modern medical pioneers who laid the foundation for holistic medicine and state the particular health/disease area of concern to each.

KEY TERMS

Androgynous
Empirical
Innovations
Ritual
Complementary therapy

Hermaphroditic
Meridians
Patriarchal
Psychopharmaceuticals

Psychophysiological
Shaman
Variables
Neurotransmitters

DEFINITIONS

Before beginning the historical overview that is the subject of this unit, certain terms used throughout this section should be explained. The literal meaning of allopathic is "utilizing drugs." Orthodox medical practice in the United States relies primarily on both drug therapy and surgery. The term *allopathic medicine* however, is used in the current literature on health care to refer to orthodox medicine as practiced in this country. In this textbook, the terms conventional and orthodox are used interchangeably with *allopathic* to refer to the existing system of medical practice in the United States. *Medical* refers to practices of a licensed medical doctor (M.D.) or osteopath (D.O.); it does not include professional practitioners such as psychologists or chiropractors. The term alternative therapy refers to a variety of therapies that are not currently used in most conventional medical practices. The phrase **"complementary therapy"** is now used by some medical practitioners who are open to nonmedical approaches. The different implications of these two phrases probably explains the preference of the medical community. *Alternative* implies "instead of," whereas *complementary* implies "in addition to" or "as an adjunct to." Because "alternative therapy" is preferred by most nonmedical practitioners, that phrase is used throughout Section VII, but does *not* mean *instead of* medical care. The decision to use an alternative therapy, either as an adjunct to medical care or as a substitute, is made by the patient, not by any alternative practitioner.

An alternative therapy may be provided by someone with a professional level of educational preparation (college degree plus professional training), someone with formal educational training leading to a certificate and/or licensure, or someone who has been trained in a specific therapeutic technique. Holistic refers to health care, medical or nonmedical, that takes into consideration the patient's total being (physical, mental, emotional, spiritual, life context, nutrition, life-style) and uses a variety of therapeutic techniques, *according to the specific needs of each patient.*

INNOVATIONS IN SCIENCE AND HEALTH CARE

The history of science and health care includes numerous examples of innovative ideas that were rejected initially by those in power at the time. Many of these innovative approaches had merit and were eventually accepted by orthodox medicine. Some innovations were premature—they required changes the culture was not yet ready to accept. **Innovations** usually conflict with existing beliefs and are usually perceived as a threat by current practitioners. Many scientists who proposed new ideas or new methods have been subjected to criticism, ridiculed, or even persecuted. Yet some of those innovators who suffered persecution are now recognized as heroes of medicine or a particular field of science.

The Scientific Model

Today, the scientific model is considered by the scientific community to be *the method* for proving the effectiveness of a specific technique, drug, or procedure. Alternative procedures are criticized by members of the scientific community because they have not been "proven effective" by the scientific method. Yet, many current medical practices have never been subjected to rigorous scientific research. At present a double standard exists, in which alternative practices are rejected or viewed with suspicion by members of the scientific community because of a lack of rigorous research, but certain long-standing medical practices that have never been subjected to such research are accepted without question.

The scientific model requires an approach in which the experimental treatment is administered to certain subjects (the experimental group), while an ineffective treatment is administered to other subjects (the control group); sometimes, there is a third group that receives no treatment. The experiment is called a "double blind study" if neither patients nor care-givers know which subjects are in the experimental group and which are in the control group. A blind study prevents patients' and care-givers' expectations from influencing the outcomes of an experiment.

Studies on the effects of drug therapy have shown that the expectations of those conducting an experiment influence the results. For example, the health care provider who knows that a patient is being given the experimental drug expects it to help the patient. This expectation can affect the patient's response to the drug. The factors that may influence the outcome of an experiment are known as **"variables."**

The scientific model requires that only one or two variables be manipulated, while all other influences are carefully controlled. After treatment, the experimental subjects (those receiving a specific treatment) are compared with subjects in the control group (those who did not receive the treatment). A treatment is considered effective only if there are significant differences between the treatment group and the control group. Research findings are considered valid (i.e., proven correct) only if other researchers can repeat the experiment and get the same results.

It is relatively easy to measure and record the effects of a precise amount of a drug on blood pressure. It is more difficult to measure an emotion such as fear and prove that minimizing a preoperative patient's anxiety results in faster postoperative recovery. It is impossible to see or measure a patient's "will to live." Yet emotions, belief systems, and factors such as intention (to get well or to escape one's present life situation by dying) are known to be powerful influences on the course of illness. Health care providers often see two patients who have the same diagnosis and are receiving the same treatment. One recovers, but the other declines and dies. The big question: What made a difference in the outcome of these two patients? These "difficult to measure" variables are ignored by researchers who are committed to the scientific model—i.e., precise measurement (quantitative data) of the effects of the specific variable being studied. Some members of the scientific/medical/healing community who are open to alternative approaches are now designing studies that adapt the scientific method to the study of intuitive diagnosis and influences on healing, such as prayer and healing touch. No one, however, has devised a method for measuring such powerful factors as the will to live, expectation, or intention.

Empirical Evidence

Empirical refers to experience and observation; *empirical data* are observations collected without the rigorous design of the scientific method. Many alternative therapies involve counseling, meditation, full body massage (also known as "body work") and other procedures that affect the emotional state, tension level, and perhaps even the beliefs of the patient. Practitioners who use various nonmedical therapies have accumulated a large body of empirical data, but their methods are criticized by members of the scientific community who demand "hard evidence" (numeral data obtained through research procedures that fit the scientific model). In spite of the difficulties, researchers are now making progress in designing such experiments.

Meanwhile, more and more physicians, seeking better results for their patients, are sufficiently impressed by the empirical data to include certain nonmedical techniques into their practice. Yet most physicians continue to practice allopathic medicine without an awareness of or interest in the potential value of alternative therapies. (The preceding statement is not intended as a criticism, but rather as a description of "what is.") Some physicians view any therapists other than medical doctors as quacks. Thus, allopathic medicine and holistic medicine represent *two very different belief systems*, which have a profound effect on each practitioner's approach to patient care.

Dilemma of the Health Care Provider

A health care delivery system in the process of significant change presents something of a dilemma for members of the health care team. What is the appropriate response for you, a health care provider, to a patient who is using an alternative therapy as a complement to medical treatment? Should you warn the patient about quackery? Should you tell the physician that the patient is not complying with the medical regimen prescribed? Does compliance mean that the patient must follow the medical protocol and forgo any other type of therapy? These questions are less relevant to the average hospitalized patient than to a patient with a chronic health problem, long-term illness or life-threatening disease. The probability of your caring for such a patient depends on your role, the particular health care setting in which you perform your role, and the extent to which you interact with each patient. It is hoped that Section VII will prepare you to handle such situations if and when they arise during your career as a health care provider.

The remainder of Unit 23 describes the historical roots of many current practices. This historical overview also reveals that a holistic approach to health care is not really new, and some therapies considered to be "alternative" in the United States have been a part of medical practice in other countries for many years.

HEALERS IN EARLY CIVILIZATIONS

In early cultures, illness was thought to be the result of supernatural forces: demons, evil spirits, or anger of the gods. The priest or **shaman** performed a **ritual** to drive evil spirits from the patient's body or to appease the angry gods so that healing would be allowed. These rituals might involve the patient, members of the family, or even the entire tribe. In addition to performing various rituals, the shaman might also use natural materials such as smoke, water, leaves, berries, bark, roots, and minerals to heal the victim.

Today there is renewed interest in shamanism, particularly the role of the shaman in Native American culture. Workshops are held to teach these natural (i.e., based in nature) healing methods. In certain Native American tribes, medicine men and medicine women are teaching younger members the healing practices of their ancestors in the hope that these ancient practices will not be lost forever.

The role of shaman requires many years' apprenticeship to a practicing shaman. The trainee must learn the healing properties of natural elements, plants, and animal products and must also become sensitive to human behavior and cultural influences on health. The shaman treats each patient with full awareness of the patient's life-style and the context within which the patient's symptoms developed—a form of holistic therapy without technology!

Ancient Cultures

Over thousands of years the healing practices of each culture were handed down from one generation to the next. The role of healer was highly respected;

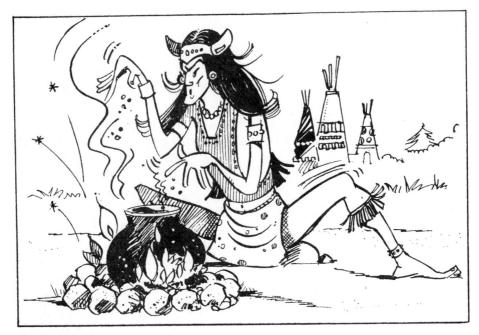

The role of the medicine man, or shaman, was an important role in many cultures.

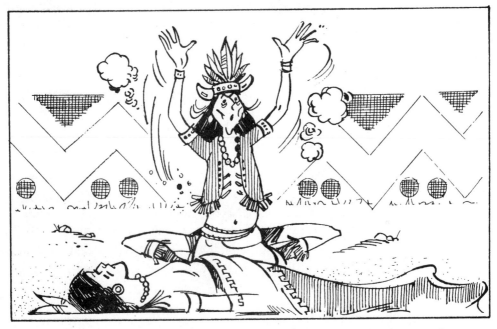

A shaman uses a variety of healing techniques, including healing rituals.

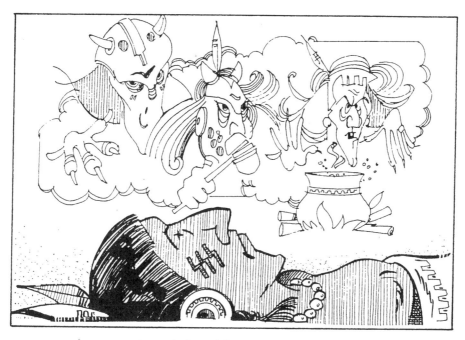

Primitive cultures believed that angry spirits cause illness.

possession of the secrets of healing conveyed power second only to the power of the ruler. In ancient civilizations, healers were primarily women and religions were centered around worship of the goddess. Large temples erected to various goddesses served as centers of healing, as well as centers of worship. The priestesses performed religious services and were also guardians of healing secrets. Dr. Jeanne Achterberg states in *Woman as Healer*:

> *Women have always been healers. Cultural myths from around the world describe a time when only women knew the secrets of life and death, and therefore they alone could practice the magical art of healing.*

Dr. Achterberg notes that women have been free to practice healing only when the reigning deity has been feminine, **hermaphroditic** (having reproductive organs of both sexes), or **androgynous** (having both male and female characteristics). Sometimes during the second millennium before the birth of Christ, the Great Goddess, whose power was believed to be derived from Earth, was replaced by a male deity, the god who reigned from above. Thereafter, the goddess religions were condemned as pagan; they either disappeared or went underground to continue their practices in secret. This shift in beliefs about the nature of god was accompanied by a shift in beliefs about healing and healers. The role of healer was a power role. With the growth of **patriarchal** religions, power shifted to the father/male figure, and the right to heal was claimed by male figures—priests, shamans, witch doctors.

Greece and Rome

Although early Greek mythology attributed illness to supernatural causes, it was the Greeks who eventually separated healing from religion and the role of physician from that of priest. Hippocrates, a Greek physician who lived during the period 460–377 B.C., is known as "the Father of modern medicine." Hippocrates insisted upon careful observation and the collection of factual information, thereby establishing a systematic approach to diagnosis of illness. His treatments included diet, fresh air and sunshine, and healthful personal habits and living conditions—what we today refer to as "a healthful lifestyle." Hippocrates demonstrated that illness results from natural causes, rather than evil spirits or the anger of the gods. This established medicine as the healing profession. Thereafter religion was the domain of priests, and care of the sick was the domain of physicians. Hippocrates also emphasized a code of behavior for physicians—the beginnings of medical ethics. The Hippocratic Oath is still used by many medical schools as part of the graduation exercise for medical students.

Early Judeo-Christian Period

Jews and early Christians believed in a divine cause for illness and divine intervention as the basis for healing. The Greeks and Romans, with their many gods, could attribute illness to the wrath of one god and healing to the kindness of another god. Jews and Christians, however, believed in one God. This raised an important question: How could the same god who causes illness also heal the sick? This dilemma was resolved by associating illness with sin. If a person became sick, then certainly that person had sinned and was being punished. These beliefs are reflected in some religions today. A current example is the view of some people that Acquired Immune Deficiency Syndrome (AIDS) is divine punishment for homosexuality, sexual promiscuity, or drug abuse.

Biblical References to Healing

Although the Bible does not describe a specific system of health care, there are many references to healing. The healing might be a ritual to cleanse the person of sin, or it might involve touch—the "laying on of hands." Were these biblical healings due to faith? purification (of sin)? or divine intervention? Did the healers of biblical times utilize some form of energy to bring about instantaneous healing?

Today, a number of healing techniques are based on influencing the flow of energy through the body. There are healers whose ability to heal, either by touch ("laying on of hands") or by "sending energy" has been thoroughly documented. A scientific organization, The International Society for the Study of Subtle Energies and Energy Medicine (ISSSEEM), has recently been established to set up research projects and seek scientific explanations. It is intriguing that early civilizations may have used energy transfer for healing, and that we are now trying to relearn (or to prove by means of the scientific method) what healers of biblical times and earlier civilizations knew and accepted as natural.

CHINESE MEDICINE

The practice of medicine in China is characterized by the use of herbs and acupuncture, a technique that has been practiced by the Chinese for at least 5,000 years. Acupuncture is based on the theory that life energy, known as Ch'i, flows through channels located throughout the body. Twelve major channels, known as **meridians,** are associated with specific internal organs. There are numerous branches and connections, so that the cells in every portion of the body receive this flow of energy. Any blockage in the flow of energy results in disease until such blockage is removed or clears up spontaneously. Each meridian has its own pulse, which is different from the arterial pulses of the circulatory system. The acupuncturist uses these twelve pulses to locate any blockage in energy flow. The location of the blockage determines what organ or body part is affected.

Modern researchers are now using sensitive electronic equipment to trace these energy pathways and locate the points of energy concentration, thus using scientific methodology to validate the underlying theory of acupuncture. Such research is a major focus of "energy medicine," an emerging specialty in medicine. The energy pathways and significant points located throughout the body provide the basis for a number of alternative therapies, such as Shiatsu, Touch for Health, Acupressure, Trigger Point Therapy, and Reflexology, some of which are discussed in Unit 26.

Acupuncture was relatively unknown in the United States until 1971, when an American surgeon reported to the American Medical Association his observations of acupuncture in China. At about the same time, an American journalist who was traveling in China developed appendicitis. His postoperative pain was controlled by acupuncture, rather than by drugs. His report of this experience, published in the *New York Times,* brought acupuncture to the attention of the American public. Although acupuncture had been an established medical specialty in France for about twenty-five years, the initial reaction of the medical community in the United States was unfavorable. In spite of that

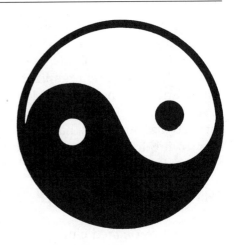

Chinese medicine and philosophy emphasize
unity and harmony among parts of the whole.

initial rejection of acupuncture, there has been growing acceptance by the general public and by some members of the medical community. Over the past twenty years the number of licensed acupuncturists has steadily increased. Needless to say, the pharmaceutical industry is particularly threatened by a drugless approach to pain management.

EVOLUTION OF MODERN HEALTH CARE

The Middle Ages, also known as the Dark Ages, lasted over a thousand years, from the fall of the Roman Empire to the Renaissance. Throughout this period, epidemics and plagues recurred, especially in crowded cities. But there was no organized health care system as we know it. Many monasteries had gardens in which various therapeutic herbs were cultivated; the monks performed simple healing procedures. In communities far from a monastery, an older man (the village "wise man") or woman (the village "crone" or "wise woman") served as healer for the community. Perhaps these healers possessed natural healing abilities. It is likely that they possessed secrets of healing that had been passed down from one generation to the next. Eventually, the influence of the wise man or the crone was perceived as a threat to the power of the local priest. A healer who was especially successful might be condemned as a heretic or witch. Many were tortured, then hanged or burned at the stake. Persecution of any healers who were neither priest nor physician continued up to the 1800s. Once a system of medicine had become established, natural healers were condemned as charlatans or quacks.

The Renaissance (French, meaning "rebirth") followed the Dark Ages and lasted about 400 years. There was renewed interest in science, art, music, and literature and less emphasis on religion. This was a period of discoveries, new insights and theories, many of which provided the foundation for the scientific methods of research that are an integral part of modern medical research.

Development in the Sciences

During the 1500s, Vesalius studied the human body and made accurate anatomical drawings. Existing beliefs about human anatomy were based on dissection of animals, since it was illegal to dissect a human body. In order to obtain cadavers for his anatomical studies, Vesalius removed bodies from the gallows at night. As a result of these secret studies of human anatomy, Vesalius corrected many misconceptions about the structure of the human body. Vesalius was ridiculed by his colleagues for proposing that their beliefs about human anatomy were erroneous, but today he is credited with establishing anatomy as a science. His book of anatomical drawings is a classic and reprints are available even today.

Just as dissection of human bodies was necessary to identify internal structures, the development of the microscope was a necessary prelude to the discovery of bacteria, the study of cell and tissue structure, and the identification of chromosomes and genes—the basis for modern genetic research. Zacharias Janssen is thought to have invented the compound microscope around 1590. But it would be over two hundred years before refinements in lens-making made it possible to magnify objects without distortion. Meanwhile, Anton Van Leeuwenhoek (1632–1723) used a simple microscope to study a wide variety of subjects, including various body fluids. As an amateur scientist, Leeuwenhoek systematically recorded his observations and made detailed drawings. His work provided the foundation for the science of microbiology, even though he was widely criticized when he first published his observations.

The Germ Theory and Antisepsis

It was not until the 19th century, less than two hundred years ago, that handwashing was proposed as a means of preventing infections. A Hungarian physician, Ignaz Philipp Semmelweiss (1818–1865) noticed that women who were assisted in childbirth by doctors who had just come from the autopsy room invariably developed "childbed fever." He proposed that doctors should wash their hands after completing an autopsy, to protect their patients. For making this suggestion, Semmelweis was persecuted by his colleagues to the point that he eventually had a nervous breakdown.

Ironically, in the year of Semmelweis' death, Joseph Lister introduced antisepsis to the practice of surgery. This was a *major event* in the history of medicine, the beginning of surgical asepsis. Dr. Lister was such a renowned surgeon that his innovation was accepted, and he did not experience rejection and persecution by unconverted colleagues. Lister's use of antisepsis introduced control of infection as an integral part of medical practice. It is noteworthy that Lister's introduction of antisepsis preceded any proof of the existence of microorganisms. Two other scientists, working separately, were to provide proof that microorganisms are present on hands and all objects, thus providing the scientific basis for both handwashing and medical asepsis.

Robert Koch (1843–1910), a German scientist, was responsible for a scientific breakthrough that we now know as the Germ Theory. Through his study of microorganisms, Koch determined the specific cause of several infectious disease, including tuberculosis. He also established the rules for proving that a specific organism was the cause of a particular infection; this provided the foundation for the field we know today as bacteriology. Development of the germ theory was a major event that established the scientific basis for asepsis, immunization, and modern sanitation.

Many scientists had observed microorganisms under a microscope, but it was Louis Pasteur who established that those tiny objects were living things that reproduced themselves. He demonstrated that wine could be preserved by destroying the microorganisms present. The process he used is known as "pasteurization" and is still used today to ensure that milk and various other foods are safe.

Later, Pasteur developed a vaccine to prevent rabies in people who had been bitten by a rabid animal, thus sparing them a horrible death. Pasteur's contributions are numerous, yet he, too, was subjected to ridicule by his colleagues, even though he was a highly respected scientist. His contributions were recognized prior to his death, however. The Pasteur Institute, founded in 1888 in his honor by the French government, continues to conduct research on the causes, treatment, and prevention of disease.

Prevention of Infectious Diseases

The work of Koch and Pasteur led to the development of vaccines to protect people against certain diseases, especially the group of infections known as the "childhood diseases." But three of the most devastating diseases are caused by viruses, rather than bacteria: smallpox, poliomyelitis, and, currently, AIDS.

In 1796, an English physician by the name of Edward Jenner developed a method of protecting people from smallpox, a serious disease with a high mortality rate. Smallpox victims were seriously ill for two to three weeks. Those who survived had numerous small scars, known as pockmarks. Widespread use of smallpox vaccine eliminated the disease in Europe and North America by 1950, but epidemics killed thousands of victims in other parts of the world. Between 1950 and 1970, intensive world-wide efforts to vaccinate the total population of any country where smallpox occurred resulted in eradication of this disease.

Up until the present outbreak of AIDS, the viral scourge of the 20th century was poliomyelitis, also called "infantile paralysis" because children were very susceptible and many were left with permanent paralysis. During the 1940s and 1950s, polio epidemics occurred with increasing frequency, especially during the spring and summer months. The mortality rate was high; many survivors were handicapped by paralysis. In 1953 Dr. Jonas Salk's vaccine became available. The Salk vaccine was widely administered and is now required in some states for admission to the public schools. Polio has not been completely eradicated, as has smallpox, but cases are relatively rare now.

Jenner and Salk made it possible to protect entire populations against two serious viral infections. As a result of immunization procedures and improved sanitation, infectious diseases are no longer the major health problem they once were. But the modern scourge, AIDS, is not yet under control. It remains for one of today's scientists to find a vaccine to protect against this virus that is so destructive to the immune system.

The Discovery of Radiation

Two physicists in France, Pierre and Marie Curie, laid the foundation for radiation therapies. Together they studied radioactive substances and identified two previously unknown elements: radium and polonium. After her husband's death, Marie Curie discovered that nearby radium had created an image of a key on a piece of film. This discovery revealed what is now basic knowledge—namely, that radioactive materials give off invisible rays that affect nearby substances.

Marie Curie and her daughter, Irene, then only seventeen years old, took a portable X-ray machine to the front lines during World War I to make X rays available to doctors treating wounded soldiers. After the war, Irene did research on radioactive substances with her husband and her mother for many years. The dangers of radioactivity were not recognized at that time; both Marie Curie and Irene died of leukemia. The contributions of the Curies are basic to various diagnostic and therapeutic procedures in current medical use.

Concurrently with the work of the Curies in France, a German physicist by the name of Wilhelm Konrad Roentgen accidentally discovered X rays. After conducting some experiments that involved passing an electric current through a special type of glass tubing, Roentgen noticed that some nearby photographic plates had become fogged. His investigation of the cause led to further experiments that resulted in the identification of invisible rays that could pass through soft tissues, but not through bone or metal. This discovery revolutionized diagnostic practices in medicine. Again, the dangers of radiation and X rays were not known in the beginning. Many radiologists died of leukemia before it was recognized that health care providers must have adequate protection when they are working around any type of radiation.

The Beginnings of Psychiatry and Psychosomatic Medicine

The pioneers discussed above all contributed to medicine as it pertains to physical health. Psychiatry, the medical specialty concerned with mental illness, began with the work of Sigmund Freud, an Austrian physician who first recognized the power of subconscious memories to affect health. Freud developed psychoanalysis, a technique for helping patients explore the unconscious part of the mind. Although many of Freud's theories are not accepted by modern practitioners, his writings and those of his students provided the foundation for psychotherapy. He was truly a pioneer, daring to explore territory that had never before been explored by physicians. Freud made the mind and emotions a concern of medicine, which had previously limited its focus to the physical body.

Now there is a merging of physical medicine and psychiatry, as the powerful influence of mind and emotions on the physical body are being acknowledged. Psychosomatic medicine is a medical specialty concerned with physical disorders that have a mental or emotional component. Although the term "psychosomatic" (psycho—mind; soma—body) is still in common use, it is slowly being replaced by the term **"psychophysiological"** (psycho—mind; physiology—body functions).

Brain Chemistry

The division between physical illness and mental illness has been clouded further by the discovery of a biochemical factor in several "mental" illnesses, especially depression, manic depressive illness, and schizophrenia. Several chemicals, known as **neurotransmitters,** are produced by certain cells within the brain. These chemicals affect mental alertness, memory, ability to concentrate, thought processes, judgment, mood, sleep patterns, sexual behavior, irritability, energy, and other factors that influence behavior and ability to perform one's daily activities. An increase or decrease in certain neurotransmitters may have a profound effect on behavior. The discovery of differences in certain neurotransmitter levels of psychiatric patients versus "normal" individuals has led to the development of a new class of drugs. These **psychopharmaceuticals** influence either the production of a specific neurotransmitter or its transmission from one cell to another. The availability of psychopharmaceutical drugs has had a radical effect on the psychiatric field. The majority of psychiatrists have abandoned "talk therapy" and limit their practice to diagnostic evaluations and prescription of one or more psychopharmaceutical drugs to manage a patient's symptoms.

Psychologists, clinical social workers, and counselors now provide most of the psychotherapy, often in conjunction with a psychiatrist who prescribes the psychopharmaceutical drugs. Individual therapy is often combined with group therapy sessions, which seem to be especially beneficial for those patients who need the interaction and support that group sessions can provide.

The Genetic Factor

The line between "physical" and "mental" illness has also been eroded by sociological studies and gene research that demonstrate a genetic tendency toward certain "mental" illnesses. These findings give weight to the hereditary aspect. At the individual level, biorhythms, exposure to light, sleep patterns, REM (rapid eye movement) sleep and dreams have been found to differ from "normal" in psychiatric patients. One relatively common problem, Seasonal Affective Disorder (SAD) occurs during the winter months, when daylight hours are decreased and cloudy days occur frequently. This disorder is a depressive state precipitated by the seasonal decrease in light. Victims of SAD tend to become depressed in the late fall, then improve as winter draws to an end and spring approaches. These individual patterns and environmental factors further cloud the question of what is a physical illness and what is a mental illness.

Multiple Causation

The discussion above indicates the fallacy of the "mental illness stigma," still quite pervasive in American society. That bias is no more justified than a bias against diabetes, a disorder involving faulty sugar metabolism. But diabetes, hypertension, autoimmune disorders, and many other "physical" illnesses are now considered to have an emotional and/or stress-related component. Even the infectious diseases, once blamed on the causative bacteria or virus, are now viewed in terms of numerous factors that impact an individual's immune system.

With increasing evidence of multiple causation of disease, the allopathic approach to treatment of symptoms is being replaced by emphasis on removal or treatment of *causes*. The search for causes leads naturally to a holistic approach to the care of each patient as an individual with a particular life style, stressors related to occupation and family dynamics, and behavior patterns developed over a lifetime. Any of these could be contributing to the current health problem.

A new breed of physician-pioneer is emerging, calling for treatment of *causes* of illness, rather than management of symptoms. These practitioners focus on the total patient. They insist that treatment must include the mental, emotional, and spiritual aspects of the person, as well as the physical aspects—a *holistic* approach to health care. This approach presents a special challenge. Holistic medicine requires taking time to identify and deal with causes, rather than treating symptoms only. A holistic approach requires taking a detailed history—both family and individual—and conducting a lifestyle inventory.

Genetic clues to the patient's illness may be found in the family history. Individual clues may be found in the individual's own history, such as abuse or neglect on the part of the primary caregiver, or the existence during childhood of Attention Deficit/Hyperactive Disorder, now considered to be a precursor of Bipolar Disorder (manic depressive illness). A description of the patient's home life and work situation may yield clues to whether or not stress is a contributing factor. The lifestyle inventory may reveal additional symptoms, such as sleep disturbances, and may also provide clues to the causation puzzle. Such a detailed study of the patient's individual situation is time-consuming. Obviously, a complete study would also include the technological approaches used in allopathic medicine, but only as needed to provide essential information for establishing a clinical diagnosis.

Treatment of the patient in a holistic setting can begin even before a final diagnosis has been established. If stress is obviously a causative factor, the patient can be taught stress-management techniques. If emotional factors are revealed, appropriate therapy for constructive use of emotions can be planned. Assertiveness training can be recommended to help a patient learn to cope with life problems more effectively. If faulty dietary habits are revealed, instruction in healthful eating may be given. Thus, each possible causative factor is dealt with in order to *heal the total patient*. Holistic health care utilizes the skills of many different therapists; it includes the techniques of allopathic medicine as appropriate, but extends the role of the physician into areas beyond orthodox medical practice.

MODERN PIONEERS IN MEDICINE

Increasingly, the powerful influence of emotions and stress on health is being recognized. The onset of diseases such as cancer is now considered to be most likely to occur when the immune system is depressed. It is well-known that disorders such as ulcers and high blood pressure have an emotional component. Now it appears that the emotional component may be the result of long-term stress. The remainder of this unit focuses on several practitioners who acknowledge the roles of stress and emotional factors in the onset and course of illness. Their innovations and searches for more effective treatment may someday be viewed as another giant step in health care.

Innovation in Cancer Therapy

Dr. O. Carl Simonton is an oncologist who noted that the cancer patients who met with him regularly for group counseling seemed to "hold their own" better than cancer patients who did not participate in the group sessions. Some members of the group actually improved. In 1976 the Institute of Noetic Sciences sponsored a project in which Dr. Simonton and his wife Stephanie (a counselor) provided psychological counseling to cancer patients who had been labeled "terminal" by their own physician. Only patients who had received orthodox medical therapies for their cancer were accepted into the project. In addition to participating in counseling sessions, each patient was encouraged to write three sets of objectives, one set for three months in the future, one set for six months, and one set for 12 months. Each set of objectives had three components.

1. Meditate for 20 minutes at least twice a day

2. Exercise for 20 minutes five days each week

3. Have one hour of play per day, seven days per week

Play time could not be accumulated; if a patient played two hours on Saturday, there still must be an hour of play on Sunday. Time spent watching television could not be counted as play time. Patients had to specify their play activities in writing. In regard to exercise, the patient would choose something he or she was capable of doing safely. One patient might be able to walk a mile. Another, confined to bed, might be limited to flexing and extending the fingers and arms periodically. Obviously, Dr. Simonton helped his patients *program themselves for living,* as opposed to programming themselves (or allowing others to program them) for dying.

Long-term follow-up of these patients indicated that about one-third lived longer than expected, some experienced complete recovery, and those who did not survive experienced a higher quality of life up until the time of death. "Higher quality" means less pain, increased activity, slower decline, and increased participation in family and community life, as opposed to lying in bed helpless and in pain for weeks prior to dying. According to Dr. Simonton, the patients who improved the most were those who were willing to get in touch with any negative aspects of their lives during the counseling sessions.

The Simonton's believed that their approach had a positive effect on the patient's "will to live."

> *. . . we are unaware of any systematic, widely-accepted approach developed specifically to deal with the fear and the emotional needs of the patient with cancer.*

Publication of the results of this therapeutic approach met with skepticism and criticism from the medical community. Does this rejection of an innovative treatment sound familiar? Some of the historical figures discussed earlier did not live to see their innovations accepted into common practice. The Simontons are more fortunate. Their approach emphasizing psychological factors was premature. Medicine was not yet ready to give up the notion that cancer is a *physical* disease or to accept the powerful influence of mind and emotions on physiological processes. But within ten years numerous physicians had accepted the Simonton's approach and were incorporating purposeful, regular counseling into the treatment protocol for cancer patients.

Innovations in Pain Management

Dr. C. Norman Shealy is a neurosurgeon who practiced the conventional methods of his specialty until he became aware that many of his patients gained only temporary relief of symptoms, even from extensive surgical procedures that were supposed to correct the problem. Dissatisfied with these results, and especially concerned about the number of neurosurgical and orthopedic patients with chronic pain, Dr. Shealy searched for more effective methods. Collaborating with a young electrical engineer, he spent two years designing a low-voltage electrical unit that could short-circuit pain by preventing the pain sensation from traveling up the spinal cord to the brain. This research led to a device now known as the Transcutaneous Nerve Stimulator (TNS unit). It is widely used for control of acute temporary pain and also for long-term, chronic pain. When this technique was first developed, it was an example of "alternative medicine." Because Dr. Shealy was able to demonstrate the effectiveness of both devices to the satisfaction of other neurosurgeons, this example of "alternative medicine" quickly assumed a place within conventional medical practice. Dr. Shealy, the first physician to specialize in management of pain, coined the term "dolorologist" for this new medical specialty. (*Dolor* is the Latin word for "pain.")

Later Dr. Shealy introduced the use of microsurgery for intracranial surgical procedures, thus eliminating the need to remove part of the patient's skull to access the brain. He trained many other surgeons in the use of this technique, thereby making another important contribution to conventional medicine. But his search for better results—control of pain, correction of causes, improvement in a patient's well-being—led him to explore other alternatives to conventional medicine. He now advises patients with chronic pain to meditate. Through meditation and identification of unresolved emotions, many of his pain patients gain control over their pain. Some are able to discontinue their long-term use of pain medication.

Innovations in Diagnosis and Therapy

Dr. Shealy's search for answers led him to study psychic healers such as Olga Worrall, whose healing ministry in Baltimore resulted in hundreds of documented cures, and Henry Rucker of the Psychic Research Foundation in Chicago. Dr. Shealy's research skills enabled him to design scientifically sound projects to study the performance of these psychics. These studies of healers led him to conclude that there is some type of energy transfer from healer to healee. The patient's body then utilizes that energy for healing. Dr. Shealy's

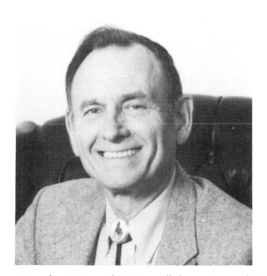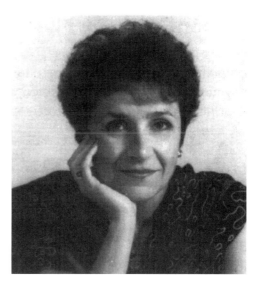

Carolyn Myss, Ph.D. in collaboration with C. Norman Shealy, M.D., has demonstrated the ability to diagnose disease intuitively with 93% accuracy. (Courtesy of C. Norman Shealy, M.D., founder, Shealy Institute for Comprehensive Health Care, Springfield, MO 65803 and Carolyn Myss, Ph.D.)

research with the Rev. Henry Rucker and seven of his associates, none of whom had medical training, showed a high level of accuracy in making an "intuitive diagnosis." These eight psychics were allowed to see, but not speak to, seventeen patients for whom a medical diagnosis had already been established. The psychics each wrote their impressions on separate sheets of paper and gave them to Dr. Shealy. All eight gave a correct diagnosis on eleven patients; at least two presented a correct diagnosis on each of the other six patients. As a result of this high level of accuracy, Dr. Shealy has continued to explore the potential of gifted "intuitives" to assist in diagnosis. (**Note:** Dr. Shealy selected the psychics to participate in this experiment according to strict criteria. He now uses the term "intuitive" rather than "psychic." Since psychic phenomena have recently caught the public interest and become something of a fad, many people claim to have psychic powers for the purpose of making money. Genuine psychics consider their special abilities to be a gift and use this gift very selectively to help others.)

Since 1985, Dr. Shealy has studied the ability of Carolyn Myss to make an intuitive diagnosis. Dr. Myss is a journalist who holds advanced degrees in Religious Studies, with specialization in the Psychological Dimensions of Spirituality. She has spent many years consciously developing her intuitive abilities, with a special focus on medical diagnosis. The research based on the collaboration of Dr. Shealy and Dr. Myss indicates that intuitive diagnosis can be a valuable aid to a physician. The tools of medicine provide essential data for the diagnosis, and the intuitive's contribution provides additional data for completing the "big picture" of the patient's problem. When physical, emotional, mental, and spiritual factors in a patient's illness have been clarified, a treatment plan for "healing the whole person" may be developed.

Dr. Shealy believes that physicians who are especially successful in diagnosis are, either consciously or unconsciously, using intuition in addition to their clinical skills. Dr. Myss believes "the skill of intuition is a natural attribute of the human spirit that can be developed and disciplined to benefit one's life." Perhaps eventually educational programs for all health care providers will include instruction in developing one's intuitive skills to enhance the effectiveness of patient care!

Another physician who has applied the scientific method to the study of "difficult to measure" variables is Dr. Larry Dossey. Many people believe that the power of prayer has a direct effect upon healing, and some can offer anecdotal evidence as "proof." The scientific community, however, does not accept anecdotal evidence. Dr. Dossey's interest in identifying various influences on the course of an illness has led him to explore alternative healing. Influenced by his scientific training, he used research methodology to study the effectiveness of prayer under a variety of conditions. His conclusions: prayer can and does have a measurable effect, regardless of whether or not a patient knows that prayers are being offered on his or her behalf.

Dr. Dossey successfully demonstrated that the scientific method can be adapted to the study of some nonmedical healing variables. By becoming Executive Editor of *Alternative Therapies in Health and Medicine,* he has assumed a leadership role in the scientific study of various healing modalities. The mission of this new professional journal is to provide a forum for the sharing of information on the use of alternative therapies. There is emphasis on "disciplined inquiry methods, including high-quality scientific research. The journal encourages the integration of alternative therapies with conventional medical practices in a way that provides for a rational, individualized, comprehensive approach to health care." (Alternative Therapies, July 1996) It is likely that this publication, with its involvement of nationally recognized authorities from a variety of disciplines, will accelerate the incorporation of some alternative therapies into conventional medical practice.

Innovation in the Management of Hypertension

Dr. Herbert Benson, a professor at the Harvard Medical School, became concerned about increasing evidence that heart attacks, strokes, and hypertension are occurring in men approximately thirteen years earlier than in their fathers. Believing the stress of modern life to exact a high price, both psychologically and physiologically, he studied approaches to stress management outside conventional medicine's use of tranquilizers and/or sedatives. Drugs can be effec-

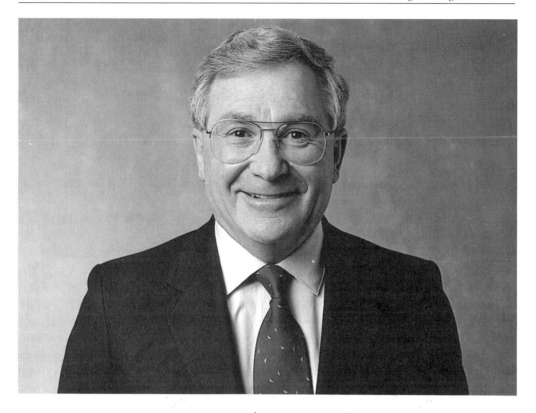

Dr. Herbert Benson

tive in controlling some symptoms related to stress. But drugs do not eliminate *sources* of stress, reverse the physiological effects of prolonged stress, or correct an underlying psychological problem.

Harvard research studies have shown that control of involuntary body processes, such as blood pressure, heart rate, and flow of blood to a specific part of the body, may be learned through the use of biofeedback. After reviewing research related to conscious control of body functions, Dr. Benson raised the question, "Can we influence our own physiological reaction to stress through individually controlled mental practices?"

Biofeedback requires many practice sessions using sophisticated equipment. Accordingly, Dr. Benson began his search for a practical, *easily learned* means of physiological control. He found that people who used Transcendental Meditation experienced certain body changes within a few minutes after achieving the meditative state. These changes were different from the physiological changes that occur during sleep and hypnosis. Eventually, Dr. Benson and his research team were able to demonstrate that hypertensive patients could lower their blood pressure by using a simple meditative technique twice a day. Many patients were able to discontinue their blood pressure medication and maintain a normal blood pressure simply by incorporating meditation into their daily routines. The choice for hypertensive patients became, "Meditation or medication?"

Concurrently, these three modern medical pioneers—all seeking more effective therapy for their patients—arrived at the conclusion that meditation, practiced at least twice a day for twenty minutes, has therapeutic effects. Dr. Simonton found that this simple practice benefitted cancer patients, even those considered to be terminal by their own physicians. Dr. Shealy found that meditation could be used to manage pain, especially chronic, long-term pain. And Dr. Benson demonstrated that meditation enabled many hypertensive patients to control their blood pressure. Each of these physicians used an alternative practice to enhance the therapeutic benefits of conventional medicine for their patients. Their findings are widely accepted now; in fact, many health care agencies now offer wellness programs that include meditation instruction.

These innovators are influencing the practices of some physicians and the breadth of services offered within some health care agencies. The effect on the roles of various health care providers remains to be seen, however. Ultimately, each health care provider's open-mindedness and willingness to change will determine whether or not he or she can adapt successfully to the role changes required by a holistic approach to health care. Many of these new ideas, some of which are explored in greater detail in the following units, have the potential to enhance each health care provider's performance in patient care, enrich personal and family life, and improve mental, physical, emotional, and spiritual health.

CHARACTERISTICS OF TODAY'S HEALTH CARE SYSTEM

You are preparing to assume an important role in today's healthy care system. But that system couldn't exist were it not for the many significant contributions of scientists, physicians, and others throughout history. Some of those contributions were initially rejected and their proponents ridiculed. Today, health care innovations and new theories, or new viewpoints regarding accepted theories, are appearing frequently. Some are rejected by orthodox medicine as quackery or, at best, "not scientifically proven." Some are tried by the more open-minded members of the orthodox medical establishment and, upon proving to be clinically effective, are incorporated into an established medical practice.

Physicians tend to be judge and jury regarding innovations and trends in health care. But what is the appropriate attitude toward such innovations for you in your role as a health care provider? What is an appropriate attitude if an innovative therapy is provided by nonmedical personnel (i.e., someone whose practice is not under the immediate direction of a medical doctor)? Eventually you will need to deal with these questions.

Technological Advances

Today's health care system is a dynamic (i.e., every-changing) system. Many current innovations are technological—new, sophisticated equipment for laboratory tests, new techniques for identifying and mapping physical changes occurring in the patient's body, modifications in therapeutic devices, complex machines for maintaining various vital functions. These technological innovations tend to be readily accepted into the existing system, though the high cost of some equipment may limit its use to large facilities. Some technological innovations require additional training for health care providers. The expanded role or time-saving features of some innovations results in ready acceptance. This is especially true of equipment and techniques that contribute to diagnosis.

Emerging Therapies and Roles

Other innovations—primarily therapeutic approaches—are less readily accepted. Rejection by medical personnel often is based on the fact that a particular technique is performed by someone who is not under the direction of a physician (i.e., "carrying out doctor's orders"). Certain techniques (i.e., acupressure, Shiatsu, Structural Integration, Therapeutic Massage, Craniosacral Therapy) require highly specialized training. Others, such as acupuncture and chiropractic require completion of a lengthy formal educational program. In addition, professional counselors from various fields (i.e., psychologists, social workers, guidance counselors, pastoral counselors) are assuming a greater role in treatment. Many of these have completed a doctoral program (i.e., Ph.D., Ed.D., D.C.) as lengthy as medical education. Some of these nonmedical practitioners are required to be licensed by the state. But education or training, certification or licensure do not guarantee acceptance by all allopathic physicians.

In fact, some techniques and some therapists may be perceived as a threat to certain existing roles within the health care system (i.e., allopathic physician, physical therapist, pharmacist). The usual reaction is to label such practices as quackery, thereby implying that the practitioner is a fraud and the technique worthless. Many patients would testify otherwise, however, having obtained benefits from an alternative therapy that they did not get from orthodox medical treatment. Since public acceptance of these alternative therapies is increasing, you are encouraged to keep an open mind, listen to patients, and withhold judgment until you have enough information to make a rational evaluation.

Actually, many of today's roles within the health care system did not exist ten or twenty years ago. For the most part, these new roles emerged as a result of fragmenting existing roles, specializing in a specific technique or group of techniques, or specializing in a specific type of patient. In the orthodox system of health care, all of these roles are performed under the direction of a physician. Many of the alternative therapies are performed by practitioners who are not working under the direction of a physician. Yet, some of these practitioners are licensed by the state; their practice, therefore, is completely legal. This makes it all the more important that health care providers be informed and able to evaluate a given therapy, without arbitrarily labeling everything that is unfamiliar as "quackery."

Also, keep in mind that some of these alternative therapies are "innovative" only from the perspective of health care in the United States. The Chinese have been using acupuncture for at least 5,000 years. Homeopathic medicine has been practiced throughout Europe for two hundred years. Chiropractic techniques were developed in the early 1900s. Being approximately eighty years old, chiropractic no longer qualifies as "innovative." It is one of the alternative therapies now widely accepted by the American public, though not by many allopathic physicians, especially orthopedic surgeons.

Major Issues in Health Care Delivery

Many issues now confront society and the health care system: abortion, AIDS, organ transplants, prolonged use of life support systems, patients' rights (including the right to refuse treatment), a patient's right to die, the Living Will, malpractice litigation. Some of these are moral and ethical issues; some have direct implications for certain roles, and therefore are of special concern to the health care providers who are most affected. Many of these issues are highly emotional; the proponents of one side or the other may base their arguments on catch phrases that arouse strong emotional reactions in the listener.

A full discussion of these issues is beyond the scope of this book; they are mentioned here because every health care provider should be informed about them. Being informed makes it possible to avoid emotionalism and examine the issue thoughtfully. You are encouraged to read, attend meetings, consider various viewpoints, and use every opportunity to become well-informed; then, decide what *you* believe instead of blindly adopting the opinion of someone else. Strive to keep an open mind, combined with a healthy dose of skepticism.

Changing Patterns in Health Care Delivery

For a large segment of the population, the major issues in health care are *accessibility* and *cost*. For providers of health services the major issue relates to the patient-physician relationship and *who should make decisions about health care options*. For third-party payers (i.e., insurance companies) the major issue is maintaining greater income (through insurance premiums) than is paid out for health care services—*making a profit*. There is currently no national health care policy to resolve the many issues related to costs. Because the health care system is evolving and the mechanism for delivery of health services affects the roles of all health care providers, an overview of trends in delivery of services and types of payment plans is provided below.

Any effort to develop a national health care policy must deal with these issues and resolve many questions, such as:

- Who is entitled to health care?

- What is *essential* health care and what is *nonessential?*

- Who should decide whether a specific service for a specific patient is essential or nonessential?

- What is a reasonable cost for each type of service?

- What is a reasonable income for each health care provider?

- Who will pay for essential services? Who will pay for services that are deemed nonessential, but are desired (or demanded) by a patient?

Health Insurance

Until the mid-1900s, health care was provided under a fee-for-service arrangement between physician and patient. Then insurance companies began to offer hospital insurance, which could be purchased directly from the insurance company or through a group plan arranged by the employer. Later, insurance companies added Major Medical benefits, which paid a portion of medical costs that did not involve hospitalization. Health insurance has served the needs of many people, but a large percentage of the population cannot afford insurance and does not have access to a group plan. In an effort to broaden insurance coverage, the U.S. Congress in 1995 passed legislation requiring employers of five or more people to provide a group health plan. While this has increased the percentage of people with access to health insurance, a large segment of the population continues to be without the protection of health insurance.

Many insurance companies negotiate with physicians and health care agencies to obtain a discount for services provided to their policy-holders. A list of Preferred Provider Organizations (PPOs) is sent to the policy-holders, with a request that the services of PPOs be utilized. Usually, there is no penalty if the insured obtains services from a provider who is not on the PPO list.

Some insurers now require "precertification" for certain procedures. This means that an employee of the insurance company must approve the physician's recommended treatment; otherwise, the insurer will not pay. This is an example of a trend that is gaining momentum during the 1990s—*medical decisions made by an employee of a business* (in this case, an insurance company), rather than by the physician.

Health Maintenance Organizations

During the 1970s, a different approach developed in California and slowly spread throughout the nation. The Health Maintenance Organization (HMO) was proposed as a group plan that would emphasize health maintenance and prevention of illness, in addition to providing health services to the sick and injured. The HMO is a membership organization. For a specific annual fee, members receive whatever health services are needed. One member may use the services of the HMO only for an annual physical examination, while another may require extensive services for a catastrophic illness. The original thinking was that the HMO, by enrolling thousands of healthy members, would be able to pay for the services needed by those members with health problems. Ideally, the HMO would promote and maintain good health for the majority of its members by emphasizing prevention, providing health education, and detecting health problems in the early stages. Although the ideal was admirable and seemed good in theory, in actuality most HMOs soon were having to focus on meeting the demands of members for health care.

Some HMOs function as mediator between the membership and health care providers by contracting with physicians and hospitals to provide health care. The largest HMO of this type in the eastern United States is U.S. Healthcare, with 65,000 doctors under contract and 2.3 million members. Other HMOs *are* the providers of health services; they own hospitals and clinics and employ physicians and staff for various clinical services. Characteristics of both types of HMO include:

- Limited panel of health service providers

- Members assigned to a primary care physician ("gate-keeper") who directly provides care and may make referrals

- Members required to use providers on the panel, except for emergency care and out-of-area care

- Penalty for utilizing providers other than the panel

- Physicians on the panel are provided financial incentives for "managing utilization of services"

Beginning in 1996, the practices of some HMOs have been under fire. An article in the January 8, 1996 issue of *Time* asserted that some HMOs require physicians to withhold important information from their patients. It is also claimed that physicians are rewarded for minimizing referrals to specialists and ordering only routine diagnostic procedures and therapies. Dr. Elliott Dacher describes his disillusionment with HMOs as a young, idealistic physician.

> *"Working as an internist in a Health Maintenance Organization (HMO), I discovered I was expected to see twenty-five to thirty patients each day, complete paper work, answer and return phone calls, and attend meetings. This left an average of six to ten minutes for each patient." (Dacher, 1991)*

It is likely that there will be continued debate about the pros and cons of HMOs for the next several years.

Managed Care

In 1996, "Managed Care" began emerging as another approach to controlling health costs. Managed Care is a *business* concept with a *profit* motive, as opposed to a *service-to-the-sick* approach that has been the basic philosophy of health care for many years. The fundamental philosophy of any business is that there must be a profit—income must exceed expenses. If the business is publicly held (i.e., has issued stock), then the goal is to make enough profit to pay every stockholder a dividend one to four times a year.

Managed Care is a network of providers, organized and managed by persons with business training and experience. The network includes Primary Care Physicians (PCP), specialists, pharmacists, hospitals, clinics, and laboratories. Each patient's care is coordinated by the PCP; the patient can see a specialist only if referred by the PCP.

The major criticism of Managed Care is that *nonmedical persons (people with a business background) make medical decisions.* Physicians may be told that they must prescribe a drug that is less expensive than the one the physician prefers, or that a depressed patient may have up to ten, but no more, sessions with a psychiatrist or psychotherapist. One group of psychotherapists had been scheduling their patients for a full hour of therapy. When they contracted to become part of a managed care network, they were told that their sessions could only be 50 minutes. Who should make that decision? The business view is that by cutting ten minutes from each of six sessions, each therapist could be scheduled to service one more patient per day.

National Health Care/Insurance

For a decade or more there have been calls for a national plan that would provide universal health care. In the richest country in the world, a large segment of the population should not be deprived of health care because of inability to pay. Many people object to national involvement in health care, crying "socialized medicine." But the reality is that the federal government and the states are already heavily involved in health care. *Medicare* is health insurance for the elderly; premiums are deducted from social security payments, and providers are paid according to a Medicare fee schedule. The patient is responsible for 20% of the fee allowed by Medicare and for a $100 deductible each year. Medicare does not pay for prescription drugs, nursing home care, or home health care. *Medicaid* is a program of health care for those whose income is below a certain level and those who are unemployed because of disability. Members of the military and their dependents are provided medical care. Veterans of all military services can obtain health care through the Veterans Administration, which has many hospitals throughout the country. All members of the U.S. Congress, their families, and their staff members can obtain free health care. Many federal employees have access to free care, and all have health insurance through the federal government.

In spite of these programs, a large percentage of the population does not have access to health care because of no insurance, not belonging to a special "covered" group, or not being able to pay. There is need for a national plan that would ensure access to health care for every citizen of the United States.

Universal Health Care—Can It Happen in the United States?

A number of plans have been submitted to the U.S. Congress in recent years. Some offered piece-meal solutions; others proposed universal coverage. In March, 1993 HR-1200 was introduced in the Congress by Rep. James McDermott (D-Washington) and Rep. John Conyers, Jr. (D-Michigan); by January, 1994 the bill had 92 co-sponsors. This bill proposed a single-payer plan, meaning that health service providers would submit bills to *one* agency for payment of services according to a specified fee schedule. All citizens would be entitled to health care without the need for private insurance. This bill was not passed; there was powerful opposition from the insurance industry.

An editorial in the *New York Times,* January 6, 1996 discussed the benefits of a single-payer system, citing the insurance industry's contributions to health care costs.

- Insurance industry profits

- Insurance industry reserve funds (large sums that must be held in reserve for payment of claims)

- Insurance industry overhead, which includes skyscrapers and large office complexes, plus thousands of employees

- Hospital and physician expenses—costs of billing for services, completing claim forms, fulfilling various bureaucratic requirements like utilization review

The requirements for any plan to eliminate these added costs of health care would have to include:

- Universal coverage and universal access to health care;

- Comprehensive benefits

- Quality assurance

- Cost controls

- Equitable financing

Under Single-Payer plans, health care providers are paid through a government-funded National Health Care System, but they *are not government employees.* Physicians, hospitals, and other health service providers are private; the government "buys" their services. Anyone, regardless of income, is entitled to receive health care. Patients choose their physicians and, in cooperation with the physician, decide on treatment options. The only need for private insurance would be to assist with the costs of nonessential services, such as cosmetic surgery. A single-payer plan would replace both Medicare and Medicaid.

A report issued by the Congressional Budget Office stated that a single-payer plan would reduce general medical costs by $114 billion. A report from the General Accounting Office in January, 1994 detailed how the Canadian health care system (a single-payer system) could be adapted to the United States.

At present there are 1,200 private insurance companies selling $192.6 billion in health insurance per year. Of every $1 of "health care costs," 26 cents goes for the costs of administering this complex insurance system. Needless to say, the insurance industry is opposed to single-payer. With one of the most powerful lobbies in Washington, the insurance industry has successful lobbied members of Congress to oppose any type of single-payer plan. But support for a national health care plan is growing at the grass-roots level. The elections of November, 1996 are likely to determine whether or not any congressional action to provide universal health care will be taken before the year 2000.

You may be wondering why you should be concerned about the issue of private insurance versus HMOs versus Managed Care versus National Health Care. The system that eventually emerges from the present conglomeration of plans may affect your working conditions, but the full implications are a matter of conjecture at this time. Certainly, any plan whose top management is concerned primarily with profit may limit employee benefits and salary increases, but that will vary from one organization to another. Certainly, you and your family have personal concerns about the system that will eventually serve your own health care needs. As you interact with patients who are dissatisfied with the benefits their own health care plan provides, you may be the object of displaced anger. Do not take complaints of this type personally. Be a good listener, and keep in mind that many people may believe their health care plan does not provide services to which they are entitled or does not allow them the choices they want to make.

References and Suggested Readings

Dacher, Elliott, S. M.D. *PNI:Psychoneuroimmunology: The New Mind/Body Healing Program*. New York, NY: Paragon House, 1993.

Dossey, Larry, M.D. *Healing Words*. New York, NY: Harper Collins Publishers, 1993. Introduction, pp. 1–10; Preface, pp. xv–xxi.

Editorial, *The New York Times*, January 6, 1996.

Editorial, "Single Payer Health Care System Would Save $114 Billion by 2003," *The Washington Post*, February 1994.

Gray, Paul. "Critics Charge that some HMOs Require Physicians to Withhold Vital Information from their Patients," *Time*, January 8, 1996, p. 50.

Shealy, C. Norman and Myss, Caroline M., Ph.D. *The Creation of Health: The Emotional, Psychological, and Spiritual Responses that Promote Health and Healing*. Walpole, NH: Stillpoint Publishing, 1993. Chapter 1, "Shifting our Thinking about the Cause of Illness," pp. 3–40; Chapter 2, "Traditional Medicine Draws Closer to the Holistic," pp. 41–58.

(Note: The following books are "classics" in the sense that they opened the door to new or different beliefs and attitudes toward health care.)

Achterberg, Jeanne. *Woman as Healer*. Boston, MA: Shambhala, 1990.

———. *Imagery in Healing: Shamanism and Modern Medicine*. Boston, MA: Shambhala, 1985.

Benson, Herbert, M.D. *The Relaxation Response*. New York, NY: Avon Books, 1975.

Shealy, C. Norman, M.D. *Occult Medicine Could Save Your Life*. New York, NY: The Dial Press, 1975.

Simonton, O. Carl, M.D., Matthews-Simonton, Stephanie, & Creighton, James, *Getting Well Again*. Los Angeles, CA: J.P. Tarcher, Inc., 1978.

REVIEW AND SELF CHECK

1. Complete the following statements.
   a. Two reasons that innovations in science and health care are often rejected, or possibly judged to be quackery, are:

   _____ and _____.
   b. The difference betweens scientific data ("hard data") and empirical

   data is _____.

2. Place the letter of each discovery listed below beside the appropriate name in the column on the right.

   a. The Germ Theory   ___ von Leeuwenhoek
   b. Handwashing   ___ Semmelweiss
   c. Use of antiseptics   ___ Koch
   d. Rabies vaccine   ___ Roentgen
   e. Microscope   ___ Salk
   f. Smallpox vaccination   ___ Curie
   g. Polio vaccine   ___ Lister
   h. X rays   ___ Freud
   i. Radium   ___ Pasteur
   j. Role of the unconscious ___ Vesalius
      mind   ___ Jenner
   k. Accurate human anatomy

ASSIGNMENT

1. Write out the meaning of the following terms, using the text, Glossary, and a dictionary as needed.

Allopathic	Androgynous	Conventional
Empirical	Innovation	Orthodox
Patriarchal	Psychosomatic	Quackery

2. Select a topic from this chapter and prepare a five-minute report to present in class, as scheduled by the instructor.

3. Participate in a discussion of one of the following topics:
   a. Beliefs about the causes of illness and recovery
   b. Innovations that have been introduced into our local health care system within the past five years.
   c. An alternative therapy or innovation that you have heard someone label as "quackery"
   d. An alternative therapy that someone you know is using

4. Participate in a role-play where you are a health care provider; your patient has just told you that he or she has enrolled in a class to learn how to meditate.

Unit 24

What Is Healing? Who Is the Healer?

OBJECTIVES

Upon completion of this unit, you should be able to:

- Explain "placebo" as used in orthodox health care systems and in a holistic health care system.
- Describe the relationship of emotional states to the immune system.
- Explain the meaning of "multiple causation."
- Compare "curing" and "healing."
- List six factors that influence healing (holistic view).
- Explain the importance of love to the healing process.
- Explain "intention" as a factor in healing.
- List five differences between the holistic approach to health care and the orthodox approach.
- Explain the importance of stress management to health.
- State two challenges of health care providers who wish to contribute to a patient's healing process.
- Name one professional association that provides educational seminars about holistic health.

KEY TERMS

Causation	Intention	Multiple causation
Palliative	Placebo	Placebo effect

Every health care provider has wondered at times why one patient recovers from a serious illness, while another patient with the same disease and therapy slowly declines and eventually dies. What triggers the healing process in some patients, even when the prognosis is grim? Is there some subtle, unseen influence that makes a difference in the course of illness?

PLACEBO EFFECT

Another puzzle is **placebo effect**—improvement or recovery when the "drug" administered to a patient is actually an inert substance, such as a sugar pill. Why does the patient improve, even though the "treatment" administered is known to be ineffective? Studies of placebo effect have led to recognition that "expectation" or "being special" (i.e., being part of a research project) may influence the outcome of treatment. Expectation applies to both patients and health care providers; if either or both believe that a treatment or drug is going to cure the patient's illness, improvement usually occurs. Placebo effect is a problem for researchers who are trying to test the effectiveness of a new treatment because it is difficult to control. This is why double blind studies are used to test the effectiveness of a new drug. Placebo effect is also used as a defense against accepting an innovative therapy. Anyone who does not want to give serious consideration to a new therapy may simply dismiss any positive results of the innovation as "just placebo effect."

THE IMMUNE SYSTEM—PROTECTOR AND DEFENDER OF THE BODY

Despite years of discussion, there is no satisfactory explanation for *why* placebo effect occurs. Also puzzling is the fact that in an epidemic some people get sick and some, even members of a victim's family, do not contract the infection. This raises questions about the immune system. Why does it protect sometimes, but not always?

It is now known that all of us have cancer cells in our bodies, but certain components of the immune system destroy those abnormal cells with great efficiency until . . . what? Why does the immune system stop destroying those abnormal cells? What change permits those cancer cells to reproduce and form a tumor?

These questions have led to a number of discoveries about what affects the immune system. Physicians in ancient cultures observed that a grieving person was likely to develop cancer within a year or two following a significant loss. But at that time, the existence of the immune system was completely unknown. Modern clinicians and researchers have established the validity of that ancient observation. Certain emotional states, especially grief, depress the immune system and render it less capable of destroying abnormal cells already present in the body. The result is a favorable climate for the growth of cancer cells.

This particular body/mind/emotions relationship is now widely accepted. Yet much research on cancer still involves searching for an external intervention. Sometimes the mass media mentions a possible vaccine to protect people against cancer. This type of thinking denies the powerful mind/body relationship, clinging instead to the "old" way of attributing both the cause and the cure of disease to external influences.

Much of our knowledge of the immune system has been gained during the past forty years. Even though today's research techniques enable scientists to study the immune system more effectively, there are still many unanswered questions.

WHO GETS SICK?

Some clinical practitioners and researchers are proposing new theories, new ways of looking at the causes of disease. One such theory is that of **multiple causation:** there are *several* contributing causes in any illness, rather than a single cause. Some of the causative factors lie *within* the individual:

- Immune system function (specifically resistance and susceptibility)

- Emotional states, which we now know to have powerful effects on the immune system

- Physiological changes due to chronic stress

- Subtle factors such as beliefs, attitudes, will to live, and, possibly, an unconscious desire to escape one's life situation

In *The Creation of Health,* Dr. Shealy lists six major causes of illness and death.

- Smoking
- Consumption of alcohol
- Obesity
- Consumption of excessive fat, salt, sugar
- Lack of exercise
- Failure to wear a seatbelt and speeding

All of these contributors to illness involve *choices,* and the choice each individual makes is based on a combination of beliefs, values, and attitudes that influence behavior. From a holistic perspective, those persons who choose unhealthful practices are also knowingly or unknowingly choosing to be sick or injured at some time in the future.

The concept of multiple causation leads naturally to the view that *true healing* requires thinking of the patient as an entity (a whole being) within the context of family life, occupational setting, community, and culture—the holistic approach. In order for true healing to occur, one must modify beliefs and attitudes and make healthful life choices.

Numerous books explaining and emphasizing the need for holistic medicine/health care were published during the 1980s. A full discussion is beyond the scope of this textbook, but the remainder of Unit 24 provides an overview of this advancing frontier in health care.

THE MYSTERY OF HEALING—WHO GETS WELL?

Perhaps one of your textbooks explains the healing process in terms of the physiological events that replace damaged, unhealthy tissues with whole, healthy tissues. As a health care provider, you need to know about that process so you can provide a therapeutic environment that will facilitate the healing process. You have already learned that a therapeutic climate includes physical comfort and strict observance of correct technique in performance of procedures. But is something else required for a truly therapeutic climate?

Perhaps you have noticed that the patients of some physicians and some therapists seem to recover more readily than the patients of other physicians and therapists. Perhaps the same surgery was performed, the same drugs prescribed, the same therapeutic techniques used. What makes the difference in results? Does the difference lie within the patient, or can it be attributed to some characteristics of the health care providers?

Dr. Shealy believes that some physicians are "natural healers." In addition to their medical skills, they unconsciously convey healing energy to their patients. Perhaps this "energy" is a natural love for humanity, especially for those who are suffering. Dr. Shealy states,

> *Certainly there have always been miracles in medicine and at least part of the miracle, I continue to be convinced, is love. . . . what made the old-fashioned family doctor . . . such a beloved and hallowed figure was simply the love he gave so freely. . . . But the patient brought something too—faith in the doctor.*

Dr. Shealy's emphasis on the healing power of love is now reflected in numerous books by other physicians who have found that loving, caring relationships, especially in group therapy settings, have a positive effect on their patients.

It is possible that many health care providers, not only physicians, are "natural healers." A well-known example is Dolores Krieger, a registered nurse and professor of nursing who developed a system of healing known as Therapeutic Touch. Dr. Krieger has taught this system to hundreds of nurses.

The Power of Love

A recent publication, *Healers on Healing,* addresses the mystery of healing through a collection of essays by healers from a variety of disciplines. Some of the section titles imply that far more is involved in healing than the therapeutic modes of traditional medicine.

- Love is the healer

- Returning to wholeness

- The healer within

- The healing relationship

- The healing attitude

- Consciousness and the healing response

The editors' introduction to Part I begins, "Love is seen as one denominator that underlies and connects all successful healing. Without it, there can be no true healing."

Many of the chapters emphasize that love is essential to healing. *Love for self* influences the patient's body response to illness; a *loving attitude on the part of health care providers* establishes a healing climate. And *loving relationships* provide the emotional support that facilitates healing. In Chapter 1, Dr. Bernie Siegel states, ". . . I believe that love is the golden thread that unites the many forms of healing." Dr. Siegel gained much public attention following the publication in 1986 of his book, *Love, Medicine and Miracles: Lessons Learned About Self-Healing from a Surgeon's Experience with Exceptional Patients.* Numerous other publications during the 1980s emphasized the importance of love—self-love as well as love from others—to health and well-being.

Several chapters address wholeness and harmony as being essential to a natural state of health. Dr. Simonton's chapter, entitled "The Harmony of Health," begins:

> *Health is the natural state of humanity. It means being in harmony with ourselves and our universe. When we are in harmony, we feel better, feel more joy, and feel healthier. If we don't recognize that state, we need to. That is what healing is all about.*

Healing Versus Curing

Part III of *Healers and Healing* focuses on the role of the patient in healing—the healer within. Dr. John Upledger makes a clear distinction between healing and curing: **healing** refers to "what is done *by* the patient (or the patient's body) in order to resolve a problem of the body, mind, or spirit. Curing usually refers to what is done *to* the patient by the physician or therapist." Clarifying this difference is important, Dr. Upledger states, because:

> *Effective therapy—whatever its outer form—initiates, facilitates, and supports the patients self-healing efforts, whereas the 'curing' process is one that provides a more temporary and perhaps only **palliative** effect.*

Noting that many healing systems and techniques facilitate the patient's self-discovery, which promotes self-healing, Dr. Upledger lists as particularly effective a number of very different techniques: meditation, nutritional therapy, herbal therapy, homeopathy, acupuncture, Rolfing, chiropractic, Alexander-Feldenkrais technique, rebirthing, counseling, biofeedback. If you are like most health care providers, many of these terms are totally new to you. It is not necessary to know about them all, but you need to know that these methods, among others, are being found effective by a large segment of the public. When you encounter a patient who has used or is using one of these methods, view it as your opportunity to learn about the technique from your patient.

HEALTH CARE PROVIDERS AS HEALERS

The second half of *Healers on Healing* addresses the roles of health care providers as healers. Dr. Dolores Krieger comments:

> *. . . I have found two characteristics to be consistent in the committed healer: compassion and intentionality. The case for compassion speaks for itself. Intentionality implies that the healer not only exerts his or her will to heal an individual, but also perceives a context in which that healing can take place. This assures that the healing practice will be done in a conscious and conscientious manner.*

Dr. Janet Quinn, also a nurse, notes that the word *heal* means "to be or to become whole." She states:

> *. . . the locus of healing is within the patient. Healing, no matter what the intervention, is not something that can be given or owned by the practitioner or the therapist. All healing, without exception, is self-healing.*

This view that the role of healer includes helping a patient to become **"whole"** is a basic premise of holistic medicine/healing, which also acknowledges that all healing is self-healing.

Intention of the Health Care Provider

Current thinking, then, emphasizes both the role of the patient and the role of loving, supportive relationships in determining the outcome of illness.

This presents a *new dimension* to the role of health care provider. Patient care that consists of carrying out the physician's orders or performing assigned procedures is a limited role. The challenge to health care providers is to perform patient care with love and with the *conscious* **intention** of helping the patient to heal. This does not require additional time or effort. It does require concentration—*giving full attention to the patient* and *focusing on loving, positive thoughts throughout a procedure* to provide a truly healing climate.

Would this make a difference? There is no *proof* at this time, but a wealth of literature provides tentative theories and case histories, with extensive evidence that *intention does make a difference.* Each health care provider must make a personal decision about whether or not to strive for creating a truly healing climate in each contact with a patient.

The Patient's Intention

Be aware also that true healing occurs only when the patient has the *intention* to get well. Intention, in turn, is affected by such factors as belief systems, faith, and will to live. A newly recognized challenge for health care providers is acceptance—*nonjudgmental acceptance*—of a patient who does not intend to get well.

This view of healing and healers may be more acceptable to you after you have become familiar with some of the research that demonstrates the interrelatedness of body, mind, emotions, and spirit. If this overview piques your interest, read one or more of the books listed at the end of this unit.

THE HOLISTIC APPROACH TO HEALTH CARE

As a student preparing to become a health care provider, you have already learned about many of the factors that influence a person's health. Your study has probably emphasized that individual choices also affect health. The belief that illness is the result of outside influences (i.e., germs, accidents that "just happen") affects the choices people make. Thinking, "other people get sick or have accidents, but I don't" may result in carelessness. How people feel about themselves influences their choices and self-care. Behaviors that indicate lack of self-care and unhealthy choices include:

- Being a workaholic

- Not allowing oneself time to play (not using leisure time for re-creating oneself)

- Eating "on the run" or eating mostly convenience meals

- Ignoring bodily sensations that may be early warning signs of illness

- Ignoring the effects of stress on body, mind, and emotions

- Ignoring safety precautions in the workplace

- Driving fast or recklessly

- Not wearing a seatbelt

Life choices are increasingly recognized as contributing causes of illness or accident. Modern living exposes us to many stresses not known by earlier societies. Each day we encounter air pollution, food additives, building materials and home furnishings that give off toxic fumes—the list is almost endless. But the greatest stressors for many people are time pressures and interpersonal relationships.

Job responsibilities plus home responsibilities plus commuting time plus errand-running leave little leisure time for many people. Time pressures interfere with the development of satisfying and mutually supportive relationships, even within a family setting. Relationship problems may continue for years because "there just isn't time to work on it." People are risking their health when they fail to make time to cope with stress and improve relationships. As a counselor stated after talking with a highly-stressed client, "The people who need meditation the most are the ones who say they don't have time. Yet, taking 20 minutes a day to meditate could make a world of difference in how their day goes."

The Mind/Body Connection

Dr. Kenneth Pelletier works with chronically ill patients in a hospital-based clinic. In addition to clinical expertise developed through the years, Dr. Pelletier has extensive knowledge of stress and psychosomatic disorders, based on a comprehensive review of the literature and research reports. He summarizes this voluminous body of literature in *Mind as Healer, Mind as Slayer.* According to Dr. Pelletier, illness is the result of "a complex interaction of social factors, physical and psychological stress, . . . personality . . . , and the inability of the person to adapt adequately to pressures." With this broad view of **causation,** he then presents evidence for classifying most of today's major health problems as psychosomatic and/or stress-related disorders.

In orthodox medicine, an illness is generally labeled psychosomatic when no organic pathology has been found. In holistic medicine, according to Dr. Pelletier, psychosomatic is defined as "a fundamental interaction between mind and body which is involved in all diseases and all processes affecting health maintenance." Such a definition mandates that diagnosis and treatment of illness take into consideration the mind/body relationship.

Placebo also has different meanings under these two systems of health care. In orthodox medicine, placebo refers to a treatment or procedure that has no therapeutic value. In the holistic view, placebo effect includes factors that could affect the healing process.

1. The patient's belief system

2. The patient's will to live

3. Patient/health care provider relationships

4. Family relationships

5. Changes in life-style

6. Ability (or willingness) to make life changes in order to reduce and manage stress

Dr. Pelletier cites several conditions under which stress (the General Adaptation Response or the fight-or-flight reaction) becomes chronic, rather than serving as an alarm response that is dissipated once the emergency has passed.

1. The source of stress is ambiguous, meaning that the individual is not really clear about who or what stressors exist in his or her life situation

2. The stress continues over a prolonged period of time

3. There are several sources of stress in the individual's life situation

The prolonged semi-alert physical state that results from this combination of circumstances eventually produces physical and/or physiological changes—a disease or, in the holistic view, a psychosomatic disorder.

Our modern lifestyle includes a wide variety of stressors, many of which we cannot escape. Dr. Pelletier maintains, therefore, that every individual must develop a regular pattern of stress-reducing activities as a means of health protection. The alternative is psychosomatic illness or dependence on a crutch such as alcohol or tranquilizers. In his practice, Dr. Pelletier uses biofeedback to help patients learn to control certain body processes and minimize or reverse the effects of stress. The clinic also emphasizes the use of meditation as a stress-reducing activity. According to Dr. Pelletier:

> *Practicing stress-reduction techniques such as meditation and biofeedback is a great step forward in the prevention of psychosomatic disease. Teaching people meditative skills . . . is one of the greatest challenges in the field of holistic preventive medicine.*

Patients must learn to differentiate between a healthful level of stress and a pathogenic level that can lead to disease. Since some serious stressors cannot be eliminated, the only healthful choice is to learn how to minimize the effects of those particular stressors. Dr. Pelletier believes the health care system must focus on prevention of stress-related disorders. This would require teaching people to identify stressors, make lifestyle changes to eliminate as many stressors as possible, develop body awareness, and learn effective stress-management techniques *before* the onset of symptoms.

Characteristics of Holistic Health Care

It is generally acknowledged, even within orthodox medicine, that approximately eighty-five percent of the patients seen in a physician's office have a psychosomatic disorder. Yet orthodox medicine continues to rely heavily on drugs and surgery as the primary treatments. At this point, it is desirable to contrast the philosophical differences between orthodox medicine and holistic medicine. The following chart is excerpted from the concluding chapter of *Mind as Healer, Mind as Slayer.*

Basic Philosophical Assumptions	
HOLISTIC MEDICINE	ORTHODOX MEDICINE
All disease is psychosomatic in origin	Disease is generally caused by external factors, such as pollution, germs.
Disease has multiple causation; each person has a "weak point" (i.e., respiratory system, heart, lower back); when that person is subjected to stress over a long period of time, disease or disability is most likely to appear at the weak point.	Most diseases have a specific cause. Infections are caused by microorganisms; there are no other causative factors.
The healing process is psychosomatic; a person's will is a primary factor in getting sick or getting well.	Good medical care produces better health.
A single factor approach to health (to healing, to prevention of illness) is too narrow.	A specific therapeutic agent can cure most diseases.
Patients have some responsibility for the course of an illness.	Healing is the responsibility of health care providers.
All states of health (including sickness) are psychosomatic.	If you are not sick, then you are well.

The holistic philosophy recognizes that each individual is unique. Health, sickness, and healing are related to a balance or imbalance among body, mind, emotions, and spirit. The holistic philosophy also emphasizes that disease is the result of multiple factors, not just one. When a patient's treatment is based on a single cause and other contributing factors are ignored, the patient is likely to experience a sequence of illnesses. The ultimate example is the patient who has undergone one surgical procedure after another, until no more internal organs can be spared. Then the patient develops a systemic disorder, such as diabetes, arthritis, hypertension or systemic lupus erythematosis. In such a case, symptoms were treated but the underlying causes of illness have been ignored. A partial *cure* was effected with each surgery, but the patient was not *healed.*

Diagnostic and Therapeutic Approaches from a Holistic Perspective

At the Psychosomatic Medicine Center of Gladstone Memorial Hospital in Berkeley, California, the physical effects of normal, stressful, and resting activities are measured to develop a patient's stress profile. The profile indicates what area of the patient's body is most affected by stress. That area is most likely to become diseased or dysfunctional if the patient's stress is not managed effectively. These findings enable the staff to predict which type of disorder the patient will eventually develop if stress is not controlled. The patient is then taught to control these physical reactions to stressors, thereby preventing physical and physiological changes that are precursors to disease.

This approach to preventive medicine recognizes *unmanaged stress as a major contributor to illness.* It also recognizes that *healing* in modern society requires the learning of stress management techniques.

In Unit 23, you learned that Dr. Simonton, Dr. Shealy, and Dr. Benson have all recognized the importance of stress management. The Simontons' research with cancer patients revealed a distinctive personality profile that includes habitual repression of anger. For that reason, each patient's therapy also includes counseling, to assist the patient in dealing with suppressed anger and other negative emotions. Patients are taught to meditate and incorporate at least two, but preferably three, meditations into their daily routines.

At his pain rehabilitation center, Dr. Shealy teaches patients to meditate and take responsibility for their health. A high percentage of his chronic pain patients, most of whom have been on pain medication for many years, eventually are able to manage their pain through meditation and other self-regulatory techniques. Dr. Shealy also emphasizes good nutrition and an exercise program appropriate for each patient.

Dr. Benson teaches hypertensive patients to meditate as an integral component of their treatment. Since meditation requires considerable self-discipline, a certain percentage of patients become "dropouts"—they do not make meditation a part of their daily routine. Of those who do practice meditation regularly, many are able to reduce their dosage of antihypertensive drug, and some are able to discontinue it completely. The potential of meditation to lower blood pressure is so powerful that Dr. Benson emphatically warns new meditators to let their physicians know that they have started meditating. The blood pressure should be monitored, so that the antihypertensive drug can be reduced as blood pressure approaches normal levels, usually within a period of two to six months.

From these few examples, several approaches emerge as essential to true healing.

1.   Concern for the patient's total being (emotional, mental, spiritual as well as physical aspects)

2.   Having the patient participate in a planned program of health care, which probably includes lifestyle changes.

3.   Teaching the patient stress-management techniques

4.   Helping the patient face and resolve emotional issues that are contributing to the health problem

5.   Helping the patient assume responsibility for his or her illness, health, and well-being

It may take weeks or months to make all the changes needed, to deal with emotional issues that may underlie the illness, or to experience the full benefits of therapy. Many patients are not willing to take responsibility for their own health. And therein lies the problem. Even those who are willing to take some responsibility may find it hard to change their lifestyle, deal with painful issues, or even to persist in a long-term plan until the benefits become apparent.

There is also a problem from the standpoint of health care delivery. The holistic approach is time-consuming. It requires going beyond the physical examination and related diagnostic studies to study the "whole patient" and the life context within which that patient lives and works. It involves teaching people, rather than providing a quick cure. It requires patience and persistence to help people identify underlying causes of illness and make significant lifestyle changes. It also requires that health care providers maintain a loving, caring attitude toward their patients.

THE AMERICAN HOLISTIC NURSES' ASSOCIATION

The American Holistic Nurses' Association (AHNA) was organized in 1980. (The American Holistic Medical Association was organized in the early 1970s,

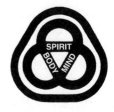

The logo of the American Holistic Nurses' Association reflects the interrelatedness of body, mind, and spirit. (From American Holistic Nurses' Association.)

with Dr. Shealy as its first president.) Membership in AHNA is open to nurses, other health care professionals, and anyone who supports the philosophy, purpose, and objectives of AHNA. Activities of AHNA include establishing criteria for holistic nursing practice, offering seminars and conferences on holistic health care, honoring nurses to contribute to holistic health principles, awarding an annual scholarship to individuals who wish to pursue a career in holistic nursing, and the formation of local groups to foster holistic health principles.

FUTURE HEALTH CARE SYSTEMS

It is possible that we will someday have two health care systems.

1. The existing system for two types of patient:
   a. Those whose illness requires orthodox medical care
   b. Those who are not willing to take responsibility for their own health

2. An alternative, holistic system for people who want to participate in their care, are willing to make lifestyle changes, and are willing to practice health maintenance techniques to the fullest extent possible

Just as there are patients who prefer orthodox medical care to holistic care, there are also health care providers who would find greater job satisfaction in one system than in the other. As a health care provider, you may eventually have the opportunity to pursue your career in either type of health care setting. Your own beliefs about health and healing should be considered when you are faced with such a choice.

SOURCES OF ADDITIONAL INFORMATION

*American Holistic Nurses' Association, 4101 Lake Boone Trail, Suite 201, Raleigh, NC 27606: (919) 787-5181.

References and Suggested Readings

In the list below, * indicates a "classic" reference, meaning that it *introduced* one or more concepts related to holistic health care.

Benson, Herbert. *Timeless Healing: The Power and Biology of Belief.* New York, NY: Scribners, 1996.

*Borysenko, Joan. *Minding the Body, Mending the Mind.* New York, NY: Bantam Books, 1987.

Borysenko, Joan & Borysenko, Miroslav. *The Power of the Mind to Heal.* Carlsbad, CA: Hay House, 1994.

*Carlson, Richard and Shield, Benjamin (eds.) *Healers on Healing.* Los Angeles, CA: Jeremy P. Tarcher, Inc., 1989.

*Jaffe, Dennis T. *Healing from Within.* New York, NY: Simon & Schuster, 1980.

Keegan, Lynn. *The Nurse as Healer.* Albany, NY: Delmar Publishers, Inc., 1994.

Krieger, Dolores. *Accepting Your Power to Heal.* Santa Fe, NM: Bear & Company Publishing, 1993.

*Krieger, Dolores. *The Therapeutic Touch.* New York, NY: Prentice Hall Press, 1979.

*Locke, Steven and Colligan, Douglas. *The Healer Within: The New Medicine of Mind and Body.* New York, NY: E. P. Dutton, 1986. (Appendices provide extensive lists of references, resources, organizations related to specific disorders, and alternative treatment centers.)

*Pelletier, Kenneth R. *Mind as Healer, Mind as Slayer: A Holistic Approach to Preventing Stress Disorders.* New York, NY: Dell Publishing Co., 1977.

*Shealy, C. Norman. *90 Days to Self-Health.* New York, NY: Dial Press, 1977.

*Siegel, Bernie S. *Love, Medicine & Miracles.* New York, NY: Harper & Row Publishers, 1986.

REVIEW AND SELF-CHECK

Complete the following statements, using information from Unit 24.

1. As commonly used in orthodox medicine, "placebo effect" means _____

   _____ .

2. Some factors included in placebo effect in a holistic view are:

   _____ , _____ , _____ , _____ .

3. An extreme emotional state, especially grief, tends to _____ the immune system.

4. Multiple causation of illness means _____ .

5. Intention as a factor that influences healing refers to both the _____
_____ and the _____ .

6. Love as an influence on healing involves both the patient's self-love and
loving attitudes on the part of _____ .

7. Some physicians differentiate *curing* and *healing;* the primary difference
is that

_____ .

8. According to the holistic view of health care, six factors that influence
healing are _____ , _____ , _____ ,
_____ , _____ , and _____ .

9. List five differences between holistic and orthodox health care.

_____   _____

_____   _____

_____   _____

_____   _____

_____   _____

10. Stress-management is a critical factor in preventing illness because

_____ .

11. One factor that is essential to healing, according to recent literature on
the subject, is _____ .

12. Two challenges for health care providers who wish to contribute to a
patient's healing process are _____ and _____ .

13. An organization of health care providers that offers seminars on holistic
health topics is _____ .

ASSIGNMENT

1. Describe from your own experience an example of placebo effect.

2. Participate in a class discussion of one or more of the following statements:
   - Love, including self-love, is essential to health and well-being.
   - Harmony among body, mind, emotions, and spirit is essential to health and well-being.
   - Life choices increase the probability of illness.
   - Life choices increase the probability of an accident.
   - Life choices promote health and well-being.
   - The power of the mind influences the course of an illness.
   - Health-related behavior may indicate lack of self-love.

3. List stressors in your life situation (include your various roles as student, health care provider, family member).

4. Beside each stressor above, indicate with a checkmark those stressors that could be eliminated by a relatively minor life change. (Example: getting up 15 minutes earlier in order to prepare for the day in a leisurely manner.)

5. Review the list and checkmarks, then list three stressors you plan to eliminate; beside each, state a specific life change you will make, beginning today (or not later than tomorrow).

6. The next time you encounter a difficult situation involving a patient (or co-worker, teacher, friend, family member), consciously project positive feelings for that person. Continue to think and feel positively as you deal with the situation. Afterward, when you are no longer in that person's presence, consider the following questions:
   a. What was the effect on you? Are you calmer, less angry than you might have been? What is your physical condition—relaxed or uptight?
   b. What was the effect on the other person? Was there an improvement in attitude or behavior as you projected positive feelings?

7. Your classmate comments, "That love stuff is stupid. It's all I can do to complete my assignment. I don't have time to go around feeling love for my patients." How would you respond?

8. Drawing on your personal experience (relatives, friends, acquaintances) and your clinical experience, list examples of people who:
    a. Recovered from a life-threatening illness, contrary to the expectation of their physicians
    b. Recovered from a serious illness through medical intervention, such as surgery, only to develop symptoms of another serious illness within the next year

9. Refer to one example in 8-a above and consider: What factors may have contributed to recovery? What traits characterize that person?

10. Refer to one example in 8-b above and consider: What traits characterize that individual?

Unit 25

Managing Stress with Relaxation/Meditation

OBJECTIVES

Upon completion of this unit, you should be able to:

- Define "mind-talk" and "mindfulness."
- Define Relaxation as a process.
- State two reasons why relaxing by means of a recreational activity is not adequate as a stress management technique.
- Describe the primary physiological change that occurs during Relaxation.
- Name the primary physiological change that occurs during meditation.
- State three psychological changes that may occur as long-term effects of meditation.
- Name two reasons a health care provider should use a stress management technique at least once a day.
- Name the major disadvantage of meditation as a therapeutic tool.
- Use a specific technique for Relaxation.
- Use a specific technique for meditation. (Optional)

KEY TERMS

Adjunct	Affirmations	Autonomic
Blood lactate	Deterrent	Guided imagery
Visualize		

In the previous unit, you learned that most health care providers acknowledge the role of stress and psychosocial factors in the onset of illness. It is not within the role of nonphysician health care providers to *prescribe* stress management for a patient, since diagnosis and prescription of a therapeutic plan are the domain of medicine. In some circumstances, however, it is appropriate for any health care provider to talk with a patient about the importance of stress management. Your participation in helping a patient learn about stress management is more likely if you are working with a holistically oriented medical practitioner. In the meantime, you, as a health care provider, have a responsibility to yourself and your family to maintain the best possible state of health. That includes learning about stress management and modifying your daily routine to include one or more specific stress management techniques. This unit, then, is for *you*.

STRESS MANAGEMENT

Unit 25 presents two specific techniques for managing stress: Relaxation and meditation. The word *Relaxation* is capitalized to remind you that we are discussing a *specific process* with *specific effects*. This is quite different from the customary use of the word "relaxation."

There are many ways of coping with stress. Some people have a daily exercise program that significantly reduces their stress level. Others participate in a sport at least once a week. Sports may or may not reduce stress, depending upon one's level of competitiveness. If winning is very important, then losing a game may increase stress, rather than reduce it.

Certain activities that people think of as "relaxing" do *not* have stress-management value. For example, watching television, partying, going to the beach, a weekend skiing trip, and other such recreational activities are **diversions**—escapes from the daily pressures of the job and routine home responsibilities. Though pleasant and possibly self-renewing, recreational activities do not bring about the physical and psychological changes that are essential to effective stress management.

MIND-TALK AS A SOURCE OF STRESS

Dr. Elliott Dacher describes two basic activities of the mind, mind-talk and mindfulness, that cannot occur simultaneously. When one is active, the other is inactive. Mind-talk is active most of the time; in fact, it is **autonomic.** *Mind-talk* involves thoughts, feelings, mental images, and various sensations. It is the ongoing mental chatter that we all experience, especially when engaged in an activity that does not require conscious mental effort. Household tasks, many job tasks, walking, riding an exercycle—these types of activities are accompanied by a stream of mind-talk *unless it is consciously controlled.*

Stored memories provide the content for mind-talk; it may be factual or psychological, useful or destructive. When mind-talk arouses negative feelings associated with a past experience, we relive some bad experience that cannot be changed. Thus, mind-talk may be the source of ongoing stress. Mind-talk can be so engrossing that a person is out of touch with what is happening at the moment. In Dr. Dacher's words, "The more aware we become of mind-talk, the more we realize how little we attend to the present moment—the only experience that is actually happening at that time" (Dacher, 1993). By taking conscious control, however, an individual may learn to avoid stressful feelings associated with past experiences and anxiety related to some anticipated (or feared) future event.

MINDFULNESS

In contrast to mind-talk, *mindfulness* must be learned, is self-initiated, and requires conscious effort. Mindfulness has three aspects that occur in sequence: attention, concentration, and meditation. One *consciously chooses* to enter a state of mindfulness, primarily by giving full attention to what is happening at the present moment. Full attention to an ongoing activity quickly becomes concentration. A state of mindfulness may be experienced while reading, enjoying some aspect of nature, being involved in an artistic pursuit, cruising the Internet, or being totally absorbed in relating to another person. By shifting from mind-talk to mindfulness, then, one attends to what is happening at present.

Dr. Kabat-Zinn, director of the stress management clinic at The University of Massachusetts Hospital in Boston, describes mindfulness as a means of fully living in the present, which is all we have. The past cannot be changed; the future is yet to be. So we should make the most of the present, which is best done through mindfulness. Dr. Kabat-Zinn teaches mindfulness and meditation to patients as a means of coping with the stress of their illnesses.

RELAXATION AND MEDITATION

The physical and psychological effects of Relaxation and meditation have been thoroughly documented by clinical practitioners and researchers. Although the therapeutic value of these two techniques is now widely accepted, the preventive potential has only been explored in limited settings, such as psychosomatic medical practices, psychological services, and corporate health maintenance programs.

Background

Historically, meditation has its roots in various religions, especially those of the East (i.e., India, China, and Japan). There are numerous references to meditation in the Bible, and many people use a prayerful form of meditation. The monks of various religious traditions use meditation as one means of spiritual development. But meditation is not prayer. In fact, many meditators do not consider their meditations to be a religious activity. Each meditator determines the extent to which his or her meditation has religious significance.

The technique known as Relaxation is a relatively new therapeutic procedure, however. It seems to have originated around 1929 with Dr. Edmund Jacobson, a Chicago psychiatrist who believed muscle tension and anxiety to be significant factors in the onset of illness. He developed a technique known as "Progressive Relaxation."

Concurrently with Jacobson's research on muscle tension, a German psychiatrist, Dr. J.H. Schultz, developed a therapeutic technique for helping patients learn to control certain autonomic functions. This technique is known as Autogenic Training, or AT. The work of these two physicians has led to the development of numerous relaxation techniques, most of which are based on either progressive relaxation or AT.

Physical and Psychological Effects

Relaxation and meditation are two different processes. You can practice a relaxation technique without meditating. However, meditation brings about physiological changes and, for habitual meditators, has long-term effects that do not occur with Relaxation alone.

Both Relaxation and meditation result in a feeling of being rested; the twenty-minute procedure may dissipate fatigue or sleepiness as much as a two-hour nap. Many people not only feel rested, but also experience increased energy at the completion of either procedure.

The primary physiological change that occurs with Relaxation is *release of tension in the skeletal muscles,* accompanied by a *decrease in **blood lactate.*** A high level of blood lactate is associated with anxiety. Relaxation training emphasizes learning to *control* muscle tension. The Jacobson method emphasizes learning to *recognize* the presence of muscle tension, then *consciously let go of the tension.* Most other methods focus on the "letting go" phase, on the assumption that the individual is already able to recognize the presence of muscle tension. Those who have achieved heightened awareness of muscle tension through the Jacobson method tend to question that assumption. Learning to recognize the presence of muscle tension, or the onset of muscle tension, is essential to successful use of Relaxation.

Some of the benefits of Relaxation can be experienced within a few practice sessions, but the full benefits are realized after the procedure has been performed at least once a day over a period of several weeks. One who has mastered the technique can recognize muscle tension as it begins (usually around the eyes or in the neck), then can quietly use Relaxation to relieve that tension within a few minutes. Obviously, anyone who works or lives in a stressful situation may benefit from using Relaxation intermittently throughout the day, to avoid a build-up of muscle tension.

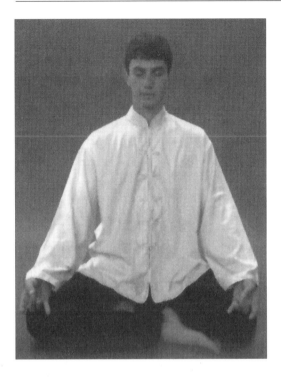

One meditation posture.

In contrast to Relaxation, meditation affects various body processes, essentially slowing the pace of bodily activity: respiratory rate and pulse rate decrease, blood pressure lowers, and the metabolic rate, as measured by the body's oxygen consumption, slows. Some therapists believe the meditative period helps the body establish balance and harmony among the various systems, a state that promotes healing and optimal functioning of the immune system.

Meditation is also characterized by a change in brain activity. In 1929, Dr. Hans Berger, a German psychiatrist, published a report in which he described a distinctive pattern of brain waves (9–13 cycles per second) that occurs when a person is in a quiet state, not actively thinking or reacting to various stimuli. Dr. Berger labeled this pattern "alpha rhythms." Subsequent research confirmed Dr. Berger's findings and identified other brain wave patterns. Beta rhythms (13–18 cycles per second) predominate during the fully conscious state. Theta rhythms (5–8 cycles per second) and delta rhythms (less than 5 cycles per second) occur during sleep.

Sleep researchers have found that brain wave patterns during sleep go through cycles, with the deepest stage of sleep characterized by delta rhythms and the lightest stage of sleep by alpha rhythms. Dreaming occurs during light sleep and is accompanied by rapid eye movements (this stage is often referred to as "REM sleep"). Although alpha rhythms occur during REM sleep and also during meditation, the meditator is awake, conscious of surroundings but not interacting through sensory, mental or emotional responses. The meditator can return to full beta consciousness at will.

The benefits of continued meditation over a prolonged period (at least two years) are psychological (i.e., mental and emotional) and spiritual. The latter term is used here, not in the religious sense, but to refer to that mysterious aspect of being human that is beyond body and mind and emotions. For many people the spiritual aspect is related to the Divine; for others, it is being in touch with the collective unconscious, cosmic forces, or other metaphysical concepts. Whatever one's personal belief regarding the spiritual, it does appear to be an aspect of individuality that must be in harmony with mind and emotions in order for the body to experience optimal well-being. The long-term effects of daily meditation include:

- Changes in perception of self, others, and life events

- Re-evaluation of values and beliefs

- A freeing of emotions, especially suppressed emotions

- Greater compassion

- Increased capacity for self-love and love for others

- Greater readiness to accept love

- Improved ability to cope with life situations

- Increased awareness of "self"

Advantages and Disadvantages

Relaxation and meditation can be viewed in the light of an investment and its dividends. For an investment of about twenty minutes a day, the potential dividends include prevention of stress-related illness, therapy for an existing illness or injury, and increased energy for daily activities as chronic muscle tension is relieved. The long-term meditator does risk the pain of dealing with suppressed emotions and of changing beliefs, values, and perceptions as a result of meditative insights. But one who completes the process of dealing with such unresolved issues is thereafter free of their restrictive, negative influence.

The disadvantages pertain to the learning process, the length of time required to experience full benefits, and competing demands for one's time. It is not easy for a busy person to incorporate a twenty-minute routine into an already full day. But it is very easy to rely on the "I just don't have time" excuse. Dr. Simonton dealt quite effectively with this excuse when he asked a conference group, "What is so important that it cannot wait twenty minutes for you to do your meditation?" Most of us, trying to answer that question honestly, cannot list anything other than a true emergency.

It takes time to learn Relaxation. It takes even more time to learn to meditate. After about two weeks of consistent practice, you begin to experience the benefits. But it takes persistence over a period of months, perhaps even one or two years, to experience the long-term benefits. Many people who learn a meditation technique do not use it consistently or for a long enough period of time to experience the long-term payoff. It is too easy to give in to competing demands on one's time.

At this point, you may be tired of reading about Relaxation and meditation. Perhaps you are ready to get involved! The remainder of this unit introduces you to three different Relaxation techniques, then to two types of meditation. Information about each is followed by a step-by-step procedure. You may want to tape record each procedure; use the tape to learn the steps of one specific procedure until you can practice without the tape. An alternative approach is to read through the instructions several times, then practice the procedure. Afterward, reread the instructions. Thereafter, read the instructions before and after each Relaxation. Soon, you will be able to go through the procedure on your own. *Learn one procedure thoroughly before going on to another.*

RELAXATION TECHNIQUES

You already know that a skill is developed through practice. *Mastery* of a task or technique is achieved by continuing to practice a skill regularly over a period of months or years. Relaxation is a special type of skill that involves control of muscle tension throughout the body. You can develop skill in controlling muscle tension only by practicing at least once a day for about twenty minutes; skill will be achieved more quickly by practicing twice a day.

One who has *mastered* Relaxation can release tension within a minute or two just by thinking, "Relax." Achieving that level of mastery enables one to manage the stress of modern living.

Some people find that Relaxation alone meets their needs. Others, after experiencing the benefits of Relaxation, develop an interest in learning to meditate. The primary emphasis here is on learning Relaxation, which requires less time than meditation. An introduction to meditation and two examples of a simple meditation follow, for those who wish to go beyond Relaxation.

Principles

There are many techniques for achieving Relaxation. No one method is right for everybody. Some people find that one method is more comfortable or more effective than others. To find the technique that works best for you, try a specific method once a day for at least two weeks. Then try another method once a day for two weeks. After you have tried the three methods described below, select the one with which you are most comfortable and practice it daily for a month. At that point, you should be able to recognize muscle tension as soon as it develops. Then, you can withdraw from a stressful situation and devote two to five minutes to "letting go." You will no longer need a full twenty minutes to reduce muscle tension. This does not mean that you discontinue your daily use of the full twenty-minute procedure; the short procedure helps you get through a stressful day with less tension build-up. Continue your daily routine for total Relaxation—a time for re-establishing balance and harmony—and accept it as a healthful part of your daily routine for the remainder of your life.

Preparation

It is important to make certain preparations before starting a Relaxation procedure.

1. Decide on the time of day and the location for your Relaxation. Then, be consistent so that time and location become associated with Relaxation. The location should be a particular room and chair (or pillow, or area of the floor) that is used only for Relaxation. Select a time when you can be alone for at least 20 minutes, preferably before eating a meal. Early morning is a good time—it gets your day off to a good start. Late afternoon is also good, to release the day's accumulated tensions before you have dinner.

2. Inform anyone in the area that you are not to be disturbed for the next 30 minutes. (Actually, you will probably use only 15–20 minutes.) If you are alone, unplug the phone or let your answering machine handle incoming calls.

3. Prepare the environment by closing the door, dimming the lights, and eliminating distractions. Put the dog and cat out.

4. Loosen any tight clothing, such as a belt or necktie; remove your shoes.

5. Assume a comfortable sitting position with the spine straight from head to hips, feet flat on the floor, hands resting on the thighs. If you have back or neck problems you may lie down. But be aware that in the lying position you may fall asleep as you become relaxed. Sleep is not the same as Relaxation! If you do choose to lie down: use the floor (your bed is for sleeping); keep the legs parallel (not crossed at the ankles); keep the arms parallel to the body but not touching it. The tendency to fall asleep passes after you have practiced the procedure several times.

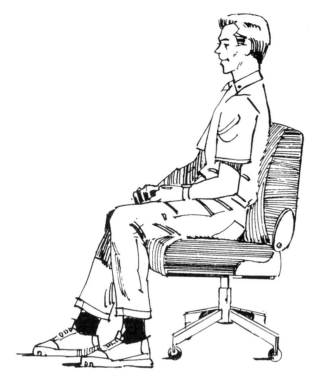

One typical relaxation posture.

6. Take several deep breaths, allowing the abdomen to expand as you inhale and to contract as you exhale.

7. Feel your body "letting go." Feel your hips and buttocks settling into the chair or floor.

8. Consciously put aside your thoughts and feelings, your worries and concerns of the day, as the final step in preparing for Relaxation.

After about 20 minutes, the body seems to signal that it is ready to resume activity. If you do not trust your ability to recognize this signal, include setting a timer in Step 3. Use a timer that sounds only once, rather than repeatedly. Then, if you choose to continue to enjoy Relaxation after the timer sounds, you can do so without having to get up and turn the timer off.

With practice these preparation steps become automatic. Now it is time to learn Relaxation.

Methods

Three different Relaxation procedures are presented below. Each has its particular advantages. With practice, each will result in the release of muscle tension throughout your body.

Progressive Relaxation

The following steps are based on a method developed by Dr. E. Jacobson, a physiologist and physician. This method is designed to help you become aware of the feeling that accompanies muscle tension, then become aware of how a relaxed muscle feels. Learning to differentiate these sensations—tension versus relaxation—increases body awareness and prepares you to recognize the need for Relaxation during the day. With practice, you will be able to Relax almost anywhere (even without sitting or lying down) and get results within a few minutes. As you do the following steps, try to keep the rest of your body relaxed while you work on a specific body part.

1. Flex the toes of both feet; observe how the toes and feet feel in this tightened state. Now, let go and observe the feeling that accompanies this release.

2. Tighten the legs (calves and thighs) and observe the tension; let go and observe the feeling of relaxation.

3. Tighten the buttocks, hips, and abdominal muscles and observe. Relax these areas and observe.

4. Tighten the muscles of the chest and upper back and observe. Relax these areas and observe.

5. Tighten the hands by making a fist and the arms by flexing at the elbow; observe the tension. Relax the hands and arms and observe.

6. Tighten the shoulders (raise them toward the ears) and observe; let go and observe.

7. Tighten the entire head area—throat and neck, jaw, face, eyes, forehead, scalp—and observe the feeling. Relax and observe the difference as tension flows out of these areas. Let the jaw relax until the lips part slightly.

8. Raise and lower the eyebrows several times. Pull the eyebrows together, as though you are frowning, then release and observe.

9. Tighten the entire body, from toes to scalp. Hold the tightness as long as you can. Let go. Become as limp as a rag doll. Observe.

10. Say to yourself, "I am relaxed. I am relaxed. I am relaxed."

11. Scan your body for any areas of tightness. If you find such an area, mentally "look at" the area and send it an order, "Relax." Repeat for any other areas of tightness.

12. Conclude the procedure by sitting (or lying) quietly for several minutes. Enjoy your state of Relaxation.

As you get up to resume activity, try to maintain the feelings of peace and relaxation. But when you do feel a group of muscles beginning to tighten, think "I am relaxed." You may find it more effective to send the order "Relax" to the specific part of the body where you tend to hold tension, such as the jaw or neck muscles. Your goal is to be able to control stress-related muscle tension just by telling yourself, "I am relaxed" several times. But that goal can be achieved only if you have your body practice "letting go" regularly over a period of time.

Autogenic Training

Autogenic Training was developed by a German physician, Dr. J.H. Schultz. It is usually referred to as "AT" or "the Schultz method." With his patients in a state of deep relaxation, Dr. Schultz used positive statements to "program" his patients for healing.

Dr. Schultz emphasized that each step be practiced until the desired effect occurs. Then and *only then* should the learner go on to the next step. The procedure includes the repetition of one or more positive statements, such as "I am at peace" or "I am in a state of well-being." A person who has learned to go through all the steps of AT reaches a state of *deep relaxation.* The combination of deep relaxation and **affirmations** (positive statements) is especially beneficial.

The following steps are based on The Schultz method. Initially, you will practice only Steps 1 and 2, then terminate the procedure. For that reason, the termination step (Step 9) is presented after Step 2 as well as following Step 8. Regardless of how many steps you perform, *always terminate the session by performing Step 9.* Now, after making the usual preparations, do the following steps:

1. Think, "I am relaxed." Repeat several times.

2. Think, "My right arm is heavy." (If you are left-handed, substitute "left" for "right" throughout this step.) Continue to think, "My right arm is heavy" while focusing your attention on your right arm. When you begin to experience heaviness in the right arm, think "My right arm is heavy and warm." When you experience both heaviness and warmth in the right arm, think "My arms are heavy and warm." Focus your attention on both arms. Experience the heaviness and warmth. When both arms are warm and heavy, think "My arms and legs are heavy and warm." Mentally focus on your arms and legs; consciously experience the heaviness and warmth. Terminate your practice by performing Step 9.

9. Bring yourself out of the relaxed state by opening your eyes, yawning, and stretching for about ten seconds; flex and extend your arms several times.

Practice Steps 1 and 2 for several days. *Do not go to Step 3 until you feel heaviness and warmth in both arms and both legs.*

3. Think, "My heartbeat is strong and regular. My heartbeat is strong and regular."
    Proceed to Step 4 only after you have practiced Steps 1 through 3 for several days. Remember to terminate the procedure with Step 9.

4. Think, "My breathing is free and easy. My breathing is free and easy." Be aware of your breathing, but do not try to control it. As you become more relaxed, your breathing will be shallow and the rate will slow. Your body is using less oxygen, but you will not experience air hunger.
    Practice Steps 1 through 4 for several days before adding Step 5. Terminate the procedure with Step 9.

5. Think, "My abdomen is warm. My abdomen is warm." Focus your attention on the abdominal area. Be aware of the warmth. You may feel this warmth spreading to the hips and around to the low back.
    Practice Steps 1 through 5 for several days, always ending with Step 9.

6. Think, "My forehead is cool. My forehead is cool." Envision a cool breeze blowing lightly across your forehead.
    This is a difficult step for many people. It is an important step, however, so *practice Steps 1 through 6 until you do experience coolness over the forehead.*

7. Think, "My mind is still and quiet. My mind is still and quiet." Experience a period of mental blankness; if any thoughts pop into your mind, mentally repeat "My mind is still and quiet."

8. Think one or more positive statements related to peace, serenity, health and well-being, happiness or joy; if you prefer, use a statement related to your religious beliefs.

9. When you are ready, bring yourself out of the relaxed state by opening your eyes, yawning, and stretching; flex and extend your arms several times. Sit quietly for a few minutes before returning to your day's activities.

Remember, never terminate Autogenic Training without performing Step 9. The circulatory system changes during deep relaxation. It is important that you perform Step 9 to *restore normal circulation to the muscular system before you become physically active.*

Self-directed Relaxation

The most widely used technique for Relaxation is probably some variation on this third method. While learning the procedure, allow at least one full minute for each step; eventually, you will be able to go through Steps 1 through 8 in one to three minutes. After making the usual preparations, mentally direct the process as follows.

1. Think, "My toes and feet are warm." Repeat until you experience warmth in the toes and feet.

2. Think, "My legs are warm." Experience the warm sensation creeping up from the toes and feet.

3. Think, "My hands and arms are warm." Repeat until you can feel the warmth in your hands and arms.

4. Think, "A warm feeling is moving up my spine." Experience this sensation.

5. Think, "The warmth is spreading up the back of my neck and into my scalp." Experience the spreading warmth.

6. Think, "My forehead, face, jaws, and throat are getting very warm." Experience and enjoy this warmth.

7. Think, "My chest is warm." Experience the warmth spreading across your chest and around to your upper back.

8. Think, "My abdomen is warm." Experience the warmth spreading over the abdomen and around to the lower back.

9. Think, "My entire body is warm and totally relaxed."

10. At this point, simply enjoy Relaxation for 20–30 minutes. If you wish, use an affirmation to accomplish some positive result, such as healing or good feelings about yourself.

After mastering Steps 1 through 9, you will experience deep relaxation for almost the full twenty minutes. Afterward, you will be refreshed and energized as you resume your activities.

MEDITATION METHODS

Meditation is a process for achieving a state of mental quietude. It is accompanied by brain waves that are significantly slower than in the thinking/sensing state, but not as slow as in sleep. The meditator is alert, aware of the immediate surroundings but not actively engaged in thinking, planning, analyzing, or other mental activities. Regular meditators find a sense of peace, increased awareness, a greater sense of self, and guidance toward solutions for current problems.

For health care providers, a significant aspect of meditation is its potential as a therapeutic tool. Meditation has a calming effect, which is itself therapeutic. Drs. Shealy, Simonton, Benson and others have found that patients who make meditation a part of their daily routine tend to improve the quality of life. Some of them get well. Many of those who do not become completely free of disease do show marked improvement. Some can be maintained on a lower dosage of medication, while others improve enough to discontinue medication. Needless to say, no patient should abandon medical therapy in order to take up meditation. Rather, meditation is best used as an **adjunct** to other therapies prescribed by the patient's physician.

The therapeutic value of meditation may be enhanced by combining the meditative state with mental imagery (visualization). Cancer patients can be taught to meditate, then mentally visualize the cancer cells being destroyed by the immune system, or visualize a tumor gradually shrinking in size. A patient with an ulcer can visualize the edges of the ulcer healing, gradually decreasing the size of the ulcer until it no longer exists. Some patients learn to control chronic pain through meditation. Meditation and visualization may be learned through reading, cassette tape recordings, or one-on-one instruction accompanied by regular (at least once daily) practice.

Principles

Since physical tension is a **deterrent** to achieving the meditative state, the first task of a beginning meditator is to learn Relaxation. Otherwise, a beginning meditator may spend the first ten to fifteen minutes releasing muscle tension, with only a few minutes spent in meditation.

There is no point in doing a meditation only once. Meditation is a *learning process*, one that must be continued at least several weeks to experience the desired effects. One reason for this lengthy learning period is that meditation requires concentration. The beginning meditator quickly discovers how hard it is to keep attention focused on the meditation itself. After a momentary "good" beginning, various thoughts or feelings surface and suddenly the meditator is thinking, planning, or remembering instead of meditating. These random thoughts and feelings are sometimes referred to as the "inner dialogue" that must be controlled in order to achieve the meditative state. Because complete control comes slowly and *only with practice*, the first challenge is learning to concentrate. This is also one of the early benefits of meditation—increased powers of concentration.

As you begin your first meditation, you will quickly experience this intrusion of thoughts. As soon as you recognize that some thought has captured your attention, gently dismiss it and return to your meditation. Some teachers of meditation suggest ways to avoid the trap of becoming involved with a particular thought. One such technique is considering these thoughts to be leaves floating on the surface of a river or creek. You, sitting on the bank, simply note each passing leaf (thought), but do not become absorbed in observing any one of them.

Do not expect immediate or dramatic results. Meditation is a discipline. Some beneficial effects will be apparent after a month or two of consistent practice. A therapeutic meditation, used faithfully two or more times a day, may begin to have effects after two or three weeks. But meditation for such purposes as stress management, personal growth, personality integration, or spiritual development is a long-term process.

Types of Meditation

There are several types of meditation and many meditative techniques. No one technique is suitable for everyone. The best approach for a beginner is to try a simple meditation for at least two months, and then try a different method for two months. After learning about several types of meditation and trying various methods, the beginning meditator will find one approach that seems "right."

The test of whether or not a meditation is right for you is how you feel afterward. Following a meditation, sit quietly for several minutes, being aware of how you feel. If you feel better than before the meditation, then that method is right for you. If you do not feel good (tired or feel strongly that something is not right), then do not use that particular technique again. Simple meditations seldom have an adverse effect, but you need to be aware of the possibility. Certain advanced meditative techniques are more likely than the simple meditations to prove inappropriate for some people.

Meditation methods can be classified as structured or unstructured. A structured meditation requires the meditator to attend to only one thing at a time: a particular thought, word or phrase, or object. The purpose of this focus is to develop the powers of concentration. Often, an additional effect is some new perception or new understanding. A structured meditation clearly defines what the meditator is to work on; any wandering is corrected and attention returned to the prescribed task.

An unstructured meditation is one in which the meditator identifies facts pertaining to a chosen subject, then focuses on *feelings* about those facts. This type of meditation primarily affects emotions. It is especially useful in a counseling situation, where the meditator can receive professional guidance in dealing with a troublesome area.

Procedures

Both of the meditations described below are structured meditations. The first is designed to build the powers of concentration; the second is a **guided imagery** meditation that should result in a sense of well-being.

Do not try a meditation until you have learned Relaxation; otherwise, you will not get the full benefit of the meditation experience. If you begin to slump during the meditation, pull yourself erect. If you have an itch and cannot ignore it, then scratch. It is better to take care of such a distraction than to spend your entire meditation trying to ignore it.

Breath Counting Meditation

1. Follow the preparation instructions for Relaxation. Set a timer and place it where you cannot hear the ticking or sit where you can see a clock.

2. Sit in a comfortable position. This may be the cross-legged position of Yoga. Otherwise, sit in a straight-backed chair with both feet flat on the floor. Place your hands on your thighs; palms may be down or up. The spine should be straight from head to low back.

3. Take three or four deep breaths. As you inhale, let your abdomen expand, then let the chest expand. As you start to exhale let the chest contract, then let the abdomen contract. Feel your body beginning to relax.

4. Now, give your full attention to counting. Do not try to regulate your breathing; let your body regulate the depth and rate. Inhale, then as you start to exhale think "1." As you start the next exhalation, think "2." Continue up to 4, then start over with 1. You may think "and" during each inhalation if that helps to keep your attention on counting. Do not focus on the breathing itself. Focus on counting, but coordinate the count with exhaling.

5. Continue breath counting for 5 to 10 minutes the first time, gradually increasing the total time to 20 minutes. As your concentration improves, you will have fewer distracting thoughts and the time will pass more quickly. When you have achieved a high level of concentration, you will be surprised when the timer sounds—"I can't believe 20 minutes have passed already!"

6. Sit quietly for a few minutes. As you get up to resume your activities, try to maintain the meditative sense of peace and harmony.

A Guided Imagery Meditation

The purpose of this meditation is to balance body energies and promote a sense of well-being. Follow the preparation steps for Relaxation to put yourself into a relaxed state.

1. Imagine that you have a pipeline running from the end of your spine down through the chair, through the floor, and through the ground right to the center of the earth.

2. Now focus your attention on your feet and their contact with the earth. (Actually, they are probably in contact with the floor, but think of this as being in touch with Mother Earth.) **Visualize** energy rising from the earth and passing through your feet and up your legs. Feel this energy passing into your body, up the abdomen and chest, up the face and over the head, then down the spine and into the pipeline. Visualize this swirling energy picking up any aches and pains, any anger or grief, any and all negativity as it flows through you and into the pipeline. (Yes, you are "flushing" the negativity out of your body!) Continue to run earth energy until your body begins to feel lighter; this could take from one to five minutes.

3. Now visualize a brilliant white light coming from above and entering the top of your head. Let this light flow through your torso, down your legs and into your feet and toes. Let more light flow into your neck and shoulders and down your arms into the hands and fingers. Feel this light filling your entire body and spreading out from your body about 18 inches, so that you are within a capsule of healing, protective light. Experience the light until you are ready to end your meditation.

4. Open your eyes and sit quietly for several minutes. You should feel refreshed and energized. Try to maintain the meditative sense of peace and harmony as you resume your activities.

CONCLUSION

You have now learned several methods for managing stress. As students in a health care educational program, you experience the stress of assignments and tests. As you carry out clinical assignments, you experience the stress of the health care setting, which may be somewhat overwhelming to you at this point. In addition, you experience the stress associated with your other life roles. Recognize that you are subject to many stressors and be good to yourself. Eat right, sleep right, take time to play and use a stress management technique at least once each and every day!

References and Suggested Readings

Carrington, Patricia. *Freedom in Meditation.* Garden City, NY: Anchor Press/Doubleday, 1977.*

Dacher, Elliott S., M.D. *Psychoneuroimmunology: The New Mind/Body Healing Program.* New York, NY: Paragon House, 1993.* Chapter 3, "Mindfulness," pp. 30–56; Exercises: "Mind-talk," pp. 41–44; "Mindfulness," pp. 45–50; "Training Yourself in Mindfulness," pp. 51–52; "A Modified Mindfulness Training Exercise" (For individuals with a restless mind), p. 53; "Mindfulness" (In daily living), p. 54.

Davis, M., Eschelman, E.R. & McKay, M. *The Relaxation and Stress Reduction Workbook; Fourth Edition* Oakland, CA: New Harbinger Publications, 1995.*

Dass, Ram. *Journey of Awakening: A Meditator's Guidebook.* New York, NY: Bantam Books, 1978.*

Gawain, Shakti. *Creative Visualization.* New York, NY: Bantam Books, 1982.*

Kabat-Zinn, Jon. *Wherever You Go, There You Are.* New York, NY: Hyperion, 1994.* "Sitting Meditation," pp. 103–126; "Walking Meditation," pp. 145–148.

Jacobson, E. *Progressive Relaxation.* Chicago, IL: University of Chicago Press, 1938.*

———. *You Must Relax.* New York, NY: McGraw-Hill, 1957.*

———. *Anxiety and Tension Control.* Philadelphia, PA: J. B. Lippincott, 1967.*

Samuels, Mike, M.D. and Samuels, Nancy. *Seeing with the Mind's Eye.* New York, NY: Random House, 1975.* Chapter 9, "Visualization Techniques," pp. 120–133.

REVIEW AND SELF-CHECK

Complete the following statements in your own words, but using the ideas presented in this unit.

1. The expression "mind-talk" refers to _____ .

2. "Mindfulness" is a mental state in which _____ .

3. Two effective techniques for stress management are _____

   _____ , and _____ .

*These references contain instructions for Relaxation and/or meditation. Also, some of the books listed under Suggested Readings in Units 23 and 24 contain meditations; see Shealy, Simonton, Benson, Borysenko, and Siegel.

4. Relaxation (the process) may be defined as _____ .

5. Two reasons recreational activities are not adequate for effective stress management are: _____

    and _____ .

6. The primary physiological effect of Relaxation is _____ .

7. The primary physiological effect of meditation is _____ .

8. Relaxation (the process) differs from the generally accepted meaning of "relaxation" in the following ways: _____

    and _____ .

9. The long-term effects of meditation include the following psychological changes: (1) _____ , (2) _____ ,

    and (3) _____ .

10. A disadvantage of meditation is that the long-term benefits are not experienced unless _____ .

11. Two reasons a health care provider should use a stress management technique at least once a day are _____

    and _____ .

ASSIGNMENT

1. Explain in your own words each of the following terms. If the term is not defined in Unit 25, use your knowledge gained from other courses, a dictionary, or the Glossary to obtain a definition relevant to the content of this unit.

Adjunct	Affirmation	Autonomic
Blood lactate	Visualization	Deterrent
Guided imagery		

2. For one week, list the stressors you experience in class, in the clinical area, at home, and in your various relationships.

3. Indicate with an "A" the stressors that arouse anxiety.

4. Use the following two procedures, adapted from exercises in Dr. Dacher's book *Psychoneuroimmunology*. (For the full exercises, see pages 41–51.) Use a clock or watch, preferably with a second hand, to time certain steps as indicated below.

   a. To become aware of the power of mind-talk to control your mind:
   - Settle into a comfortable position, note the time, then close your eyes.
   - For three minutes, be aware of any thoughts that occur to you.
   - Notice how one thought leads to another, in endless procession.
   - Begin to label each thought as it occurs: a memory, expectation about a future event, a judgment about an event or someone, something you like or dislike.
   - Become aware of any feelings that arise as certain thoughts occur: fears, anxieties, anger, guilt, pleasure.
   - For the next two minutes, count the thoughts that occur. Open your eyes and note the position of the second hand and the minute hand. Now, give your full attention to your breathing, excluding all thoughts of any type. As soon as a thought occurs, note the positions of the second hand and minute hand. How long were you able to focus on your breathing, without any thought occurring? You probably maintained the focus on your breathing for only a few seconds, certainly for less than a minute. This illustrates the power of mind-talk.

   b. To learn how mindfulness can control mind-talk:
   - Observe your breathing—the movement of air in and out of your nostrils, the movement of the chest wall, or the expansion and contraction of the abdomen during inspiration and expiration.
   - When a thought occurs, be aware that your attention has shifted from focusing on the breath to focusing on mind-talk. Without trying to control it, just quietly observe your mind-talk. Note that as you observe without getting involved, your body becomes more relaxed.
   - Gently return to focusing on the breath. Each time a thought occurs, repeat these two steps. The length of time you can maintain your focus on the breath will increase with practice. Now, you should also be more aware of how mind-talk automatically controls your attention, *unless you take conscious control.*

NOTE: The previous exercise introduces you to the first stage of mindfulness—attention. The next two stages, concentration and meditation, may be achieved as you practice Relaxation and, if you choose to do so, one or more meditation exercises.

5. For the next two weeks, use a Relaxation technique either before breakfast or dinner.

6. For the following two weeks, try a different Relaxation technique.

7. After you have completed Activity #6, try a third method. Then plan a long-range stress management program using the method you prefer.

8. Optional: After you have mastered one or more Relaxation techniques, try a simple meditation once a day for at least one month. If you find meditation beneficial, read about meditation as you continue to practice. You may eventually outgrow the simple meditations and want to explore some of the more complex types of meditation. Many of the references listed under Suggested Readings in Units 23–26 provide guidance and/or meditation procedures.

Unit 26

A Broadening View of Health Care

OBJECTIVES

Upon completion of this unit, you should be able to:

- Name two defenses against being exploited by a quack.
- List four possible indicators of quackery.
- Explain the primary characteristic of a holistic approach to health care.
- State the focus of the specialized areas known as psychoneuroimmunology and energy medicine.
- State one characteristic of osteopathy, chiropractic, hypnosis, psychotherapy, biofeedback, and homeopathy.
- Name two alternative therapies that influence energy flow through the body.
- Name three therapies that use pressure points to stimulate energy flow and relieve energy blockage.
- State the primary difference between acupuncture and acupressure.
- Name five effects of therapeutic massage.
- State two responsibilities of a health care provider to someone who asks advice about an alternative therapy.

KEY TERMS

Dogma	Dysfunctional	Thermograph
Misalignment	Invasive	Malalignment
Subluxation	Paradigm	Posthypnotic
Autohypnosis		

As pointed out in previous units, numerous changes are occurring in medical practice and the delivery of health care. Some of these changes affect the roles and responsibilities of various health care providers—for example, people are utilizing a variety of alternative therapies to assist in stress reduction or to alleviate a specific health problem. Unit 26 is designed to help you differentiate between possible quackery and legitimate alternative therapies, identify some of the changes occurring within orthodox medicine, and know the characteristic features of some common alternative therapies.

WHAT IS LEGITIMATE THERAPY? WHAT IS QUACKERY?

A legitimate health care provider does not make false promises. A legitimate health care provider employs appropriate therapies and encourages each patient, even in the presence of serious illness, to maintain hope and a positive attitude. On the other hand, the possibility of quackery exists if a practitioner:

1. *Promises* a "cure"

2. Claims to have a *secret method* not available to other practitioners

3. Demands a large payment "up front"

4. Becomes defensive or evasive about his or her qualifications

Recognizing unrealistic claims of curative power is the first line of defense in protecting oneself from a fake healer. The second line of defense is determining the qualifications of the practitioner.

The recognized roles in health care services require some type of formal education. Qualified professional practitioners display in their offices at least two college or university degrees and a license from the state or a certificate from a recognized professional organization. Qualified practitioners of an alternative therapy also have documentation. Educational programs that prepare a specific type of practitioner issue a certificate or diploma to those who successfully complete the program of study. In some states, certain alternative practitioners must be licensed by the state.

If such documentation is not displayed, ask to see written evidence of the practitioner's qualifications. A potential client has the right to know the qualifications of a practitioner, especially when a fee is involved. If questions regarding licensure, certification, or educational preparation make the practitioner defensive, evasive, or even uncomfortable, it may be better to seek help elsewhere.

A field that does not require educational preparation and licensure is psychic healing. Dr. Shealy and Dr. Elmer Green at the Menninger Institute have studied psychic healers, such as Olga Worrall. They were able to demonstrate in a scientifically controlled experiment that Mrs. Worrall could affect another person by what she called "sending energy." Dr. Dolores Krieger has demonstrated that Therapeutic Touch may actually change the composition of blood (i.e., an increase in hemoglobin). Actual changes in body structure or function

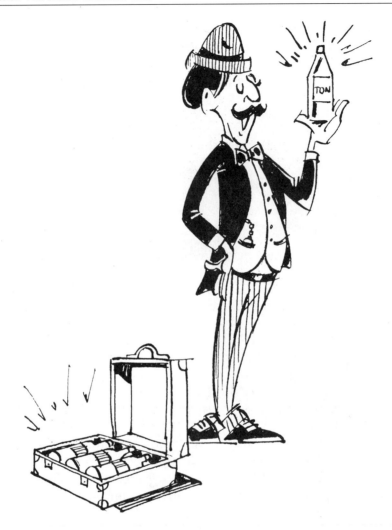

resulting from "energy transfer" from one person to another have now been demonstrated, but the *how* and *why* are not fully understood at this time. Be aware that true psychic healers such as Mrs. Worrall are relatively rare. Mrs. Worrall considered her ability to heal others a divine gift, and she used that gift with humility and compassion to benefit others. Most psychic healers do not charge, although they may accept a contribution to a church or charitable organization that sponsors their work.

Implications for Health Care Providers

As a health care provider, you may be asked for a recommendation or opinion about an alternative therapy or a particular practitioner. Exercise caution in

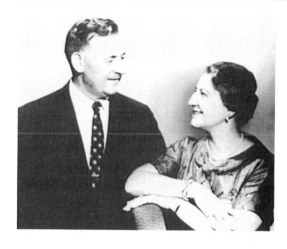

Olga Worrall with her husband, Ambrose, who was also a psychic healer.

responding to such a request. Your best and safest approach is to help that person obtain the information needed for (1) evaluating the proposed therapy or practitioner, and then (2) making his or her own decision. Do not make such a decision for someone else. Instead, point out the educational, licensure, or certification requirements for the therapy being considered. You should also know what is a legitimate title. Anyone may call themselves "counselor," "therapist," or "healer." But the terms "licensed" and "certified" can be used legally only if the practitioner has been granted that title by the state, an educational program, or a professional association.

Each person who considers the services of any nonmedical therapist has a responsibility to evaluate the qualifications of the practitioner, then make a *conscious decision* based on information about that specific therapy and that particular practitioner. After a reasonable trial period, another *conscious decision*—to continue or not continue—should be based on whether or not the therapy is beneficial. The need for careful evaluation of a therapy and provider is less critical, however, if the therapy is offered through a holistic health center headed by a physician or other health-related *professional* practitioner. The employing agency has a responsibility to check credentials and determine if the practitioner is competent.

THE HEALING PROFESSIONS

Changes in health care during the past two or three decades include changes in medical practice and roles. Health care was once the sole domain of the medical doctor and the dentist, but numerous other professional practitioners are now involved in some aspect of health care. The growth in holistic medicine has contributed to greater involvement of nonphysicians (i.e., psychologists, counselors, nutritionists, and exercise physiologists) in health care, with increasing emphasis on individual responsibility of the patient to participate in decisions regarding his or her health care program.

Holistic Medicine

According to Donald Ardell, author of *High Level Wellness*, "holistic" means:

> . . . *viewing a person and his or her wellness from every possible perspective, taking into account every available concept and skill for the person's growth toward harmony and balance. It means treating the person, not the disease. It means using mild, natural methods whenever possible. For the person, it means engaging in a healthier lifestyle to enjoy a higher level of wellness. The holistic approach promotes the interrelationship and unity of body, mind, and spirit. It encourages healthy, enjoyable activity on all these levels of existence. A holistic approach differs from simply following an "alternative" therapy. It is not an alternative to conventional medical practice. Rather, it includes judicious use of the best of modern western medicine combined with the best health practices from East and West, old and new. (p. 5).*

Although this description may seem idealistic or even impractical, the holistic approach simply requires that the patient's mental, emotional, and spiritual aspects be considered, in addition to the physical functions that are the focus of orthodox medical practice. Further, the patient's total life situation is considered, with special attention to stress factors and to any **dysfunctional** attitudes and beliefs. Treatment includes whatever orthodox medical interventions are indicated, plus measures to decrease the effects of stress and to correct any dysfunctional attributes that have been identified. The total treatment plan may include one or more unconventional therapies, such as acupuncture, biofeedback training, or neuromuscular massage therapy. Some of these unconventional therapies are provided by nonmedical health care providers.

In *The Creation of Health*, Dr. Shealy and co-author Carolyn Myss describe the characteristics of a holistic health care practice. Table 26–1 lists some characteristics that may be considered to form a theoretical foundation for the holistic approach to health care. Note that the patient's willingness to assume responsibility for his or her health is not only acknowledged, but viewed as essential to healing. This *involvement of the patient in decision-making* is difficult for many allopathic physicians, who are accustomed to a *dominant* role in the doctor/patient relationship. The holistic physician, however, is comfortable in a *cooperative* doctor/patient relationship. Dr. Shealy states, "Any physician who denies the patient the right to choose or who pushes a given therapy is, by definition, not holistic." (Shealy, 1993)

In emphasizing the spiritual aspects of illness and health, Dr. Shealy is not speaking of religion, but rather of the subtle aspects of *being human*, such as feelings, beliefs, will, intuition, compassion, and tolerance for other beings,

TABLE 26–1
Theoretical Basis for Holistic Health Care*

- Every illness or physical malfunction is complex and has multiple causation.
- Illness is the result of mental, emotional, physical, attitudinal, and spiritual stress, in addition to environmental, chemical, electrical, and cosmic forces.
- Spiritual stress arises from fear, anger, guilt, frustration, anxiety, and depression.
- A healthy attitude and healthful habits are essential to a healthy body.
- Unhealthy habits represent a deficiency in love, wisdom, reason, and will.
- Resistance to disease is the result of heredity, maternal habits and nutrition, and lifetime exposure to various environmental influences.
- Treatment must be directed toward healing emotions and spirit, in addition to treatment of physical symptoms.
- Thoughts, feelings, and beliefs of the patient are tools that may be used to rebuild the body.
- The patient is actively involved in decisions: treatment, changes in lifestyle, changes in beliefs and attitudes.
- The patient is responsible for the healing process.
- Denial blocks the healing process.
- The therapist's task is to facilitate the healing process.

*Based on Shealy & Myss, *The Creation of Health,* Chapters 1 and 2.

beliefs regarding the cosmos and/or the Divine. Dr. Shealy believes that science and technology, which currently characterize the health care system, must begin to encompass spirit in order to humanize the practice of medicine. When the delivery of health care services does embrace these holistic concepts, the roles of all health care providers will be affected. There will be greater emphasis on *therapeutic interaction* as patient care procedures are performed. Table 26–2 lists some characteristics of the future health care system, as perceived by Dr. Shealy.

The belief that patients must assume greater responsibility for their health is reflected in the current activities of former U.S. Surgeon General Everett Koop. As Surgeon General, Dr. Koop was responsible for establishing policy for the U.S. Public Health Service; in that role, he represented allopathic medicine. During 1996, he began a project to develop a medical video series for the public. Explaining the need for this series, Dr. Koop stated that the best way for a patient to face a medical condition is to *take responsibility and become knowledgeable.* Only two or three decades ago doctors considered information about diseases to be their exclusive domain! This example of greater openness of

---

TABLE 26-2
Holistic Characteristics of a Health Care System of the Future*

- Patient care will be provided by a team.
- The *minimum* team will consist of a physician (M.D. or D.O.), nurse, physical therapist, psychotherapist, and the *patient.*
- Team members will consciously develop their intuitive skills as an aid to identify each patient's needs.
- Spinal manipulation and massage will be an integral part of the treatment plan.
- Acupuncture and electromagnetic forms of therapy will be used, in association with music and sound, to balance the patient's energy system.
- The patient will be taught the elements of a healthy lifestyle, including principles of good nutrition.
- The use of Relaxation techniques will be considered an essential part of a healthful lifestyle.
- An exercise program will be an essential part of the patient's healthy lifestyle.
- Naturopathic concepts and homeopathic remedies will be incorporated into medical practice.
- Spiritual healing will be encouraged to provide the framework for physical, chemical, emotional, and behavior therapies.
- Therapeutic touch and other forms of energy therapy will be accepted.
- Holistic health education will be part of the school curriculum, beginning in kindergarten.
- Parents will attend classes to improve parenting skills and learn to incorporate holistic health practices into family living.
- Patients will be expected to confront their negative beliefs and attitudes and change unhealthy habits.

---

*Based on Shealy & Myss, *The Creation of Health*, Chapter 2.

allopathic medicine to patient involvement is encouraging to proponents of the holistic approach.

A startling wake-up call to orthodox medicine was delivered when a special article to *The New England Journal of Medicine* was printed in the January, 1993 issue. A group of health professionals associated with several medical schools and major hospitals conducted a survey during 1990 to determine the extent to which the American public was using unconventional therapies. The findings clearly indicated that the American public is seeking and using numerous unconventional therapies, either in conjunction with medical care or as an alternative. Some of the major findings of this study include:

- *One in three* U.S. adults used an unconventional therapy in 1990

- Visits to providers of unconventional therapies *exceeded* the number of visits to primary care medical doctors nationally

- Out-of-pocket expenditures for unconventional therapies were comparable to out-of-pocket expenditures for all hospitalizations

- About one out of every four Americans under the care of a medical doctor for a *serious health problem* also used an unconventional therapy

- Seven out of ten unconventional therapy encounters *occurred without the knowledge of the medical doctor.*

This article in a prestigious medical journal received much attention in the medical community and was brought to the attention of the public by articles in the mass media. Subsequently, a number of significant changes began to occur. Some medical practices and health care agencies broadened their scope to include one or more alternative therapies as an option for patients. The U.S. Congress directed the National Institutes of Health to establish an Office of Alternative Medicine. Two journals of alternative medicine have been established. Numerous books by physicians and other professionals with a holistic perspective have been published. Newsletters that emphasize the holistic approach and/or the use of natural remedies are now available.

The remainder of this unit is devoted to preparing you to understand and accept some of these changes: several emerging areas in medicine, some non-medical systems of therapy, and specific therapeutic techniques. Some were among the "unconventional therapies" included in the 1990 survey; all would be included, or at least accepted as having potential value, in the holistic health care system of the future.

Psychoneuroimmunology

It has long been accepted in conventional medicine that emotional factors may affect various body functions, even to the point of changing body structure, as in an ulcer. There is now compelling evidence that mental/emotional states affect the immune system. The "mind/body connection" is being studied extensively by researchers such as Dr. Pelletier, Dr. Joan Borysenko and her husband, Dr. Myrin Borysenko, an immunologist. This area of research is called psychoneuroimmunology (PNI), an interdisciplinary field involving such disciplines as psychology, biophysics, biophysiology, and medicine. Dr. Shealy considers PNI to be "one of the most exciting and innovative fields today." PNI includes the study of mental factors (i.e., attitudes, thoughts, beliefs) and stress on the immune system. PNI research is also identifying neurochemicals that are released in association with anger, hostility, guilt, and other negative emotional states.

Dr. Elliott Dacher believes that PNI research is demonstrating the capacity of individuals for self-healing. Attaining competence in self-healing requires learning and using several techniques for regulating and directing one's life. Two essential components of self-healing are mindfulness and self-regulation. Mindfulness, achieved through meditative practices, may lead to insight and creativity, which in turn may lead to self-regulation and healing. Dr. Dacher has incorporated training in these powerful techniques in his medical practice; as a result, his patients learn how to participate in their own healing. Dr. Dacher also conducts workshops to teach these techniques to groups, especially health care providers, and has published a text/workbook for helping people learn mindfulness and self-regulation through independent study and practice.

Energy Medicine

Dr. Elmer Green, first President of the International Society for the Study of Subtle Energies and Energy Medicine (ISSSEEM), says that in 1964 he discussed with a prominent psychiatrist the kind of scientific program presented twenty-seven years later at ISSSEEM's 1991 conference. The psychiatrist, a leading researcher in psychiatry and mental health, believed that the scientific world would not be ready to accept the mind/body relationship before the year 2000. Since that discussion in the early 1960s, Dr. Green has pioneered research on the power of the mind to influence autonomic body functions and on the conscious/unconscious mind interaction.

Dr. Green believes that biofeedback research and interest in human potential have contributed to greater readiness of the scientific community "to seriously examine evidence that had long been put aside, ignored, pushed under the rug, because it contradicted the presently-accepted scientific **paradigm.**" (ISSSEEM Newsletter 2:1) The development of techniques and instruments sensitive enough to measure the body's "subtle energies" has stimulated interest among many researchers. The energy pathways of the body have been mapped, thereby validating scientifically the existence of the meridians. The electromagnetic fields of the body are being studied. By the year 2000, the knowledge that is just beginning to accumulate may well be the basis for new therapies involving techniques that influence body energies. Energy medicine is a new frontier in medicine; the discoveries that emerge will very likely have a profound effect on health care and therapeutic procedures.

Osteopathy

The first school of osteopathic medicine was established in Missouri in 1892. Originally, osteopathy was fiercely opposed by the medical establishment but was widely accepted by the public. The basic theoretical foundation for osteopathic practice is that musculoskeletal disorders, especially any **malalignment** in the vertebral column, interferes with circulation of blood, flow of body energies, and other functions essential to good health. Osteopathic technique originally consisted of manipulations to relieve tension around the spinal column. The educational preparation of osteopaths was gradually extended until it became as lengthy as medical education, the primary difference being instruction in manipulation of the spine as a therapeutic tool. Eventually, osteopaths were accepted by teaching hospitals for specialization in such areas as surgery and obstetrics. Most general hospitals now grant staff privileges to osteopaths. In addition, there are one hundred eighty osteopathic hospitals in the United States; some general hospitals have an osteopathic wing. There are now fifteen colleges of osteopathic medicine. All states and Canada have licensure requirements for osteopaths. The osteopathic physician uses the legal title "D.O." (Doctor of Osteopathy) instead of "M.D." (Doctor of Medicine).

Chiropractic

The basic theory underlying the practice of chiropractic is that any **subluxation,** or **misalignment,** of a vertebra creates pressure on one or more nerves where they emerge from the spine. This pressure interferes with proper function of the nerve, which then affects the functioning of the body part served by that nerve. The purpose of a chiropractic treatment, then, is to remove pressure from the nerve by restoring each vertebra to its proper alignment. A chiropractor uses X-ray films, various tests of body movement and muscle strength, measurements (i.e., length of the legs, level of the hips, level of the shoulders), and palpation to locate problem areas.

A malalignment of the spine may result from normal daily activities. Sitting for long periods of time, poor posture, and poor body mechanics when bending or lifting have an adverse effect on spinal alignment. Any fall, a car accident, even a sudden stop, can result in malalignment or damage to the soft tissues surrounding the spine. The most frequent symptoms are low back pain, headache, pain in the temporomandibular joint (TMJ), pain that radiates down the leg or down one arm. The injury known as whiplash involves the muscles of the neck and shoulders; once the swelling and pain of whiplash have subsided, a malalignment of one or more cervical vertebrae may be found.

The underlying philosophy of chiropractic is that correction of any problem that interferes with nervous system functioning enables the body to heal itself. Chiropractic treatment consists of adjustments at specific points to correct subluxations and relieve nerve pressure, plus a number of other techniques as needed by the individual patient: traction, cold, heat, massage, acupressure, ultrasound, or electromagnetic stimulation. As muscle spasm diminishes and spinal alignment improves, the chiropractor may recommend exercises to strengthen the affected area or to improve posture. Many chiropractors do a nutritional analysis and recommend dietary changes. Chiropractors do not recommend either prescription or over-the-counter (OTC) drugs because of the risk of side effects. Many chiropractors do recommend herbal or homeopathic remedies, especially for management of pain during the acute phase.

Chiropractic education is a four-year postbaccalaureate program, so it is equal in length of time to medical and osteopathic education. Licensure, required in every state, is based on a National Board Examination. Some states permit chiropractors to use acupuncture; other states limit acupuncture to medical practitioners. The legal title for a chiropractor is D.C. (Doctor of Chiropractic).

Psychotherapy/Counseling

The area of practice known as psychotherapy originated with the work of Freud, beginning around 1880. Freud's concern with the mind—a radical new approach in medicine—eventually resulted in a new medical specialty, psychiatry. Initially, the specific concern of psychiatry was mental illness. But during the last forty years the human potential movement emerged. People became aware that developing their full potential was hindered by such problems as poor adjustment, lack of assertiveness, inability to cope with life problems, poor interpersonal skills, and addiction. The demand for services to help people deal more effectively with their life situations led to rapid growth of the mental health field.

As a result of this expansion, mental health ceased to be the domain of medicine, specifically the psychiatrist. Professional counseling emerged as a field of practice, related to but different from psychiatric practice. Most psychotherapists work with clients who are not mentally ill, but need help in learning to cope with some type of life problem—release suppressed emotions, correct faulty thought patterns, improve interpersonal skills, or modify the dynamics within a family or work setting.

Mental health is now an interdisciplinary field involving psychologists, social workers, counselors, ministers, recreation therapists, occupational therapists, music therapists, and art therapists. The educational preparation varies from about six years (for a master's degree) to eight or more years (for a doctorate) in such fields as psychology, social work, pastoral counseling, family therapy, or counseling (clinical, addiction, rehabilitation). Titles of professional workers in the field include Licensed Clinical Psychologist, Licensed Clinical Social Worker (LCSW), Licensed Marriage and Family Therapist (LMFT), Certified Rehabilitation Counselor (CRC), and Certified Addiction Counselor (CAC). If a practitioner uses a term such as "licensed counselor" or "certified counselor" rather than one of the above legal titles, it would be wise to ask,

(1) "Licensed (or certified)by whom?" and (2) What is the special area of licensure (or certification)? Unless a license was issued by the state or a certificate issued by an educational program or professional association, the term "counselor" is meaningless.

THERAPEUTIC TECHNIQUES

Most therapeutic techniques consist of someone doing something *to* someone else. With increasing emphasis on individual responsibility for health and healing, there is greater interest in techniques people may use to help themselves, such as Relaxation or meditation to manage stress. Some of the techniques described below involve a continuing therapist/client relationship. Others are self-help techniques to be used as needed or on a regular basis as part of a health maintenance program.

Homeopathy

Homeopathy was developed as a therapeutic system by Samuel Hahnemann, a German physician who had become dissatisfied with medical practices of the early 1800s. The basic notion of homeopathy is that "like cures like." For example, the tears and runny nose of a new cold are like the tears and runny nose produced by close contact with raw onions. Therefore, allium (Latin for "onion") in *very small* doses could be used to treat a cold. Over a period of many years, Dr. Hahnemann used volunteers to determine the effects of a large amount of many substances—plant, mineral, and animal. He then matched these effects to the symptoms of various disorders and experimented to find the dilution (i.e., the minimal amount) of that substance that would control those specific symptoms. This procedure—determining the effects of a specific substance—is known as "a proving." After many years of research and clinical trials, Dr. Hahnemann's use of homeopathic remedies was so effective that he developed a large following of patients and other physicians throughout Europe.

Homeopathy has been practiced in Europe and India for over 200 years. In England, there are two levels of homeopathic medical practice. At one level, the homeopathic physician has been trained in diagnosis and treatment according to the methods of Dr. Hahnemann and his followers. Another level of homeopathic physician has completed orthodox medical training, then specialized in homeopathy. Homeopathic hospitals were included in the British National Health Service when it was established in 1947. The royal family of Great Britain has used homeopathic physicians for several generations.

Homeopathic remedies are prepared according to very precise measurements and procedures. The original solution, usually an alcoholic extract, is diluted repeatedly to produce the dilution used as a remedy. The more dilute a remedy is, the more powerful its effects. This is known as the "potency idea" or "potentiation." The extreme dilution of homeopathics is the basis for rejection of homeopathy by many allopathic physicians, even though extreme dilutions are the basis for desensitization procedures used by allopathic physicians to treat allergies. The manufacture of homeopathics is regulated by the Food and Drug Administration. The *Homeopathic Pharmacopoeia of the United States* is the official source of detailed information about every homeopathic medication. Homeopathics are available without a prescription. Consultation with a homeopathic physician is the preferred approach to using homeopathics, but may be difficult to obtain in many communities.

Homeopathy was popular in the United States during the 1800s. In 1900, there were twenty-two homeopathic colleges and fifty-six homeopathic hospitals. There were also homeopathic sanitariums, mental asylums, and children's hospitals. Increasing opposition from conventional medicine during the early 1900s led to the decline of homeopathy; the last homeopathic college closed in 1930. (Campbell, 1996) Six decades later, there is renewed interest in homeopathy in the United States. The National Center for Homeopathy teaches postgraduate courses for physicians, so acceptance and use of homeopathy is slowly spreading throughout the medical community.

Homeopathy has already gained a large following among those who wish to take responsibility for their own health. It is another facet of the broad spectrum of therapeutic alternatives. Many people prefer homeopathy not only because they have found it effective, but also because of its total safety, a notable contrast to the risk of side effects from many pharmaceuticals. Most health food stores carry a variety of homeopathics, and some national drug store chains now have a homeopathic section.

Homeopathy differs from conventional medicine in many respects. In homeopathic medicine, the totality of symptoms is considered before selecting an appropriate medicine. The individuality of the patient is important, and the individual characteristics of each illness are considered in detail. No one symptom determines the treatment; rather, the complex of symptoms presented indicate which homeopathic is indicated. Table 26–3 shows how each aspect of a headache indicates one or more homeopathic remedies, but the total picture presented by the patient's symptoms would determine the specific medication of choice. Usually, a medication is used every three to four hours, but only as long as symptoms are present. Sometimes, one or two doses will clear up all symptoms. If the patient has not recovered after two days, symptoms are reviewed and another remedy started, based on the total picture at that time. Table 26–3 illustrates an important point: not all headaches (or sore throats, coughs, or colds) are the same; each illness must be considered in regard to many specific factors before selecting a homeopathic remedy.

TABLE 26–3
Matching Symptoms to Homeopathic Remedies: Headache

	SYMPTOMS	PREFERRED HOMEOPATHIC REMEDY*
PAIN:	Intense, throbbing	Belladonna, Sanguinaria
	Sharp, knife-like	Sanguinaria
	Stinging, burning	Spigelia
	Band around the head	Gelsemium
	Steady ache	Bryonia
ONSET:	Sudden	Belladonna
	In morning	Bryonia, Nux vomica
	In back of head	Gelsemium, Sanguinaria
END:	Sudden	Belladonna
FOCUS:	Forehead	*Belladonna*, Bryonia, Pulsatilla
	Right eye	Sanguinaria
	Right side of head	Belladonna, Gelsemium, *Sanguinaria*
	Left eye	*Bryonia*
	Left side of head	Belladonna, Spigelia
	Changes frequently	Belladonna, Pulsatilla, Sanguinaria
OTHER:	Hands and feet cold	Belladonna
	Face flushed, hot	Belladonna
	Recurrent pattern	Sanguinaria
	Visual disturbances	Gelsemium
	Fatigue, looks tired	Gelsemium
	Nausea	Nux vomica
	Sensitive to light	Belladonna
	Sensitive to noise	Belladonna, Spigelia
	Sensitive to movement	Belladonna, *Bryonia*, Nux vomica, Sanguinaria, Spigelia
	Sensitive to touch	Belladonna
	Sensitive to strong smells	Belladonna
	Irritable	Bryonia, Nux vomica
	Wants to be left alone	Bryonia, Gelsemium
	Wants to be comforted	Pulsatilla
MADE WORSE BY:	Warmth or cold	Spigelia
	Motion	Belladonna, *Bryonia*, Nux vomica, Gelsemium, Sanguinaria, Spigelia
	Going down steps	*Belladonna*
	Walking briskly	Pulsatilla
	Blowing nose	Pulsatilla
MADE BETTER BY:	Firm pressure	Belladonna, Bryonia, Pulsatilla, Sanguinaria
	Sitting	*Belladonna*
	Being up & about	Nux vomica
	Gentle motion	Pulsatilla
	Walking slowly in open air	Pulsatilla

*Italics indicate preferred remedy for that symptom

(Adapted from Cummings & Ullman, *Everybody's Guide to Homeopathic Medicines*.)

Administration of a homeopathic medicine is different from pharmaceuticals. A homeopathic medicine should be taken at least twenty minutes before eating or thirty minutes after eating or drinking. Homeopathics come in the form of small globules, tablets, and liquids. The globules and tablets must not be touched; the desired number should be poured into the lid or dispenser top of the vial, then dropped under the tongue. They are very soluble, so absorption usually requires a minute or less. Liquids are dispensed in a dropper bottle; the drops should be placed on the tongue and left there until absorbed.

The practice of homeopathic medicine is regulated by the states. Most states allow the use of homeopathy by licensed health care professionals: medical doctors (M.D.), osteopaths (D.O.), naturopaths (N.D.), dentists (D.D.M. and D.D.S.), chiropractors (D.C.), and veterinarians (D.V.M.). Interestingly, because homeopathics are inexpensive, safe, and easy to use, a layperson can learn to select appropriate medications for many common illnesses. Several hours of study and possession of one or more good references can be used to cope with numerous health problems. Obviously, any acute illness or an illness that does not respond to home treatment should be evaluated by a licensed health practitioner.

Hypnosis

Hypnosis is a mental state in which the attention is fixated on an idea or problem selected by the individual or by the hypnotist. There are many misconceptions about hypnosis, due in part to theatrical depictions of its use for evil purposes or for the entertainment of an audience. Hypnosis does not give the hypnotist control over another person's will or values.

As a health care provider, you need to know that hypnosis can be an effective therapeutic tool. It is currently used by many doctors and dentists to control pain or to produce anesthesia in a particular area of the body. It is used by some psychotherapists to help patients change habits (i.e., smoking) or deal with anxiety in a specific situation (i.e., taking a test). For example, a psychotherapist accompanied a cancer patient to the oncology clinic and hypnotized her just before chemotherapy was administered. Under hypnosis, the patient was told that she would have no nausea following her chemotherapy—and she didn't! This is an example of **posthypnotic** suggestion, in which the hypnotized subject is prepared to behave in a certain way after the hypnosis session has ended.

The hypnotic state may be induced by another person, the hypnotist, or it may be self-induced once the procedure has been learned. In order to be effective, four conditions are necessary.

1. The individual is willing to be hypnotized and is ready to deal with a specific problem or gain a specific benefit from the hypnosis session.

2. The individual achieves physical relaxation, either through a specific breathing routine or a relaxation procedure.

3. The individual achieves a hypnotic state in which there is intense concentration on the problem or desired effect.

4. While the individual is in a hypnotic state, a suggestion is made that is intended to have a specific effect, either during the hypnotic period (as for a dental procedure) or at some later time following the hypnotherapy session. Some counselors teach selected clients to practice **autohypnosis** (auto = self) between therapy sessions.

Hypnosis is a powerful tool. It is not a game. It should be performed only by a trained hypnotherapist. Teachers of hypnotherapy usually only accept as trainees persons who have a valid reason for learning hypnosis. Professional practitioners learn hypnotherapy by participating in a workshop or taking a series of classes. A qualified hypnotherapist will probably have a certificate that indicates completion of hypnotherapy training. There are no state licensure requirements for hypnotherapy.

Biofeedback

Biofeedback is a method for helping a person learn to control some body function. The equipment used depends upon the particular problem, but always includes some type of feedback—lights or sounds that signal when a physiological change occurs. Some of the early work with biofeedback involved teaching patients how to relieve migraine headaches. The patient was placed in a comfortable position and instructed to warm the fingers. A **thermograph** attached to one finger could detect a slight change in temperature—too slight for the patient to be aware of. A blinking light informed the patient that he or she was getting the desired result. Patients who successfully learned to relieve the headache could not explain what they did, yet they could invoke the process as needed. This is the basis of biofeedback. Without feedback to signal onset of the desired change, patients would not know when they are gaining control—that is, doing the right thing to get the desired effect.

Biofeedback, then, is a learning tool. It is not therapy as such, but it can enhance any therapy that involves learning to gain control of some body function. A person who has tension headaches may learn to relax the muscles of the neck, upper back, forehead, and scalp with the help of biofeedback that measures muscle tension. A person who has paralysis of certain muscles can be encouraged by biofeedback equipment that measures the slightest gain in movement. A hypertensive patient can, with the help of a special type of blood pressure cuff, learn to lower both the systolic and diastolic blood pressure. A person with tachycardia may be able to learn to stop an episode within

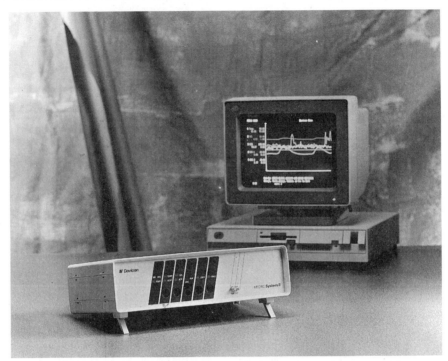

Biofeedback equipment. (Courtesy of Davicon, Inc., Boston, MA)

minutes of onset. Someone with Reynaud's disease may learn to dilate blood vessels in the area, thereby improving circulation.

Vickie was being treated for Reynaud's disease with drug therapy, but it was not effective. Circulation in the left index finger became so bad that her doctor told her the finger should be amputated. As an executive secretary whose keyboard skills were essential to her job, Vickie was opposed to amputation of her finger. She sought a less drastic alternative. A psychotherapist used biofeedback to help her learn to warm her fingers. Over a period of several weeks, circulation to the finger improved and amputation was not necessary.

Note that some of the conditions mentioned above could be reactions to stress. Some critics of biofeedback maintain that the results are due to the patient achieving a state of relaxation. Others maintain that the results are due to processes not yet understood. In spite of the fact that "why" or "how" biofeedback works is not fully understood at this time, it does help some people learn to manage a serious health problem. Because biofeedback is associated with the clinical setting, some people who would not make the effort to learn Relaxation or meditation will utilize biofeedback. For those patients who can learn to monitor and regulate a body function, biofeedback is an alternative to drugs, surgery, or having to live with a difficult problem.

Biofeedback is usually prescribed by a physician, although a patient who has heard about it may actively seek a therapist who offers biofeedback. Usually a physician or psychologist is in charge of biofeedback training, but the actual sessions may be conducted by a technician. Some training is required to learn to use the various types of equipment. Equipment vendors usually provide instruction to the staff of an agency that purchases their equipment. There is no state regulation of biofeedback at this time.

ALTERNATIVE THERAPIES

Most of the commonly used alternative (i.e., nonmedical) therapies involve a hands-on technique (as in massage), the application of pressure at specific points (as in acupressure and reflexology), or influencing the flow of body energies (as in Therapeutic Touch and polarity therapy). Some practitioners use a variety of techniques, according to a patient's specific problem. Others specialize in one particular technique and use it exclusively. Some of the alternative therapies can be learned readily by a health care provider and used to enhance basic patient care. Some may be used to enhance a practitioner's own health and well-being.

Therapeutic Touch

Therapeutic Touch is a system of healing developed by Dr. Dolores Krieger, a professor of nursing at New York University. Therapeutic Touch has its roots in an ancient practice known as "laying on of hands." Dr. Krieger has validated its effectiveness scientifically during nine years of research on healing, followed by six years of clinical application. Several thousand nurses have attended workshops to learn the procedure, which may be readily incorporated into nursing practice. It is possible to learn the procedure from a book, but supervision by an experienced therapist is better.

Therapeutic Touch involves the hands but not touching, in spite of the name. Throughout the process, the hands are held one to three inches away from the body but within the body's electromagnetic field. There are four steps.

1. Centering, that is, focusing inward

2. Assessing the client's energy field to locate areas of congestion, deficit, or imbalance

3. Mobilizing the client's energy field to establish a free flow of energy

4. Directing energy to the client to raise the client's energy level, establish balance and fill in any areas of deficit

Dr. Krieger believes that the use of the hands for healing is a "universal human act." In her words:

*Therapeutic Touch has recaptured this simple but elegant ancient mode of healing and mated it with the rigor and power of modern science; there is hard evidence that treatment by Therapeutic Touch affects the healee's (patient's) blood components and brain waves, and that it elicits a generalized relaxation response. (*The Therapeutic Touch, *p. 16)*

By "hard evidence," Dr. Krieger means data collected through a scientific experiment. Those data indicate that physiological changes occurred during the time that Therapeutic Touch was being used. She believes that the power of Therapeutic Touch lies in the ability of the healer to *direct* the flow of energy. The healing effect is due to providing a boost in energy, which in turn accelerates the body's healing capacities. She states, ". . . in almost every case there comes a moment when it must be acknowledged that it is the patient who heals himself." (p. 17)

Therapeutic Touch is especially effective in relieving pain and inducing a profound state of relaxation. Therapeutic Touch also can be used for self-healing as a meditation/visualization, in which you visualize energy from above entering your body and flowing through it. The hands can be placed over an area of discomfort, while visualizing energy flowing into the affected area. Those who wish to incorporate a religious aspect into the healing may think of the light as Divine Light.

Healing Touch

The Healing Touch Program is an energy-based system of therapy developed by Janet Mentgen, RN who has been practicing energy healing since 1980. The goal of Healing Touch (HT) is to facilitate self-healing by restoring harmony and balance in the energy system. This is accomplished by using one or more specific techniques drawn from the work of six other energy healers, including Dolores Krieger. HT is now used extensively in all clinical areas of nursing. It can be incorporated into the practice of other health care providers who are in direct contact with patients. The procedures can also be learned by persons without a medical background who wish to develop healing abilities.

HT was first offered as a pilot project at the University of Tennessee and in Gainesville, Florida in 1989. It is now offered as a multilevel program throughout the U.S., Canada, Australia, New Zealand, and the Netherlands. Upon completion of Level III, the trainee is eligible to apply for certification. Certified HT therapists can establish their own practice. The HT therapist does not diagnose or prescribe, nor does the therapist perform any medical treatment. HT does not involve actually touching the client. The HT therapist works with the electromagnetic energy field that surrounds the physical body and with the chakras—energy centers located along the spine and at other specific points along the meridians.

In 1988, Janet Mentgen was honored as Holistic Nurse of the Year by the American Holistic Nurses Association. Since that time, she and other HT instructors have taught the techniques of HT to approximately twenty thousand persons in the United States alone. During 1995, workshops were held in forty-one states and in four other countries, with over 7,800 participants. Obviously, many people are finding these techniques valuable. The power of HT can be experienced by participating in a Level I workshop, which tends to convert even the skeptical participant into a believer in the energy system of the body.

Polarity Therapy

Polarity therapy is also concerned with the transfer and balancing of energy. Dr. Randolph Stone, an osteopathic physician/chiropractor/doctor of naturopathy, developed a rather involved system for balancing body energies. His system included relaxation exercises, manipulations, diet for cleansing the body, yoga, and other techniques for maintaining a healthful flow of body energies.

A simplified system of polarity therapy is widely used today. It can be learned from a textbook or through one-on-one instruction. Receiving a polarity balancing treatment from a practitioner, or serving as the subject for someone who is learning polarity therapy, quickly increases your awareness of body energies and the extent to which they can be influenced.

Polarity therapy includes a variety of techniques designed to balance the body's energy flow and to remove any negative energy.

1. The hands are placed in a sequence of positions and held there for several minutes, until a tingling or pulsing sensation indicates that the energy is flowing.

2. The hands "sweep" the body and extremities with a light brushing motion that removes negative energies.

3. The fingers are used to apply gentle pressure at specific points, especially on the feet, to remove any blockage in energy flow.

4. Specific moves are utilized according to each patient's problems and needs.

At the completion of a polarity session, the client is relaxed and has a sense of well-being, but feels energized upon resuming activity. Polarity therapy requires that one person apply the technique to another. It is not limited to one-on-one sessions, however.

The Polarity Circle, described by Richard Gordon in *Your Healing Hands: The Polarity Experience,* is a powerful healing tool. Six people (the healers) form a circle around a seventh, who is in the dorsal recumbent position. Each person places the hands at two specific points; the positions are held until there is a "sensing" that the energy flow has been balanced. It is interesting that this sensing usually occurs simultaneously with several of the healers; it may occur after five minutes with some clients, but not for 20 or 30 minutes with another.

There is no provision for certification or licensure of polarity therapists. Schools for massage therapy include polarity in the curriculum. Any Certified Massage Therapist knows polarity, but may or may not include it in a massage session. Many massage therapists use a combination of massage and one or more energy-balancing techniques.

Stimulation of Reflex Points

A number of therapeutic techniques utilize certain points for stimulating energy flow or for releasing a blockage in energy flow. Acupuncture is an **invasive** procedure, in that the skin is penetrated. Acupressure, Shiatsu, and reflexology utilize many of the same points as acupuncture, with the advantage of being noninvasive.

Acupuncture

Dr. Borysenko tells of watching a surgeon remove a lobe of a patient's lung with the patient wide awake, talking and sipping tea. The only anesthesia being used was acupuncture. When Dr. Borysenko expressed amazement, a physician also observing shrugged his shoulders and commented that it was only "hypnosis and other crazy stuff." Dr. Borysenko uses this example to explain "blocks of reframing" or being "stuck"—ways of holding on to old knowledge, beliefs, or opinions. Someone who has a block to reframing rejects any new information that does not fit the familiar "frame," *even when evidence of the new information is observed first-hand.*

Acupuncture is a good example of new knowledge (new at least to U.S. physicians until the early 1970s) that was rejected because it conflicted with existing beliefs and with **dogma** of the medical community. But acupuncture is widely practiced in other countries and is gaining acceptance in the United States. Dr. Shealy believes that acupuncture has great potential for relief of chronic pain. Others see it as a desirable alternative to the numerous risks of rendering a patient unconscious with anesthesia.

Acupuncture is a complete system of healing governed by principles developed some five-thousand years ago in China. Having withstood the test of time, it is today an integral part of Oriental medicine. Vital body energies, known as *chi*, flow through the body along twelve meridians; blockage in this flow of body energy results in disease. Meridians are named according to the

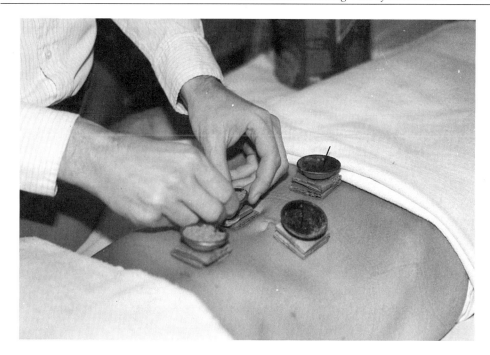

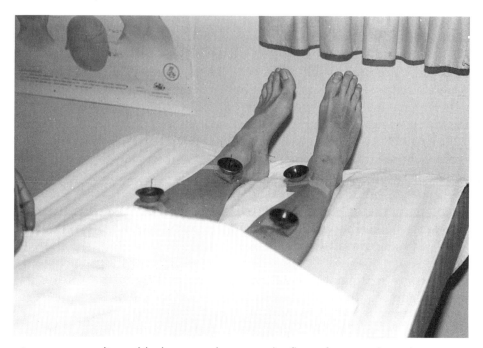

Acupuncture relieves blockages and restores the flow of energy through one or more meridians. (Courtesy of George Milowe, M.D. Photographer: Mike Nelson)

body organs; specific points along each meridian are related to some organ or area elsewhere in the body. Acupuncture technique consists of inserting one or more fine needles at appropriate points to relieve blockages and restore the flow of body energies. For example, the point for relieving neck pain is in the knee area, as is the point for the gall bladder. There is even a procedure for treating addicts by stimulating specific points in the ear lobe! The underlying theory of acupuncture is complex, and extensive knowledge is required for safe and effective use of the technique.

Most acupuncture practitioners in the United States have gone to the Orient or England for training. Some medical centers in the United States now offer training in acupuncture for medical personnel. The Traditional Acupuncture Institute in Columbia, Maryland offers a three-year course leading to the Master of Acupuncture degree. Many of the students and some faculty members are nurses.

Some states limit the practice of acupuncture to medical doctors; others license trained acupuncturists with or without a medical degree. Anyone considering the use of acupuncture should determine the qualifications of the practitioner—educational preparation *and* licensure.

Acupressure

Acupressure is widely practiced throughout China and is now gaining followers in this country. Acupressure is a noninvasive alternative to acupuncture for relief of pain or muscle tension and for boosting one's energy level. When acupressure successfully stimulates the flow of energy (i.e., relieves a blockage), it stimulates self-healing by the body. Acupressure may be learned and used by anyone, may be self-administered, and is safe. The technique involves using the fingers, knuckles, or even an elbow to apply pressure at specific locations. Points that are relevant to the problem are tender. After locating a tender point, the acupressurist applies pressure for several seconds, then releases. The pressure-release sequence is repeated for several minutes until tenderness at that point disappears.

There are numerous books from which one may learn acupressure. There are also several centers where health practitioners may learn advanced techniques. The practice is not regulated, meaning that a practitioner does not have to be licensed. Those who complete a course or workshop are awarded a certificate from the school or center that offers such training. Word-of-mouth recommendations and personal experience are about the only means of determining the effectiveness of the procedure or a particular practitioner.

Shiatsu

Shiatsu is the Japanese adaptation of acupressure. In Japanese, the word *shiatsu* means "finger pressure." Shiatsu consists of a rhythmic application of pressure

POINT LOCATION CHARTS

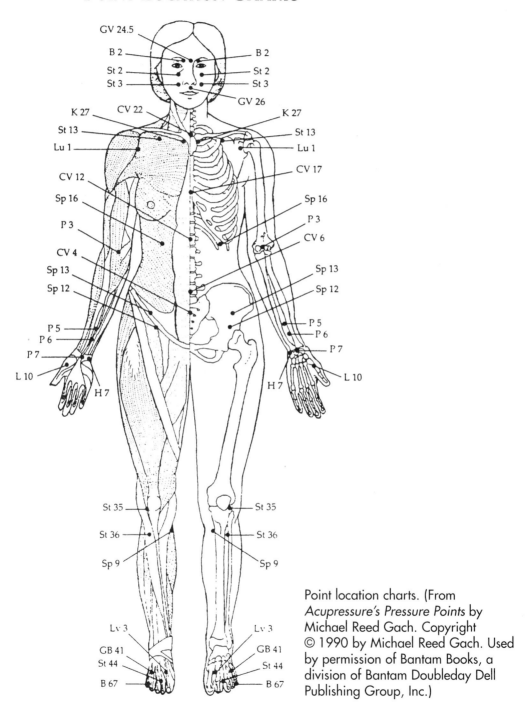

Point location charts. (From
Acupressure's Pressure Points by
Michael Reed Gach. Copyright
© 1990 by Michael Reed Gach. Used
by permission of Bantam Books, a
division of Bantam Doubleday Dell
Publishing Group, Inc.)

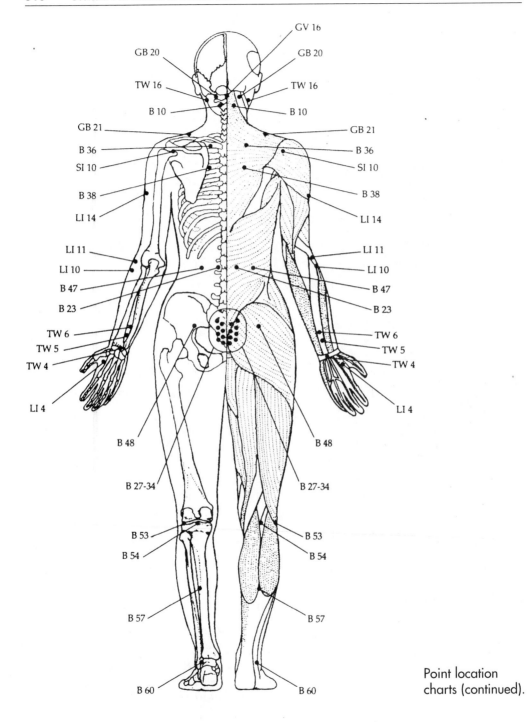

Point location charts (continued).

at specific points, using the thumbs, fingers, or palms. Detailed charts show the points at which pressure should be applied for a specific purpose. For areas above the neck, pressure is applied for no more than three seconds. In other areas, pressure is applied for seven seconds. If a particular point is painful, pressure should be light; every few minutes, pressure can again be applied to the painful spot. The point becomes less painful with each application of pressure until, eventually, deep pressure can be applied. Shiatsu can even be self-administered to relieve a headache, toothache, or other pain in a specific area. Performed by a therapist, Shiatsu is a form of whole-body therapy. Many massage therapists use selected Shiatsu points to enhance the effectiveness of a therapeutic massage.

Some schools of massage therapy include Shiatsu in the curriculum. New York state requires completion of a course in Shiatsu to qualify for the massage therapy licensure examination. Although Shiatsu is complex and best learned through formal training, the basic technique may be learned from a well-written textbook. Any therapist who wishes to use the technique on clients should participate in a workshop, enroll in a Shiatsu course, or obtain one-on-one instruction from a qualified Shiatsu practitioner. States do not regulate the practice of Shiatsu.

Reflexology

It has been suggested that the footwashing mentioned in the New Testament was actually foot reflexology—a ritual in which a host or hostess made a newly arrived guest comfortable by washing and massaging the feet. Reflexology uses specific pressure points on the hands and feet that correspond to specific organs or body areas. For example, a line along the arch of the foot corresponds to the spine. A person with neck pain has tender points toward the front of the arch; one with low back pain, toward the heel end of the arch. The reflexology points have been mapped; charts show the points on the feet and hands that correspond to specific body areas. Reflexology may be used therapeutically, but is especially effective if used once a week as a preventive measure. At the end of a reflexology session, the client is usually completely relaxed. One reflexologist says her clients always leave with "happy feet."

Massage schools include reflexology in their curriculum. The International Institute of Reflexology in St. Petersburg, Florida offers a two-week course and certifies graduates as "reflexologists." Faculty from the Institute offer workshops throughout the world, including numerous sites within the United States. Although learning the basics of reflexology from a good textbook may be adequate for self-use or for working on friends and family, anyone who claims the title "reflexologist" should be certified by an educational program. The states do not regulate the practice of reflexology. The following illustration shows reflex points on the feet from the therapist's view (i.e., the left foot is on the right side of the diagram).

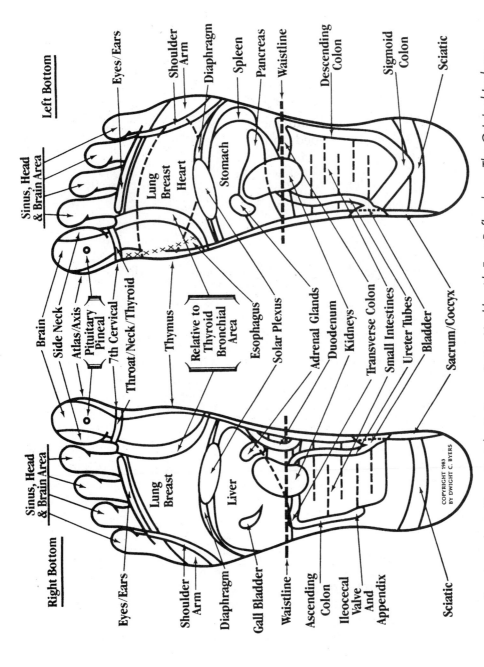

Foot reflexology chart. (From Dwight C. Byers, *Better Health with Foot Reflexology: The Original Ingham Method.* Courtesy of Ingham Publishing Company and the International Institute of Reflexology, P.O. Box 12642, St. Petersburg, FL 33733–2642.)

Massage Therapy

Massage is an ancient therapeutic technique. Swedish massage, probably the best-known type, consists of several basic techniques and specific procedures for manipulating the soft tissues. Swedish massage was originally developed as a medical treatment, performed only by a masseur (male) or masseuse (female) with extensive training. At one time, massage was the primary technique used by physical therapists; today, however, most physical therapists use a variety of techniques but very little "hands-on massage."

With growth of the holistic health movement, numerous variations on basic Swedish massage were developed and massage therapy has emerged as an effective health care alternative. Most massage therapists use some of the basic techniques encompassed by Swedish massage. Many massage therapists incorporate polarity therapy and pressure point therapy into the massage routine. A neuromuscular massage therapist also uses pressure at certain points to stimulate nerve function, which then improves muscle activity in the area.

Certain techniques are especially effective for specific problems, such as sports injuries, tension headaches, whiplash, or muscle spasm. A weekly massage is a pleasant way to release tension and an excellent stress management technique.

The advantages of massage therapy are numerous, regardless of which particular method is used. Some specific benefits include:

- Improved performance and increased stamina (for athletes)
- Accelerated healing (following muscle or joint injuries)
- Correction of body alignment (especially in conjunction with osteopathic or chiropractic adjustments)
- Improved circulation, as tense muscles relax
- Improved elimination, as increased blood flow through the muscles removes accumulated waste
- Improved balance and coordination as posture, alignment, and muscle function improve
- Decrease in anxiety, as excess lactic acid is removed from muscles and blood
- Release of suppressed emotions that may be the basis of long-term muscle spasms
- Increased energy as muscle tension is released, since tight muscles tend to trap energy
- Relief of pain and/or muscle spasm associated with such conditions as arthritis, chronic neck or back pain, asthma, multiple sclerosis, and other chronic disorders

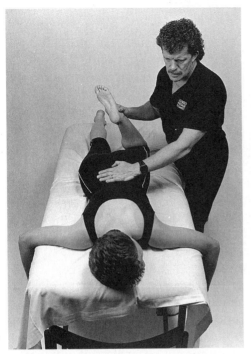
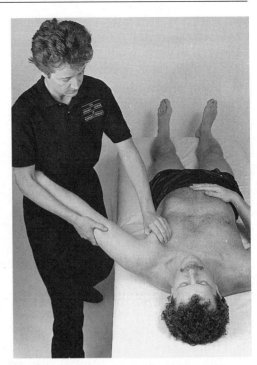

Massage therapy has numerous benefits. (Courtesy of Chicago School of Massage Therapy, Marc Harris.)

A Certified Massage Therapist (CMT) has completed a formal course of instruction. Available courses vary in length from about 100 hours to several thousand hours. A legitimate massage therapist is completely professional and respects the modesty of the client at all times. The massage therapist does not diagnose or prescribe, but does need information about any existing health problem and the reason for seeking massage therapy.

Licensure requirements vary from one state to another. In those states that do not require a license, learn the educational qualifications of any practitioner being considered as a therapist. Qualified massage therapists are willing to discuss their educational preparation. (Be aware that the term "massage parlor" sometimes means house of prostitution.) The best recommendation for a massage therapist (or any health care provider) comes from satisfied clients.

THE SELF-HELP TREND

Public interest in alternative therapies seems to have evolved out of the self-help movement. The human potential movement focused on freeing oneself from psychological and mental blocks, in order to "be all that you can be." That movement resulted in a flood of "pop psychology" self-help books on such topics as assertiveness, self-esteem, communication, interpersonal relationships, and sexuality. The result was a marked change in attitudes toward responsibility for increasing one's effectiveness in coping with life situations and improving relationships. Then various health organizations began to emphasize exercise and a healthful diet, further encouraging individual responsibility for health and well-being.

The current interest in alternative therapies seems to be a natural outgrowth of these earlier movements. Also, more and more people recognize that modern life involves high levels of stress. One can seek escape from stress and life problems through such crutches as tranquilizers or alcohol. Or, one can utilize stress-reduction techniques and modify lifestyle to eliminate some sources of stress. If a chronic health problem exists for which allopathic medicine can only offer symptomatic relief through drugs, one can follow that route or seek an appropriate alternative therapy. With the growth in self-help and individual responsibility, more and more people do opt for an alternative therapy. And many of those seek an alternative that they or a family member can administer.

Seeking Guidance and Instruction

Obviously, becoming informed about possible alternatives is the first step. Libraries and bookstores offer a wealth of information on the topics discussed in this unit, as well as numerous others. The ideal is to participate in a workshop or short course designed for the public. Some junior/community colleges and vocational/technical schools now offer such courses in their noncredit divisions. One popular course is Massage for Couples; another is Reflexology. But it is also possible to learn some techniques by reading, watching an experienced person, or even having a session with a therapist.

Techniques for Self-Management

The person who is seeking techniques for self-help probably has already assumed some degree of responsibility for health management. That does not mean that the individual fully understands all that is involved in achieving optimal health. If you have the opportunity to help such a person, encourage the individual to learn about wellness rather than to seek help for a single problem. That means considering lifestyle, stressors in the life situation, stress management techniques, nutrition, exercise, and any mental/emotional factors that may be affecting physical health. By now you surely recognize that this is the holistic approach. High level wellness (and, in the case of chronic diseases, recovery) cannot be achieved without a holistic approach. Remember the difference between "curing" and "healing"? The goal for every patient should be true healing, so that optimal health, whatever that might be *for that individual,* can be achieved.

Some self-help techniques can be learned from books and articles. Others, such as identifying emotional factors that need to be resolved, may be accomplished more readily with professional help. The person who begins a self-help program alone may experience improvement, then become aware of the need for help. Whatever the approach, most of the following will contribute to improvement in one's overall health:

- Awareness of choices that affect health

- A *conscious* choice to modify lifestyle

- Daily use of a stress management technique

- Self-study, workshops, and/or counseling to release feelings related to old traumas, unmet childhood needs, unresolved conflicts

- One or more techniques for directing the flow of body energies and releasing blockages

ROLE OF THE HEALTH CARE PROVIDER

As a health care provider, you have a responsibility to encourage a patient to have faith in the doctor and in the prescribed therapy. Inevitably, however, you will encounter someone (patient, relative, friend) who wants advice about an alternative therapy or about some self-help approach. It is not wise to give such advice. But Section VII should have broadened your view enough that you may help such a person obtain the information needed to evaluate a proposed alternative. This represents a departure from the "old" attitudes, namely that any nonmedical approach is "quackery."

It is up to you to use your best judgment in each situation. An open mind combined with a healthy dose of skepticism is a good combination. Just do not deny someone the potential benefit of an alternative therapy simply because you are ignorant about it or because it is not offered in your particular health care agency at this time.

References and Suggested Readings

Becker, Robert O., M.D. *Cross Currents.* Los Angeles, CA: J.P. Tarcher, 1990.

Byers, Dwight C. *Better Health with Foot Reflexology: The Original Ingham Method.* St. Petersburg, FL: Ingham Publishing, Inc., 1983.

Cummings, Stephen & Ullman, Dana. *Everybody's Guide to Homeopathic Medicines.* New York, NY: The Putnam Publishing Group, 1991.

Dacher, Elliott S. *PNI: The New Mind/Body Healing Program.* New York, NY: Paragon House, 1991.

Feinstein, Alice (ed.). *The Visual Encyclopedia of Natural Healing.* Emmaus, PA: Rodale Press, 1991.

Feltman, John (ed.). *Hands-On Healing*. Emmaus, PA: Rodale Press, 1989.

Gach, Michael Reed. *Acupressure's Potent Points: A Guide to Self-Care for Common Ailments*. New York, NY: Bantam Books, 1990.

Gordon, Richard. *Your Healing Hands: The Polarity Experience*. Santa Cruz, CA: Unity Press, 1978.

Krieger, Dolores. *The Therapeutic Touch: How to Use Your Hands to Help or to Heal*. New York: Prentice-Hall, 1986.

Krieger, Dolores. *Accepting Your Power to Heal: The Personal Practice of Therapeutic Touch*. Santa Fe, NM: Bear & Company Publishing, 1993.

Kunz, Kevin and Kunz, Barbara. *Hand and Foot Reflexology: A Self-Help Guide*. New York, NY: Prentice-Hall, 1982.

Lindner, Ohasi and Lindner, Vicki. *Do-It-Yourself Shiatsu*. New York, NY: E.P. Dutton Publishers, 1976.

Lowe, Carl and Nechas, James W. et. al. *Whole Body Healing*. Emmaus, PA: Rodale Press, 1983.

Macrae, Janet. *Therapeutic Touch: A Practical Guide*. New York, NY: Alfred A. Knopf, 1988.

Shealy, C. Norman & Myss, Caroline M. *The Creation of Health: The Emotional, Psychological, and Spiritual Responses that Promote Health and Healing*. Walpole, NH: Stillpoint Publishing, 1993.

Siegel, Alan. *Polarity Therapy: The Power That Heals*. Garden City, NY: Prism Press.

Ullman, Dana. *Discovering Homeopathy: Medicine for the Twenty-First Century*. Berkeley, CA: North Atlantic Books, 1991.

Journals and Newsletters Devoted to Holistic Health Care and/or Natural Healing

Larry Dossey, M.D., Exec ed. *Alternative Therapies in Health and Medicine*. Inno-Vision Communications (a division of the American Association of Critical-Care Nurses (AACN), Aliso Viejo, CA 92656. 1-800-899-1712. (Bimonthly journal)

Homeopathy Today. Newsletter of the National Center for Homeopathy.

The Institute for the Advancement of Health. *Advances*. 16 E. 53rd St., New York, NY 10022. ($39 membership fee, quarterly journal and monthly newsletter.)

Richard Leviton, ed. *Alternative Medicine Digest: The Voice of Alternative Medicine*. Future Medicine Publishing, P.O. Box K, Milton, WA 98345.

Julian Whitaker, M.D., ed. *Health & Healing: Tomorrow's Medicine Today*. Phillips Publishing Co., 7811 Montrose Rd., Potomac, MD 20854. (Monthly newsletter)

David G. Williams, N.D., ed. *Alternatives for the Health Conscious Individual*. Phillips Publishing Co., 7811 Montrose Rd., Potomac, MD 20854. (Monthly newsletter)

Sources of Additional Information

Acupressure Institute, 1533 Shattuck Ave., Berkeley, CA 94709. (Books and videotapes on acupressure.) 1–800–442–2232.

American Holistic Nurses Association, 4101 Lake Boone Trail, Suite 201, Raleigh, NC 27607.

American Shiatsu Association, 295 Huntington Ave. Boston, MA 02015.

Campbell, Anthony. The Royal London Homeopathic Hospital Trust. Internet address: ecampbell@rlhh.demon.co.uk

Colorado Center for Healing Touch, Inc., 198 Union Blvd., Suite 204, Lakewood, CO 80228. 303–989–0581.

International Institute of Reflexology, P.O. Box 12642, St. Petersburg, FL 33733. 1–813–343–4811.

National Center for Homeopathy, 801 North Fairfax St., Suite 306, Alexandria, VA 22314. email: nchinfo@igc.org (Information packet $6)

Nurse Healers and Professional Associates Cooperative, Inc., 175 Fifth Ave., Suite 3399, New York, NY 10010.

The American Massage Therapy Association, 1130 West North Shore Ave., Chicago, IL 60626.

The American Polarity Therapy Association, P.O. Box 44-154, Somerville, MA 02144.

REVIEW AND SELF-CHECK

Complete the following statements, using information from Unit 26.

1. Two ways to protect oneself against quackery are:

   _____ and

   _____ .

2. Four behaviors that may indicate quackery:

   _____ , _____ ,

   _____ , and _____ .

3. The primary characteristic of a holistic approach to health care is _____

   _____ .

4. A specialized area concerned with studying the effects of mind and emotions on the nervous system and the immune system is _____

   _____ .

5. Energy medicine is a specialized area concerned with studying _____

   _____ .

6. Two therapeutic methods that influence the flow of body energies are

    _____ and _____ .

7. Three therapies that stimulate specific points to unblock the flow of

    energy: _____ ,

    _____ , and _____ .

8. The primary difference between acupuncture and acupressure is: _____

    _____ is an invasive procedure and

    _____ is not.

9. Six beneficial effects of therapeutic massage:

    _____   _____

    _____   _____

    _____   _____

10. If someone asks a health care provider for advice about an alternative
    therapy, his or her responsibility is:

    a. _____ and

    b. _____ .

ASSIGNMENT

1. Participate in a class discussion about how a health care provider should
    respond to a request for advice about using a specific alternative therapy
    for a chronic problem.

2. Participate in a class sharing session. Those who have experienced
    an alternative therapy may share their experiences. Those who
    have *observed first-hand* (hearsay is not acceptable) the effects of an
    alternative therapy on a family member or close friend may share their
    observations.

3. As a class project, planned with your instructor, find out what alterna-
    tive therapies are available in your community. Present findings to the
    class as oral reports or, with the approval of your instructor, invite an
    alternative therapist to speak to the class and demonstrate one or more
    therapeutic techniques.

Glossary

aberrant: deviation from normal or from a specific standard.

abstinence: voluntary avoidance of a specific substance or behavior.

abuse: improper treatment; may be verbal or physical, resulting in injury to the victim; also, may be sexual, involving a child or unwilling adult.

abuse, drug: misuse or overuse of a drug, legal or illegal.

acceptance: approval or belief in an idea, someone, or something.

accusative statement: a form of blaming directed toward a particular person or group.

adaptation: the process of changing in order to fit into new circumstances.

adaptive response: physiological changes that enable a person to deal with an emotion-arousing situation; "fight or flight" reaction.

addiction: physiological dependence on a substance; cessation results in withdrawal symptoms.

adjunct: supplementary to something that is primary; the adjunctive substance, treatment or procedure tends to enhance the effectiveness of the primary substance, treatment or procedure.

adjustment: the degree to which one is dealing successfully with life situations.

adrenalin: the hormone produced by the adrenal glands during emotion-arousing situations; increases muscular strength and endurance; prepares the individual for "fight or flight."

adverse: unfavorable, harmful.

affirmation: a positive statement that fosters a sense of well-being, often used in association with Relaxation or meditation.

affluent: having an abundance; wealthy.

aggression: a form of behavior that usually indicates hostility; may take the form of verbal attack, physical attack, or refusal to cooperate.

alcoholism: physiological dependence on alcohol.

allopathic: pertaining to therapy that relies primarily on drugs; as currently used, refers to medical practice in which drug therapy and surgery are the most common forms of treatment.

alternatives: two available choices. (See *options*.)

alternative therapy: a nonallopathic therapy; term preferred by most practitioners of various alternative therapies. (See also *complementary therapy*.)

altruism: concern about the well-being of others; may lead one to perform charitable acts.

amateurish: lacking the experience and competence of a professional.

ambiguity: vagueness or lack of clarity.

amputation: removal of a body part; may be surgical or traumatic.

analgesic: substance that relieves pain without causing loss of consciousness; less potent than a narcotic.

androgynous: having both female and male characteristics.

anticipatory grieving: grieving experienced during a terminal illness, or before the death of a loved one.

appraisal: an evaluation or estimate.

aptitudes: natural tendencies, talents, or capabilities. Those who have an aptitude for a specific area (i.e., mathematics) learn material related to that area more easily than someone who does not have that aptitude.

aspiration: goal, desire for achievement.

assumption: acceptance of something as fact without evidence or proof.

attitude: disposition toward something specific; includes feelings, beliefs, and behavior.

authoritarian: relating to authority; sometimes used to imply unquestioning obedience to authority.

autism: an extreme state of withdrawal in which there is little or no interaction with others.

autohypnosis: self-induced trance, usually for a specific purpose.

autonomic nervous system: the part of the nervous system that controls the activity of vital organs.

autonomy: the state of functioning independently, without outside control or direction.

behavior: conduct or actions.

bereavement: separation from or loss of someone who is very significant in one's life.

bias: prejudice.

biorhythm: the rhythmic or cyclic patterns of various physiological processes and functions.

bisexual: oriented toward both males and females as sexual partners.

blood lactate: the level of lactic acid in the blood stream.

bona fide: genuine, in good faith.

brain death: condition in which cerebral functions, brain stem functions, or both are absent.

burnout: a state of physical and mental exhaustion due to cumulative stress.

capabilities: unexpressed traits that may be developed under the proper conditions.

causation: that which produces a specific effect.

cessation: a ceasing or stopping.

chromosomes: rod-shaped bodies that carry the genes containing hereditary characteristics; each cell (except the germ cells) has forty-six chromosomes in the nucleus.

circadian rhythms: intrinsic rhythms with a period of twenty-four to twenty-five hours; especially relevant to the sleep cycle.

clarification: explanation or qualification of something.

clarity: clear, unambiguous.

co-dependency: relationship in which the dysfunctional behavior (usually alcoholism or drug addiction) of one person meets certain needs of the other (i.e., a wife receives satisfaction from "rescuing" her alcoholic husband).

collaborate: to cooperative with, work together toward a common goal.

comatose: in a coma, unconscious.

compatible: existing together harmoniously.

compensation: (1) a defense mechanism in which a substitution of some type provides temporary relief from the discomfort of an unmet need, but does not actually satisfy the need; (2) some form of payment or reward.

complementary therapy: a nonallopathic therapy; preferred by many medical doctors over the term "alternative therapy."

condolences: expressions of sympathy.

conformity: tendency to be like others, to observe the conventions of a group.

congenital: a condition present at the time of birth.

consequence: the result of an action or behavior.

conservator: one who has been legally designated to protect the interests of a person who is unable to manage his or her affairs.

consistency: tendency toward uniformity in each occurrence.

convalescence: the period of recovery from an illness or accident.

counteract: to make ineffective, reverse the effects of something.

counterpart: having the same function or occupying the same level of position.

covert: hidden, not observable; opposite of overt.

covert noncooperation: hidden form of noncooperation; a form of passive aggression that involves deceit.

cremation: the disposal of a corpse by means of fire.

crisis: a significant event that may result in radical changes in one's life.

criterion: a standard used as a basis for a judgment or decision.

culpable: being held responsible for; guilty; being blamed.

cultural bias: a distortion of judgment about a person or group because of their cultural background or social class.

cumulative: increasing by steps.

curative: tending to cure or heal.

cynicism: distrustful of human nature or motives.

DNA: acronym for de-oxy-ribo-nucleic acid, the substance that contains the hereditary makeup of each cell.

daydreaming: a defense mechanism that involves escaping into fantasies through one's imagination.

debilitating: weakening; impairing one's strength.

defense mechanism: a mental device that helps one avoid uncomfortable feelings or makes one's behavior seem more reasonable.

denial: (1) a tendency to avoid recognizing or acknowledging a situation that, if not denied, would cause emotional pain or embarrassment; (2) the usual immediate reaction to an unfavorable diagnosis; (3) the first stage of dying, according to Dr. Kubler-Ross.

dependency: reliance on someone or something for support.

desensitize: make a person less sensitive to something; alter reactions to some situation or event.

desertion reaction: a form of withdrawal that may occur when a very young child or an elderly person is left in the care of someone other than a family member.

detachment: aloofness; withdrawal, usually associated with suppression of feelings.

deviation: a variation from normal or some established standard.

digital: using the fingers or toes.

discrimination: different treatment of a person because of some specific characteristic, such as age, gender, race, religion, national origin, or economic status.

disoriented: confused.

displacement: a defense mechanism in which strong feelings (usually anger) about one person are transferred or directed to someone else who did not initially arouse the feelings.

dis-stress: a state of discomfort that is due to long-term stress or ineffective ways of managing stress.

dogma: established opinion; a point of view proposed as authoritative without adequate grounds; a code of authoritative tenets.

drug dependence: term currently used without specifying either dependence or addiction.

dynamic: characterized by ongoing changes; energetic.

dysfunctional: faulty or disturbed function.

egocentric: concerned primarily with self.

emotions: inner feelings that are responses to life situations, memories, or thoughts.

empathy: ability to identify with another person's situation and understand the feelings and reactions of that person.

empirical: based on observation and experience, rather than on experimental data.

enabler: one who facilitates another's addictive behavior by helping the addict gain access to the addictive substance.

enunciation: the uttering of sounds; may be clear or unclear to the listener.

environment: all the physical and atmospheric conditions that surround a person; social environment includes the people with whom one is in contact much of the time.

ethics: standards of conduct, a code of behavior for a specific group; medical ethics are the standards of conduct to be observed by health care providers.

ethical: conforming to standards of conduct established for a specific group or culture.

ethnic: relating to race or nationality; groups of people classed together because of customs, traits, and common beliefs.

euthanasia: administration of a lethal substance to a person who is dying and in great pain; also called "mercy killing."

evoke: arouse, create, or elicit.

expectation: something one thinks will occur.

FAS: acronym for Fetal Alcohol Syndrome.

fantasy: unrestrained imagination; may be related to a specific aspect of life, such as sexual fantasy.

forgo: do without something by choice.

frustration: any blocking of progress toward a desired goal.

GAS: acronym for General Adaptation Syndrome.

gene: unit that carries an hereditary trait.

genetic: carried by the genes; pertaining to heredity.

genotype: the specific hereditary makeup of a person.

grief: intense emotional suffering due to a loss.

grief work: the process of working through the emotional reaction to loss; generally considered to last at least one year.

guilt: self-reproach due to the belief that one has committed a wrong.

habits: established behavior patterns; series of actions that may occur without conscious effort.

habituation: psychological dependence, need, strong desire.

hallucinogenic: causing a person to hallucinate, to perceive sights and sounds that are not actually present.

hassle: an annoyance.

heredity: the transmission of characteristics from parents to offspring.

heterosexual: sexual preference for someone of the opposite sex.

hierarchy: arrangement in a specific order or rank from lowest to highest; vertical relationships.

holistic: perceiving the whole and all of its parts; in health care, the philosophy that healing occurs most readily when all aspects of the patient are considered.

homeostasis: the balance of chemicals and hormones necessary for normal physiological functioning.

homosexual: sexual preference for someone of the same sex.

horizontal communication: communication between people on the same level; no one has authority over someone else.

hospice: facility for the care of terminally ill patients, based on a death-with-dignity philosophy.

hostility: anger, either specific or general; may be the basis for aggressive tendencies.

humane: characterized by compassion, sympathy, and consideration.

humanize: make more humane.

hypnosis: trancelike condition usually induced by another person, in which the subject is receptive to suggestions.

imminent: about to occur; may include a sense of threat.

immortality: exempt from death.

impending: to occur soon.

incapacitated: incapable of functioning.

incest: sexual intercourse between persons whose blood relationship makes it illegal for them to marry; usually involves parent/child, brother/sister, or uncle/niece; may be an aspect of child abuse.

incompatible: not harmonious.

inconsistency: differing from one occurrence to another.

individualistic: tending toward independent thinking, behavior, or beliefs.

individual worth: right to be valued and respected as a human being, regardless of personal circumstances or qualities.

inebriated: intoxicated, drunk.

inevitably: not able to be avoided or evaded.

innovations: a new and different idea, method, device.

institutionalize: place someone in an institution such as an hospital, nursing home, or psychiatric facility; may be voluntary or involuntary.

intangible: untouchable; representing value but without material being.

intention: a specific purpose (a conscious thought) for a particular action.

interment: burial.

intervention: any action performed with the intention of changing what is happening; actions to control or stop a disease process; actions to prevent harm; actions to promote healing.

invasive: (1) intrusive into or through body tissues, as by cutting in a surgical procedure or introducing an instrument into an internal organ or body cavity; (2) tending to spread or infiltrate.

invulnerable: immune to sickness, injury, or attack.

irreversible: incapable of being reversed; unchangeable, as in the direction of a process.

lethargy: abnormal drowsiness, sluggishness.

litigation: a lawsuit.

macabre: having death as a pervasive theme.

malingering: deliberate pretending of illness when there is none.

malalignment: bad alignment.

mandate: authoritative command to act.

manifestation: the way something is displayed.

manipulative: using various strategies to influence others in order to obtain something.

martyr complex: psychological condition in which a person derives satisfaction from being taken advantage of by another person.

medicalize: apply the medical model to a situation that does not require diagnosis and treatment; make a specific situation the domain of physicians.

mediocre: performance that is acceptable but not good.

meridians: (as related to Chinese medicine) twelve energy channels that extend through the body on the vertical plane.

message discrepancy: difference in meaning between the message sent and the message received; may be due to lack of agreement between the sender's verbal and nonverbal messages.

metaphysics: branch of philosophy that is concerned with the nature of being and existence.

mind set: mental readiness to react in a specific way.

misalignment: wrong alignment.

moral: standards of right and wrong; similar to ethical, but different from legal.

mortality: the nature of man or woman as a being who must eventually die.

narcotic: addictive type of drug used medically to relieve pain.

necrosis: death of tissues in a limited area.

neurotransmitter: chemical substances that transmit impulses in the brain and nerves.

noradrenalin: hormone produced by the adrenal medulla during emotion-arousing situations.

nurturing: providing nourishment and the kind of care that encourages growth and development.

omnipotent: unlimited power.

options: more than two available choices.

orientation: adaptation to a new set of conditions.

orthodox: according to established doctrine.

overt: obvious, observable; opposite of covert.

overt noncooperation: behavior in which a person is openly uncooperative.

palliative: relieving or controlling symptoms without healing the underlying disease process.

paradigm: a model, example, or pattern.

paraphilia: diagnostic term for a variety of atypical sexual behaviors.

paraphrase: restate, express a meaning in different words.

passive aggression: indirect resistance, sometimes while giving the appearance of cooperation; may be due to covert hostility.

patriarchal: attributing supremacy to the father or a father figure; lineage through the male parent.

pedophilia: sexual activity between a child under the age of thirteen and someone five to ten years older than the child; a type of child abuse.

perpetrator: those who have committed some type of offense or crime.

perversion: atypical sexual behavior that is preferred over normal sexual intercourse.

phenotype: an organism's physical type; a set of characteristics that establish physical appearance.

physiological: dealing with the functions and vital processes of living organisms; the physical aspect of being, rather than the mental, emotional, or spiritual aspects.

placebo: inactive substance administered instead of a specific therapy.

placebo effect: beneficial effect of a placebo, usually reflecting the expectations of the patient, health care provider, or both.

plateau: an elevated area or surface.

posthypnotic: the period following hypnosis.

potential: hidden or undeveloped trait, quality, or talent. (Ability is a quality or talent that has been developed. A characteristic is a trait that has been developed.)

prejudice: a preconceived opinion held without regard to the facts; generalized negative feelings toward a person or group because of race, sex, or subculture.

prepubescent: child who has not yet experienced the physical changes that accompany puberty.

probability: the likelihood that something will occur; stated numerically in science and statistics.

procrastinate: put off doing something until a later time.

proficient: skillful.

prognosis: predicted course or outcome of a disease or injury.

prosthesis: an artificial replacement for a missing body part.

proxy: one who has been designated to act on behalf of another person.

psychoanalysis: method of treating mental/emotional disorders by discovering and analyzing repressed memories, emotional conflicts, past traumas.

psychopharmaceutical: drug that has specific effects on the mind, emotions, or mood, usually by altering brain chemistry.

psychophysiological illness: physical disorder due to mental and emotional factors, usually involving an organ or functions controlled by the autonomic nervous system; also known as "psychosomatic illness."

psychosocial: pertaining to social conditions and their relationship to psychological health.

psychosomatic: relating to the interaction of mind and body.

psychosomatic illness: see psychophysiological illness.

psychotherapy: treatment of mental and emotional illness through one or more psychological techniques.

psychotic: mentally ill, out of touch with reality.

quackery: the use of ineffective techniques in the pretense of healing, for the purpose of financial gain rather than a desire to help the sick.

quality control: a system of checks to ensure that specific standards are maintained.

quality of life: the characteristics of one's life situation; may vary from extremely poor to excellent.

random: absence of a definite pattern.

rapport: a relationship in which there is mutual acceptance, understanding and respect.

rational: based on a reasoning process; sensible.

reflecting: indicating an awareness of another person's emotional state by "mirroring" their feelings.

regression: exhibiting behaviors that are appropriate to an earlier stage of development.

REM: acronym for Rapid Eye Movement.

REM sleep: the phase of sleep during which dreaming occurs.

repertoire: the complete range of skills possessed by a person; in music, the complete range of musical works a musician is prepared to perform.

repression: the storing of unexpressed feelings and the associated painful memories in the unconscious.

resentment: chronic anger that is not consciously expressed, but may be an unconscious influence on behavior.

reprimand: a stern reproof or censure for a fault or mistake.

resuscitation: the reviving of a person who is apparently dead.

revert: to go back.

rigor: challenging, difficult; strict precision.

ritual: acts that are repeated in a specific form.

role: the duties and behaviors expected of a person in a specific situation.

STD: acronym for Sexually Transmitted Disease.

satisfaction: an inner feeling of pride or pleasure.

selective observing: a tendency to notice certain details of a situation while ignoring or overlooking other details.

self-concept: all the things a person believes to be true of himself or herself; may be realistic or unrealistic.

self-confidence: results from belief in oneself as a competent person.

self-control: a learned behavior pattern for expressing feelings and dealing with life situations in socially acceptable ways.

self-esteem: the feelings about oneself at any given moment; tends to fluctuate according to the most recent experience and the feelings associated with it.

self-reliant: ability to depend upon oneself; confidence in one's own judgment, decisions, abilities, and coping skills.

separation anxiety: extreme anxiety that a child may develop when a caregiver is absent or about to leave.

sexism: belief or attitude that one sex is inferior to the other; often the basis for discrimination.

sexual deviation: often used instead of "perversion" to refer to atypical sexual behavior.

sexual variation: currently used to refer to any type of sexual deviation.

social needs: psychological, emotional, mental and spiritual needs that can only be satisfied through relationships with other people.

socioeconomic: relating to a combination of social and economic factors.

spectrum: a range or continuous sequence.

stamina: endurance, strength, staying power.

stance: a mode of standing or positioning of the body and feet.

standards of behavior: rules of conduct, beliefs about what is proper and improper behavior.

stress: physiological response (internal and adaptive) to extreme or chronic emotional states.

stressors: outside influences that arouse some type of emotional response.

subluxation: displacement of a vertebra; diagnostic term used by chiropractors.

subtle: delicate, refined, not obvious.

suppressed: not expressed, held down.

surrogate: a substitute.

survivor guilt: tendency of a survivor to feel guilty for being alive, especially when someone else did not survive an accident.

sympathy: concern for another person, especially one who is experiencing illness, trauma or crisis.

TLC: acronym for tender loving care.

taboo: forbidden.

temperament: the type of emotional state (positive or negative) that characterizes a person.

tentative: temporary, uncertain, subject to change.

teratogens: any substances that cause abnormalities in a fetus.

thanatology: the study of death and dying.

thermograph: a device for measuring and recording temperature changes in a specific area of the body.

transformation: a change in outward appearance, structure, character, or condition.

unique: one of a kind.

vacillate: waver or hesitate in making a choice, especially between alternatives or among options.

valid: true or correct; having legal force.

value systems: the importance attached to various aspects of living, such as beliefs, ideas, objects, relationships.

variability: tendency or ability to change.

verbalize: express in words; often used to indicate oral expression, rather than written.

vertical communication: communication between people at different levels of authority.

visualize: process of forming a mental image.

whiplash: injury to the muscles and connective tissues of the neck, causing severe pain, stiffness, and limitation of motion.

withdrawal: the shutting off of communication or physical removal of oneself from a situation; may serve as a defense mechanism in a specific situation; indication of emotional or mental illness when there is retreat from reality and refusal to interact with others.

withdrawal (drug-related): withholding a substance to which someone is addicted; the group of symptoms that occur as the body reacts to absence of the addictive substance.

Index

A

AADD. *See* Adult attention deficit disorder

Aberrant behavior, 204

Abuse, 161
    child, adjustment and, 164–67

Acceptance, 92–93
    during adolescence, 95
    of death, 406
    need for, 91–103
    of patient behavior, 262

Accidental death, 337

Accidents, adjustment and, 179

Accomplishment, 11

Achievement, as health care provider, 8–11

Achterberg, Jeanne, 431

Acupressure, 516
    point location charts, 517–18

Acupuncture, 514–16

Adaptation, new conditions, ability, 33

Addiction, 46, 205

Adjustment, 134–49
    cultural threats to, 159–80
    defense mechanisms and, 210–11
    defined, 134
    emotions and, 137–41
    to illness, 158–59
    improving, 142–46
    inner conflict and, 224–25
    threats to, 152–88

Adolescence
    acceptance during, 95
    changes during, 155
    conformity, acceptance and, 95
    drugs, illicit, 168
    group standards, 95–96
    losses during, 348
    peer pressure in, 168
    sexual activity, stress of, 168–69
    stressors of, 167–69
        drugs, 168
        peer pressure, 168
        sexual activity, 168–69

Adrenalin, 107

Adult attention deficit disorder, 163

Adult Children of Alcoholics, 204

Adulthood, stressors of, 169–72

Advice, giving, as communication block, 257

Aerosols, 205

Affirmations, 483

Affluence, 24

Affluent class, patient from, 25–26

Aggressive behavior
    adult of patients, coping with, 276
    child of patients, coping with, 275
    of patient, coping with, 269–71

Agreeing, as communication block, 257

Alcohol abuse, 201–4

Alcoholics Anonymous, 203

Alcoholism, 201–4

Ambiguity, in verbal communication, 317